Practical Guide in
Andrology & Embryology

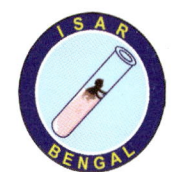

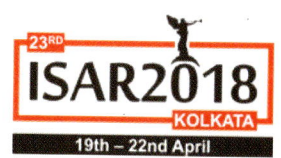

To commemorate the occasion of 23rd ISAR National Conference **ISAR Bengal** published monogram titled "**Practical Guide in 4 volumes**".
- **Infertility**
- **Assisted Reproductive Technology**
- **Reproductive Surgery**
- **Andrology and Embryology**

Practical Guide in Andrology & Embryology

Editors

Gita Ganguly Mukherjee DGO MD FICOG FICMCH FRCOG
Formerly, Professor and Head
Department of Obstetrics and Gynecology
RG Kar Medical College and Hospital
Kolkata, West Bengal, India

Gautam Khastgir MD (Cal) FRCS (Edin) FRCOG (Lond) FICOG
Medical Director and Subspecialist
Department of Reproductive Medicine and Surgery
Bengal Infertility and Reproductive Therapy Hospital (BIRTH)
Kolkata, West Bengal, India

Ratna Chattopadhyay MBBS PhD
Head (Embryology and Andrology)
Institute of Reproductive Medicine
Kolkata, West Bengal, India

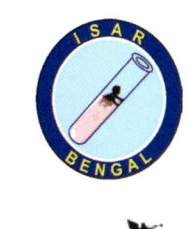

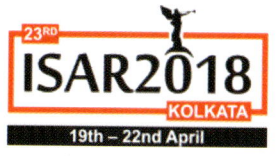

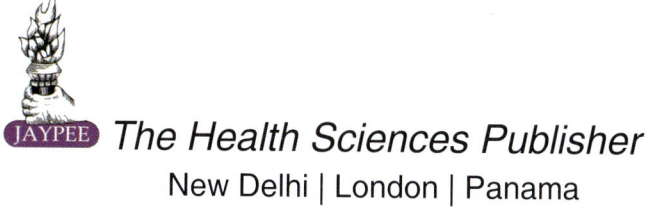

The Health Sciences Publisher
New Delhi | London | Panama

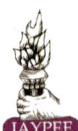 **Jaypee Brothers Medical Publishers (P) Ltd**

Headquarters
Jaypee Brothers Medical Publishers (P) Ltd
4838/24, Ansari Road, Daryaganj
New Delhi 110 002, India
Phone: +91-11-43574357
Fax: +91-11-43574314
Email: jaypee@jaypeebrothers.com

Overseas Offices

J.P. Medical Ltd
83 Victoria Street, London
SW1H 0HW (UK)
Phone: +44 20 3170 8910
Fax: +44 (0)20 3008 6180
Email: info@jpmedpub.com

Jaypee-Highlights Medical Publishers Inc
City of Knowledge, Bld. 235, 2nd Floor,
Clayton, Panama City, Panama
Phone: +1 507-301-0496
Fax: +1 507-301-0499
Email: cservice@jphmedical.com

Jaypee Brothers Medical Publishers (P) Ltd
17/1-B Babar Road, Block-B, Shyamoli
Mohammadpur, Dhaka-1207
Bangladesh
Mobile: +08801912003485
Email: jaypeedhaka@gmail.com

Jaypee Brothers Medical Publishers (P) Ltd
Bhotahity, Kathmandu, Nepal
Phone: +977-9741283608
Email: kathmandu@jaypeebrothers.com

Website: www.jaypeebrothers.com
Website: www.jaypeedigital.com

© 2018, Jaypee Brothers Medical Publishers

The views and opinions expressed in this book are solely those of the original contributor(s)/author(s) and do not necessarily represent those of editor(s) of the book.

All rights reserved. No part of this publication may be reproduced, stored or transmitted in any form or by any means, electronic, mechanical, photocopying, recording or otherwise, without the prior permission in writing of the publishers.

All brand names and product names used in this book are trade names, service marks, trademarks or registered trademarks of their respective owners. The publisher is not associated with any product or vendor mentioned in this book.

Medical knowledge and practice change constantly. This book is designed to provide accurate, authoritative information about the subject matter in question. However, readers are advised to check the most current information available on procedures included and check information from the manufacturer of each product to be administered, to verify the recommended dose, formula, method and duration of administration, adverse effects and contraindications. It is the responsibility of the practitioner to take all appropriate safety precautions. Neither the publisher nor the author(s)/editor(s) assume any liability for any injury and/or damage to persons or property arising from or related to use of material in this book.

This book is sold on the understanding that the publisher is not engaged in providing professional medical services. If such advice or services are required, the services of a competent medical professional should be sought.

Every effort has been made where necessary to contact holders of copyright to obtain permission to reproduce copyright material. If any have been inadvertently overlooked, the publisher will be pleased to make the necessary arrangements at the first opportunity. The **CD/DVD-ROM** (if any) provided in the sealed envelope with this book is complimentary and free of cost. **Not meant for sale.**

Inquiries for bulk sales may be solicited at: jaypee@jaypeebrothers.com

Practical Guide in Andrology and Embryology

First Edition: **2018**

ISBN 978-93-5270-485-9

Printed at Rajkamal Electric Press, Kundli, Haryana.

Dedicated to
*All the infertile couples and those
who are devoted to alleviate their agony*

Contributors

A Suresh Kumar
Senior Gynecologist and Obstetrician
Director
Ashoka Super Speciality Hospital and Research Pvt. Ltd.
Raipur, Chhattisgarh, India

Ahmad Majzoub
Fellowship in Andrology and Male Infertility
Department of Urology
Hamad Medical Corporation, Doha, Qatar

Alex C Varghese
Scientific Director
ASTRA Fertility Group
Village Centre Court
Mississauga, Ontario, Canada

Amita Subramanian
Consultant
Cloud Nine Hospital
Chennai, Tamil Nadu, India

Anjali Joshi
Senior Embryologist
Rotunda–The Center for Human Reproduction
Mumbai, Maharashtra, India

Arati Biswas
Professor and Head
Department of Obstetrics and Gynecology
Calcutta National Medical College
Kolkata, West Bengal, India

Arundhati Athalye
Senior Scientific Officer/Research Officer
Department of Assisted Reproduction and Genetics
Jaslok Hospital and Research Centre
Mumbai, Maharashtra, India

Ashok Agarwal
Director of the Clinical Andrology Center and Fertility Laboratory
Director of Research at the American Center for Reproductive Medicine
Cleveland Clinic, Cleveland, USA

BN Chakravarty
Director, Institute of Reproductive Medicine
Kolkata, West Bengal, India

Bindu Chimote
Consultant Clinical Embryologist
Vaunshdhara Fertility Centre
Nagpur, Maharashtra, India

Chaitra K Vannappa
Manipal Fertility
Bengaluru, Karnataka, India

Charudutt Joshi
Director and Consultant Embryologist
Gametes India Pvt. Ltd.
Indore, Madhya Pradesh, India

Charulata Chatterjee
Senior Embryologist
Yashoda Fertility and Research Institute
Secunderabad, Hyderabad, Telangana, India

Dattatray Naik
Embryologist
Jaslok-FertilTree International Fertility Centre
Jaslok Hospital
Mumbai, Maharashtra, India

Debhashree Ganguly
Consultant Embryologist
Johar IVF Centre
Kolkata, West Bengal, India

Deepak Modi
Molecular and Cellular Biology Laboratory
ICMR-National Institute for Research in Reproductive Health
Mumbai, Maharashtra, India

Dhiraj Gada
Director
Shalby Gada Life ART Center
Indore, Madhya Pradesh, India

Firuza Parikh
Department of Assisted Reproduction and Genetics
Jaslok-FertilTree International Fertility Centre
Jaslok Hospital, Mumbai, Maharashtra, India

G Manjula
Assistant Professor
Department of Clinical Embryology, Reproductive Medicine and Surgery
Sri Ramachandra Medical College and Research Institute
Chennai, Tamil Nadu, India

Gautam Khastgir
Medical Director and Subspecialist
Department of Reproductive Medicine and Surgery
Bengal Infertility and Reproductive Therapy Hospital (BIRTH)
Kolkata, West Bengal, India

Gita Ganguly Mukherjee
Formerly Professor and Head
Department of Obstetrics and Gynecology
RG Kar Medical College and Hospital
Kolkata, West Bengal, India

Gunja Bose
Consultant
Institute of Reproductive Medicine
Kolkata, West Bengal, India

Hrishikesh D Pai
Director; Consultant Gynecologist
Bloom IVF Group (Mumbai, Delhi, Gurugram, Chandigarh, Navi Mumbai, Bengaluru)
Lilavati Hospital & Research Centre
Mumbai, Maharashtra, India

Jaideep Malhotra
President– FOGSI 2018
Managing Director
ART Rainbow IVF
Agra, Uttar Pradesh, India

Julia Szeptycki
Consultant, Astra Fertility Group
Mississauga, Ontario, Canada

Keshav Malhotra
Lab Director (Chief Embryologist)
ART Rainbow IVF
Agra, Uttar Pradesh, India

Konkon Mitra
Consultant IVF Specialist
Surgy Centre
Kolkata, West Bengal, India

Kunal A Doshi
Obstetrician and Gynecologist
IVF Consultant and Centre Administrator
ProFert IVF Fertility Clinic
Mumbai
Ashish Maternity and Nursing Home
Vile Parle East
Mumbai, Maharashtra, India

Lakshmi Krishna Leela B
Medicine, Gynecology and Infertility Specialist
Consultant in Reproductive Medicine and Infertility
Yashoda Hospital, Hyderabad, Telangana, India

Madhavi Panpalia
Consultant Gynecologist and Obstetrician and Fertility Specialist
Jaslok-FertilTree International Fertility Centre
Jaslok Hospital, Mumbai, Maharashtra, India

Madhumita Roy Choudhury
Consultant Embryologist
Surgy Centre
Kolkata, West Bengal, India

Contributors

Madhuprita Agrawal
Gynecologist, Obstetrician, Laparoscopy Surgeon and Test Tube Baby Specialist
Ashoka Super Speciality Hospital and Research Pvt. Ltd.
Raipur, Chhattisgarh, India

Meenal Khandeparkar
Consultant, Jaslok-FertilTree International Fertility Centre
Jaslok Hospital, Mumbai, Maharashtra, India

Milind R Shah
Professor and Head
Department of Obstetrics and Gynecology
Gandhi Natha Rangaji Homoeopathic Medical College
Solapur, Maharashtra, India

Moumita Naha
Consultant
Department of Reproductive Medicine and Surgery
Bengal Infertility and Reproductive Therapy Hospital (BIRTH)
Kolkata, West Bengal, India

Nabendu Murmu
Senior Scientific Officer, Grade-II
Chittaranjan National Cancer Institute
Kolkata, West Bengal, India

Nandita Palshetkar
Gynecologist and Infertility Specialist
Bloom IVF Centre
Lilavati Hospital and Research Centre
Mumbai, Maharashtra, India

Nandkishor Naik
Chief Embryologist
Jaslok-FertilTree International Fertility Centre
Jaslok Hospital, Mumbai, Maharashtra India

Narendra Malhotra
Professor
Dubrovnik International University, Croatia
Director–Global Rainbow Healthcare
Agra, Uttar Pradesh, India

Natchandra Chimote
Consultant Embryologist and Scientific Director
Vaunshdhara Fertility Centre
Nagpur, Maharashtra, India

Navin Desai
Senior Embryologist
Nova IVI Fertility
Mumbai, Maharashtra, India

Neharika Malhotra Bora
Assistant Professor
Bharati Vidyapeeth University
Pune, Maharashtra, India
Consultant, ART Rainbow IVF
Agra, Uttar Pradesh, India

Niladitya Sanyal
Reproductive Medicine Scientist
Laboratory Head
Department of Pathology
Bengal Infertility and Reproductive Therapy Hospital (BIRTH)
Kolkata, West Bengal, India

Nivedita Shetty
IVF Specialist
Department of Reproductive Medicine
Columbia Asia Hospital
Mysore, Karnataka, India

Pankaj Talwar
Head of Department
ART Centre
Army Hospital (Research and Referral)
Delhi Cantonment, India

Parag Nandi
Chief Embryologist, Cradle Fertility Centre, Kolkata, West Bengal, India

Pooja Awasthi
Consultant Embryologist
Origin IVF and Fertility Centre
Ghaziabad, Uttar Pradesh, India

Pratip Chakraborty
Consultant
Institute of Reproductive Medicine
Kolkata, West Bengal, India

Prochi Madon
Honorary Geneticist
Department of Assisted Reproduction
and Genetics
Jaslok-FertilTree International Fertility Centre
Jaslok Hospital
Mumbai, Maharashtra, India

Rajeev Agarwal
Gynecologist, Infertility Specialist and
Laparoscopic Surgeon
Director–Care IVF
Kolkata, West Bengal, India

Rajvi H Mehta
Executive Body Member–ACE
Trivector Embryology Support Academy
Mumbai, Maharashtra, India

Ranjana Mangoli
Senior Embryologist
Fertility Clinic and IVF Centre
Mumbai, Maharashtra, India

Ratna Agrawal
Senior Embryologist
Director, Ashoka Super Speciality Hospital
and Research Pvt. Ltd.
Raipur, Chhattisgarh, India

Ratna Chattopadhyay
Head (Embryology and Andrology)
Institute of Reproductive Medicine
Kolkata, West Bengal, India

Rishina Bansal
Lab Manager and Embryologist
Nova IVI Fertility
Mumbai, Maharashtra, India

Rishma Pai
Gynecologist and Infertility Specialist
Bloom IVF Centre
Lilavati Hospital and Research Centre
Mumbai, Maharashtra, India

Ritu Gada
Clinical Embryologist
University of Oxford
Oxford, UK

Ritu Hinduja
Infertility Specialist
Nova IVI Fertility
Mumbai, Maharashtra, India

Rohit Gutgutia
Clinical Director
Nova IVI Fertility
Kolkata, West Bengal, India

SM Rahman
Consultant
Department of Signal Transduction and
Biogenic Amines
Chittaranjan National Cancer Institute
Kolkata, West Bengal, India

Sakuntala Banerji
Consultant
Institute of Reproductive Medicine
Kolkata, West Bengal, India

Sanketh Dhumal S
Clinical Embryologist
KS Hegde Medical Academy
Mysore, Karnataka, India

Saroj Agarwal
Chief Embryologist
Care IVF, Kolkata, West Bengal, India

Shailaja Gada Saxena
Head, Department of Molecular Medicine
Reliance Life Sciences (RLS)
Dhirubhai Ambani Life Sciences Centre
Navi Mumbai, Maharashtra, India

Shanti Roy
Formerly, Professor and Head
Department of Obstetrics and Gynecology
Patna Medical College and Hospital
Patna, Bihar, India

Shovandeb Kalapahar
FNB Trainee
Institute of Reproductive Medicine
Kolkata, West Bengal, India

Contributors

Shubhangi Gangal
Chief Embryologist
Gunjotikar Nursing Home and IVF Center
Thane, Maharashtra, India

Soumojit Paul
Consultant Embryologist
Nova IVI Fertility
Kolkata, West Bengal, India

Sreyashi Mitra
Consultant
Department of Signal Transduction and Biogenic Amines
Chittaranjan National Cancer Institute
Kolkata, West Bengal, India

Srinivas MS
Director and Chief Embryologist
Caree Fertility Pvt. Ltd.
Bengaluru, Karnataka, India

Stacy Colaco
Consultant, Molecular and Cellular Biology Laboratory
ICMR–National Institute for Research in Reproductive Health
Mumbai, Maharashtra, India

Subir Chatterjee
Chief Embryologist
Bengal Infertility and Reproductive Therapy Hospital (BIRTH)
Kolkata, West Bengal, India

Sudesh A Kamat
Senior Embryologist
Lilavati Hospital
Mumbai, Maharashtra, India

Sujatha Ramakrishnan
Fertility and Scientific Director
Department of Clinical Embryology
Cloud Nine Hospital
Chennai, Tamil Nadu, India

Sulagna Dutta
Department of Physiology
Faculty of Medicine
MAHSA University, Malaysia

Sunita Sharma
Consultant, Institute of Reproductive Medicine
Kolkata, West Bengal, India

Suparna Banerjee
Consultant
Department of Fertility
Johar IVF Centre
Kolkata, West Bengal, India

Swaminathan D
Senior Embryologist, IRM, MMM,
Scientific Director and Senior Embryologist/Geneticist
Santhathi—Centre for Reproductive Medicine
Dakshina Kannada, Karnataka, India

Sweta Agrawal
Consultant Obstetrician and Gynecologist
Raipur, Chhattisgarh, India

Varsha Samson Roy
Chief Embryologist and Scientific Director
Manipal Fertility
Bengaluru, Karnataka, India

Vijay Mangoli
Laboratory Director
Fertility Clinic and IVF Centre
Mumbai, Maharashtra, India

Vijayakumar Narayanamurthy Chelur
Consultant Clinical Embryologist
Belagavi, Karnataka, India

Virendra Shah
Embryologist, Chairman
Indian Society for Assisted Reproduction
Indore, Madhya Pradesh, India

Zeba Ali Jahangir
Consultant
Nova IVI Fertility
Kolkata, West Bengal, India

Preface

One important criterion of success following in vitro fertilization (IVF) or any assisted reproductive technology (ART) procedure is the formation of good quality embryos, which depends upon retrieval of good quality oocytes, fertilization by healthy sperms and optimal culture environment.

Forty years have passed since the birth of the first IVF baby Louise Brown, but improvement in success rate is not very promising as yet. So modification of the learning curve and changes in treatment and culture protocol are frequent phenomena in this field.

Andrology, the science of fertilization potential of the male gamete, is evolving rapidly and thus it exposes us to so many unknown facts about the real increase in male infertility and gives us an insight into the uniqueness of the human sperm cell.

Embryology is the science which helps in unravelling the miracles in embryogenesis, both in vivo and in vitro. It guides the embryologists to learn conventional methods and also to modify or upgrade our knowledge whenever it is needed.

Profound communication between the clinician and embryologist is the main pillar of success in any ART center. Understanding the IVF laboratory or embryology helps the clinician to guide the patient and for planning further treatment.

This book is, contributed by practical experience of passionate and knowledgeable embryologists, scientists and clinicians whose informative and concise chapters will help beginners to navigate and guiding the practising embryologists to follow the right track and to upgrade themselves.

The chapters regarding fertility preservation, frozen embryo transfer and mitochondrial transfer are gradually becoming more important priority-wise, and have been nicely elaborated in this guide book.

A chapter on animal laboratory will encourage the renowned ART clinics to strengthen their training and research facilities.

We are extremely thankful to all the contributors for their caring and insightful write-ups in spite of their busy and hectic schedules. Without their assistance, this book could never have been written.

We are grateful to Professor BN Chakravarty for his immense support, continuous guidance and inspiration, and also contributing very important chapter in this book.

Overlapping and lack of continuity are common in a book written by many authors. We tried to overcome these as far as possible.

We thank Shri Jitendar P Vij (Group Chairman) and Mr Ankit Vij (Managing Director) of M/s Jaypee Brothers Medical Publishers (P) Ltd., New Delhi, India, for their continuous support in making this book a reality.

We hope you will find this book useful.

Gita Ganguly Mukherjee
Gautam Khastgir
Ratna Chattopadhyay

Contents

Chapter 1.	**The Male Gamete: A Unique Cell** *BN Chakravarty, Arati Biswas, Shovandeb Kalapahar*	1
Chapter 2.	**Evaluation of Male Infertility** *Shanti Roy*	18
Chapter 3.	**Sperm Function Tests** *Keshav Malhotra, Neharika Malhotra Bora, Jaideep Malhotra, Narendra Malhotra*	24
Chapter 4.	**Screening of Male Partner before ART Procedure and its Recent Advancement** *Swaminathan D, Sanketh Dhumal S*	32
Chapter 5.	**Role of Genetics in Clinical Evaluation of Male Infertility** *Stacy Colaco, Deepak Modi*	44
Chapter 6.	**Sperm Preparation Techniques and its Modification According to Different Sperm Seminopathy** *Charudutt Joshi*	56
Chapter 7.	**Advanced Sperm Selection Technique for ART** *G Manjula*	64
Chapter 8.	**Effects of Oxidative Stress on Different Sperm Functions: How to Evaluate and Manage** *Sulagna Dutta, Ahmad Majzoub, Ashok Agarwal*	76
Chapter 9.	**Sperm DNA Fragmentation and its Clinical Implication** *Niladitya Sanyal, Subir Chatterjee, Gautam Khastgir*	89
Chapter 10.	**DNA Fragmentation Index and Magnetic Activated Cell Sorting: A Practical Approach** *Rishina Bansal, Ritu Hinduja, Navin Desai*	97
Chapter 11.	**Antioxidant or Nutraceutical Therapy as Medical Management in Idiopathic Infertility** *Charulata Chatterjee, Lakshmi Krishna Leela B*	107
Chapter 12.	**Environmental Effect on Male Infertility: Preventive Therapeutic Approach** *Sreyashi Mitra, Nabendu Murmu, SM Rahman, Parag Nandi*	117

Chapter 13.	Role of Micromanipulation in Recent Advancement of Assisted Reproductive Technology Procedures	128
	Arundhati Athalye, Dattatray Naik, Nandkishor Naik, Prochi Madon, Madhavi Panpalia, Meenal Khandeparkar, Firuza Parikh	
Chapter 14.	Intracytoplasmic Morphologically Selected Sperm Injection	142
	Sudesh A Kamat, Hrishikesh D Pai	
Chapter 15.	Male Sexual Dysfunction	149
	Milind R Shah, Kunal A Doshi	
Chapter 16.	Semen Banking	158
	Soumojit Paul, Zeba Ali Jahangir, Rohit Gutgutia	
Chapter 17.	Basic Requirement to set up an IVF Laboratory	171
	Virendra Shah, Anjali Joshi	
Chapter 18.	Recent Advancement in the Maintenance of Laboratory Quality Control	188
	Julia Szeptycki, Alex C Varghese	
Chapter 19.	Troubleshooting in the ART Laboratory from Oocyte Retrieval till Embryo Transfer	208
	Sujatha Ramakrishnan, Amita Subramanian	
Chapter 20.	Attributes and Responsibilities of an Efficient Embryologist	220
	Rajvi H Mehta	
Chapter 21.	Oocyte-Cumulus Insight	228
	Ratna Chattopadhyay, Parag Nandi	
Chapter 22.	Time-lapse Videography versus in Time Quick Analysis by an Experienced Embryologist	238
	Varsha Samson Roy, Chaitra K Vannappa	
Chapter 23.	Noninvasive Method of Embryo Selection	255
	A Suresh Kumar, Ratna Agrawal, Madhuprita Agrawal, Sweta Agrawal	
Chapter 24.	Embryo Loading: An Important Step in Embryo Transfer Technique	266
	Madhumita Roy Choudhury, Konkon Mitra	
Chapter 25.	Elective Single Embryo Transfer	270
	Gautam Khastgir, Moumita Naha	
Chapter 26.	Assisted Hatching and its Clinical Application	277
	Shubhangi Gangal	
Chapter 27.	Fertilization Failure: What an Embryologist Should Know?	288
	Vijayakumar Narayanamurthy Chelur	

Chapter 28.	**Oocyte Cryopreservation** *Hrishikesh D Pai, Nandita Palshetkar, Rishma Pai*	295
Chapter 29.	**Embryo Cryopreservation** *Hrishikesh D Pai*	300
Chapter 30.	**Blastocyst Culture and Vitrification:** **A Step Ahead for Single Embryo Transfer** *Vijay Mangoli, Ranjana Mangoli*	307
Chapter 31.	**Criteria to Select Oocytes and Embryos for Cryopreservation** *Charulata Chatterjee*	317
Chapter 32.	**Freeze-All Embryo Versus Freezing on Condition** *Rajeev Agarwal, Saroj Agarwal*	326
Chapter 33.	**Ovarian Tissue Freezing** *Pankaj Talwar, Pooja Awasthi*	336
Chapter 34.	**Role of Preimplantation Genetic Diagnosis and Comparative Genomic Hybridization in Healthy Outcome of ART** *Dhiraj Gada, Shailaja Gada Saxena, Ritu Gada*	359
Chapter 35.	**Purpose of an Animal Laboratory in Research:** **Outcomes in the Avenue** *Pratip Chakraborty, Sakuntala Banerji, Gunja Bose*	367
Chapter 36.	**Third-Party Reproduction: From Embryologist's Point of View** *Nivedita Shetty, Suparna Banerjee, Debhashree Ganguly, Srinivas MS*	376
Chapter 37.	**Understanding of ART Laboratory** **Work from Clinicians Point of View** *Sunita Sharma, Gita Ganguly Mukherjee*	385
Chapter 38.	**OMICS: Metabolomics, Proteomics, Secretomics and Genomics—Its Application in the Viability Score of Oocyte and Embryo** *Bindu Chimote, Natchandra Chimote*	394
Index		*405*

CHAPTER 1

The Male Gamete: A Unique Cell

BN Chakravarty, Arati Biswas, Shovandeb Kalapahar

▉ INTRODUCTION

Sperm is the motile male reproductive cell, which is highly specialized cell in human body. The term spermatozoon is derived from the ancient Greek word "sperma" (meaning seed) and "zoon" (meaning living being) and more commonly known as a sperm cell. It is the haploid male gamete cell.

There are three types of cells in our body, e.g. somatic cells, stem cells, and germ cells.

Spermatogonia are the immature germ cells. They divide several times during the process of spermatogenesis. The spermatogenic process is directed by genes located on the Y chromosome and takes around 70 days to complete from the spermatocyte stage. 12–21 more days are required for the transport of sperm from the testis through the epididymis to ejaculatory duct.

A uniflagellar sperm cell that is *motile* is referred to as a *spermatozoon*, whereas a nonmotile sperm cell is referred to as a *spermatium.*

Human spermatozoa have some unique characteristics which are summarized below:

- Sperm cell is the smallest cells in the body in terms of volume
- These cells (adult sperm cells) do not grow or divide
- The sperm cells are the most polarized cells; head in front and tail at the rear part of the body
- They fulfill their function outside the body, in different individuals, e.g. in female genital tract
- Unlike somatic cells, the sperm head has a large nucleus but lacks large cytoplasm. Nucleus constitutes 65% of spermatozoa head
- The sperm cells are unique among mammals for presence of plenty of abnormal forms of spermatozoa in the ejaculate.

Most tightly compacted eukaryotic DNA that is present in mammalian sperm, at least sixfold more highly condensed than the DNA in mitotic chromosomes.[1] To achieve this high degree of packaging, sperm DNA interacts with protamines to form linear, side-by-side arrays of chromatin. This differs

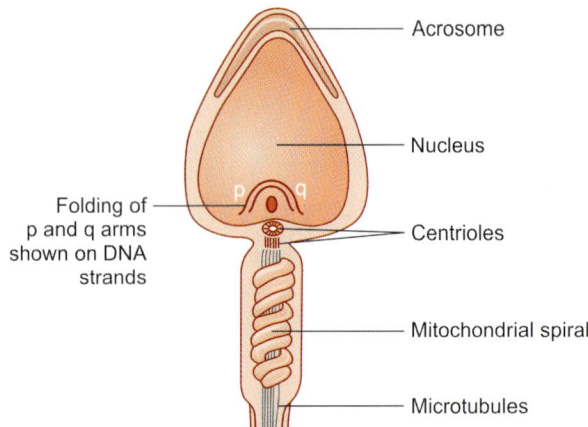

Fig. 1: Human spermatozoa.

markedly from the builder DNA packaging of somatic cell nuclei and mitotic chromosomes, in which the DNA is coiled around histone octamers to form nucleosomes. In addition to the sperm nuclear matrix, sperm nuclei contain a unique structure termed the *sperm nuclear annulus* to which the entire complement of DNA appears to be anchored.

The centromeres are located centrally and telomeres peripherally. Folding of chromosomal p- and q-arms are flexible (Fig. 1). This specific chromosomal arrangement may be responsible for increased frequency of abnormal sperm shape and increased frequency of aneuploidy.

- It has been observed that sex chromosome and G-group (chromosome 21 and 22) are more susceptible to nondisjunction during spermatogenesis.
- Morphologically abnormal sperms (large head, round head, etc.) have either numerical or structural abnormalities of chromosomes.

■ ANATOMICAL SEGMENTS OF ADULT SPERMATOZOA (FIG. 2)

A mature human sperm cell has got the following parts—head, neck, and tail. Tail is again divided into—middle piece, principal piece, and end piece.

Head

It is oval in shape consisting of large nucleus and a dome-shaped acrosome present on the nucleus. In humans, sperm cells consists of a flat, disk-shaped head which is 5 μm in length and 3 μm in width and a tail 50 μm long.[2] The tail *flagellates*, which propels the sperm cell (at about 1–3 mm/minute in humans) by whipping in an elliptical cone.[3] The spermatozoon is characterized by a

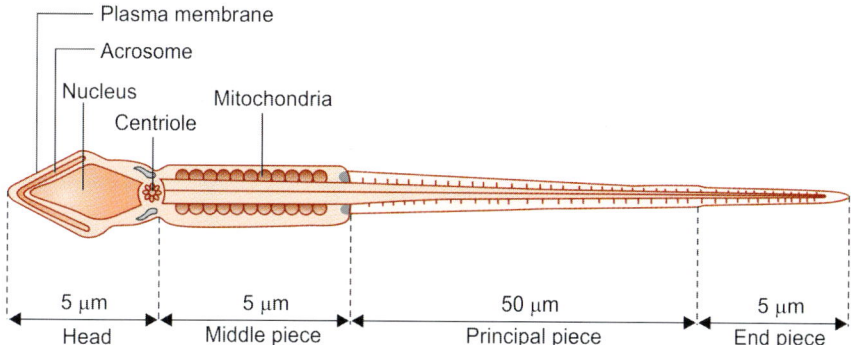

Fig. 2: Morphology of human spermatozoa.

minimum of *cytoplasm* and the most densely packed DNA. The coverings of the sperm head from outside are:
- Plasma membrane
- Outer and inner acrosomal layers of membrane
- Acrosomal sac containing enzymes
- Nuclear cap
- Nucleus.

Acrosome

This is found at the anterior tip of the sperm (derived from Greek term "akron" meaning extremity and "soma" meaning body). The acrosome forms a cap like structure called the *acrosomal cap*. This occupies the space between anterior half of the nucleus and the plasma membrane of the sperm tip. The acrosome arises from the golgi complex during spermatogenesis. The acrosome itself is bounded by a unit membrane. It consists of a number of hydrolytic enzymes such as acid phosphatase, hyaluronidase, and others. These enzymes help in tissue lysis (dissolving) and this facilitates the penetration of the sperm into the egg membrane. The enzymes are proteolytic and help in dissolving the egg membrane.

The membranes of late spermatids and spermatozoa contain a special small form of angiotensin-converting enzyme called *germinal angiotensin-converting enzyme*. The function of this enzyme in the sperms is unknown, although male mice in which the function of the angiotensin-converting enzyme gene has been disrupted have reduced fertility.

Sperm Nucleus

The nucleus occupies most of the available space of the sperm head. It is the shape of the nucleus that ultimately decides the shape of the sperm head. Structurally it is enveloped by a nuclear membrane. Sometimes, however the posterior part of nuclear membrane (towards the body of the sperm) is somewhat depressed to accommodate the proximal centriole. The nucleus consists of DNA as well as basic proteins. There is no nucleolus.

Function: Nucleus contain genetic information and half number of chromosomes. The acrosome releases a hyaluronidase enzyme which destroys the hyaluronic acid of the ovum and enters into the ovum.

Neck

It contains centrioles which are proximal centriole and distal centriole.

Function: Distal centriole gives rise to axial filament of the sperm which runs up to the end of the tail. Centrioles help the zygotic division by forming the first mitotic spindle. The posterior or the distal centriole is responsible for the formation of the microtubules of the sperm tail.

Tail

Middle Piece (Figs. 3A and B)

It is tubular structure in which mitochondria are spirally arranged. It has a pair of longitudinal fibers called beta fibers, surrounded by a ring of nine pairs of longitudinal fibers called alpha fibers. In human sperms, the alpha fibers of axial filament are accompanied on the outside by nine, much thicker fibers called gamma fibers or coarse fibers. The alpha, beta, and gamma fibers are the sites of various enzymes.

Alpha fibers have ATPase enzyme, while beta fibers have acetyl co-A succinate. These fibers are anchored to the distal centrioles. The fibers are surrounded by the mitochondria. Very often the mitochondria are fused together and form a spiral sheet that surrounds the axonemal fibers. Around the periphery of midpiece of the sperm is found a thin sheet of cytoplasm mainly composed of microtubules. This layer is called manchette.

Function: Middle piece is called power house of sperm because it gives energy to the sperm to traverse through the female genital tract.

Principal Piece

The principal piece which constitutes most of the length of tail consists of the central core made up of axial filaments with a 9+2 arrangement (2 central, 9 peripheral). The tail fibers are attached to each other by arms containing the protein dynein, which is an ATPase. Hydrolysis of ATP (adenosine triphosphate) in the adjacent mitochondria provides the energy for sperm motility, which is produced by a sliding action between the fibers in the sperm tail.

Surrounding this core is a fibrous tail sheath which often appears as semicircular ribs oriented at right angles to the long axis of the filament. Sometimes, they appear as helical coils. In human beings, two of the gamma fibers are fused with the surrounding ribs to form anterior and posterior columns extending throughout the length of the principle piece.

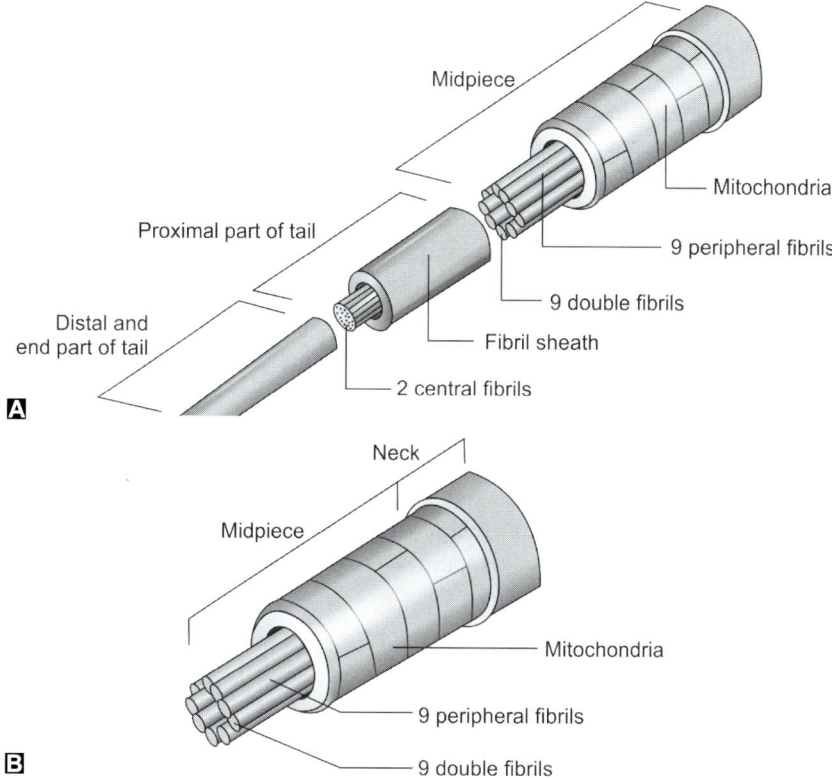

Figs. 3A and B: Morphological anatomy of midpiece, principal piece, and end piece.

This arrangement divides the principal piece into two functional compartments—one having three gamma fibers and the other containing four. This symmetry is thought to help in a more powerful stroke of the tail in one direction. This is called the power stroke. The end piece is a small tapering portion of the tail containing only the axial filament covered with cytoplasm and plasma membrane.

End Piece

This the terminal end of tail. Length is about 5 µm.

Sperms have no cytoplasmic organelles such as ribosomes and endoplasmic reticulum. There is no stored food in the sperm.[4]

■ MOLECULAR FUNCTIONS OF DIFFERENT SEGMENTS OF SPERMATOZOA

Functions of the Head

The plasma membrane which constitutes the outer coat of the head consists of a very unstable fatty acid which is known as polyunsaturated fatty acid (PUFA).

PUFA has both helpful and unwanted functions in reproduction. The helpful function consists of facilitating fusion and disintegration of plasma and acrosin membrane leading to exocytosis of the enzyme acrosin. This happens when the sperm head comes in contact with zona pellucida at the time of fertilization. This procedure is known as "acrosome reaction" and "zona penetration" which allows the sperm head to enter into the perivitelline space.

Due to presence of PUFA (unstable fatty acid) excessive fluidity of plasma membrane is seen that is very specialized character of sperm. These may be responsible for premature disintegration and exocytosis of acrosome. This may happen when many leukocytes are present in seminal plasma, or due to presence of plenty of immature sperm cells, varicocele, and excessive centrifugation.

Under normal conditions, cytoplasmic syngamy occurs when the sperm head after zona penetration comes in contact with oocyte oolemma (outer coating of oocyte cytoplasm). Cytoplasmic syngamy has two important molecular events: (a) calcium oscillation, (b) cortical reaction. This happens due to oocyte activation through sperm head contact with oolemma.

Calcium Oscillation

Calcium oscillation occurs due to calcium influx from cytoplasmic organelles (rich in calcium stores). The primary effect of calcium oscillation within oocyte cytoplasm is removal of inhibitory factor for completion of meiosis-II which gets initiated with meiosis-I of oogenesis (during intrauterine life). In other words calcium oscillation induces maturation promoting factor (MPF) within oocyte cytoplasm, which is necessary for release of second polar body (completion of meiosis-II). Following meiosis-II, the oocyte nucleus is converted into a spindle (containing half of the genetic material) and forms the female pronucleus). Before the female pronucleus is formed, calcium oscillation also helps in formation of male pronucleus. This is an interesting step. The male pronucleus is formed primarily by removal of nuclear cap of the sperm head, replacement of the special type of sperm head protein—protamine by histone migrating from the oocyte nucleus. This is followed by assembly of a new nuclear envelop—formation of male pronucleus. Pronuclear chromatin condenses to form nucleolar precursor body (NPB). These are also known as nucleoli. Arrangement and synchrony of male pronuclear nucleoli with regard to nucleoli of the female pronucleus are significant markers of good or bad pronuclei (normal or abnormal fertilization)(Fig. 4).

Function of Centriole in Sperm Neck

This helps in apposition of two pronuclei (male and female) by forming microtubules. The last stage of fertilization namely "nuclear syngamy" is completed by these microtubules.

The Male Gamete: A Unique Cell

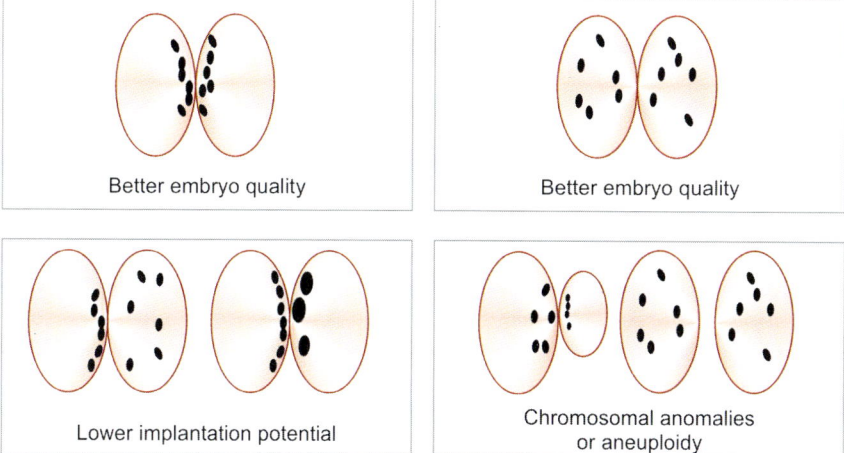

Fig. 4: Morphological assessment of fertilization through nucleolar arrangement in pronuclei.

Function of Tail

This helps the sperm to swim in the female genital tract. It is the main part of sperm that helps in movement through the female genital tract. The ability to move forward (*progressive motility*), which is acquired in the epididymis, involves activation of a unique protein called *CatSper*, which is localized to the principal piece of the sperm tail. This protein appears to be a Ca^{2+} ion channel that permits cAMP-generalized Ca^{2+} influx. In addition, spermatozoa express olfactory receptors, and ovaries produce odorant-like molecules. Recent evidence indicates that these molecules and their receptors interact, fostering movement of the spermatozoa towards the ovary (chemotaxis).

■ EXAMPLES OF SPERM ABNORMALITIES (FIG. 5)

- *Head*: Defects in shape and size—like large, small, tapering, pyriform, amorphous, and vacuolated (more than 20% of head surface is occupied by vacuoles). There may also be double head or combination defect.
- *Neck and midpiece abnormalities*: This consists of absence, non-inserted, fractured, bent and thin midpiece.
- *Tail abnormalities*: Tail abnormalities include short, multiple, hair pin, broken, coiled, and tail with terminal droplets.
- *Cytoplasmic droplets in the head*: Cytoplasmic content of the sperm head is much less than the nuclear DNA content. Cytoplasmic area greater than one-third of the area of the normal sperm head are considered abnormal.

■ SPERMATOGENESIS

This can be discussed under two broad headings:
1. Molecular consideration
2. Anatomic consideration.

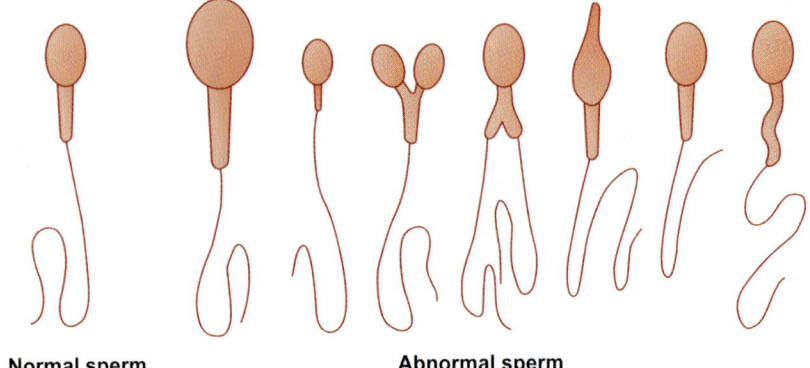

Normal sperm   **Abnormal sperm**

Fig. 5: Sperm abnormalities.

Molecular Consideration

The origin of adult spermatozoa from spermatogonial germ cell passes through three molecular phases:

1. *Mitotic proliferation*: Duplication of chromosomal DNA followed by cell division, to maintain pool of stem cells. Proliferation and differentiation of diploid spermatogonial germ cell occurs in this phase.
2. *Meiotic division*:
   – Duplication of chromosomal DNA, two cell divisions, results in haploid spermatogonia, to halve chromosome number.
   – Genetic diversity.
3. *Phase of spermiogenesis (cytodifferentiation)*: This phase consists of a series of changes involving development of nuclear DNA, acrosomal cap, tail, and ultimately resulting in development of an adult spermatozoa.

These events collectively, approximately continue for 70 days. Within this long period there may be numerous opportunities for introduction of damage to the genome of male gamete. *This knowledge provides the practical information that while performing intracytoplasmic sperm injection (ICSI) with spermatid or secondary spermatocyte, there may be a risk of injecting a damaged spermatocyte.* This may lead to failure of fertilization or development of an abnormal embryo.

Proliferation and Differentiation of Diploid Spermatogonial Cell

In the testis, the spermatogonial stem cells proliferate and differentiate producing three types of spermotogonia:
1. Population identical to spermatogonial stem cell (resting cell) and these do not differentiate towards adult spermatogonial cell.

2. Population trying to differentiate towards adult spermatogonial cell—they are the precursors of future adult spermatozoa.
3. Cells that are likely to undergo apoptosis.

During this phase, the spermotagonial cells are diploid, i.e. they contain two chromosomes each, and two chromatids (DNA strands) in each chromosome.

Phase of Meiosis

During this phase, the diploid proliferating and differentiating stem cells are converted to haploid gamete. This is a critical and unique event of genetic recombination. Primary spermatocyte (spermotogonial stem cells) with DNA content equivalent to two chromatids in two chromosomes replicate into four distinct chromatids (DNA strands) initiating meiosis (Fig. 6).

Chromosome segregation and crossing over of genes amongst DNA strands occurs during this phase. Crossing over is critical in gametogenesis—may lead to genetic defect and structural anomaly of sperm. Because, during this phase of crossing over, there may be loss or defect in the genetic material.

After chromosomal pairing and crossing over—the first meiotic division is completed, i.e. two secondary spermatocytes are formed. There is one chromosome and two chromatids (DNA strands) in each secondary spermatocyte. Therefore, the DNA content in each secondary spermatocyte is still diploid.

The second meiotic division (Fig. 7) starts where there is separation of two DNA strands in each chromosome—resulting in formation of four spermatids, each spermtaocyte having a haploid number of chromosome and a haploid DNA.

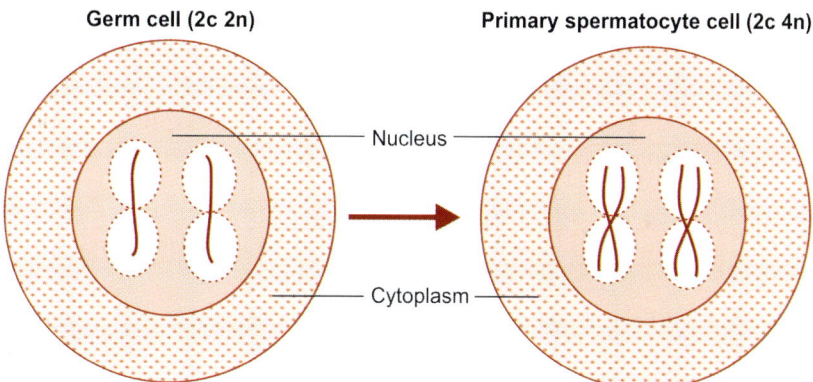

Fig. 6: Phases of meiosis.

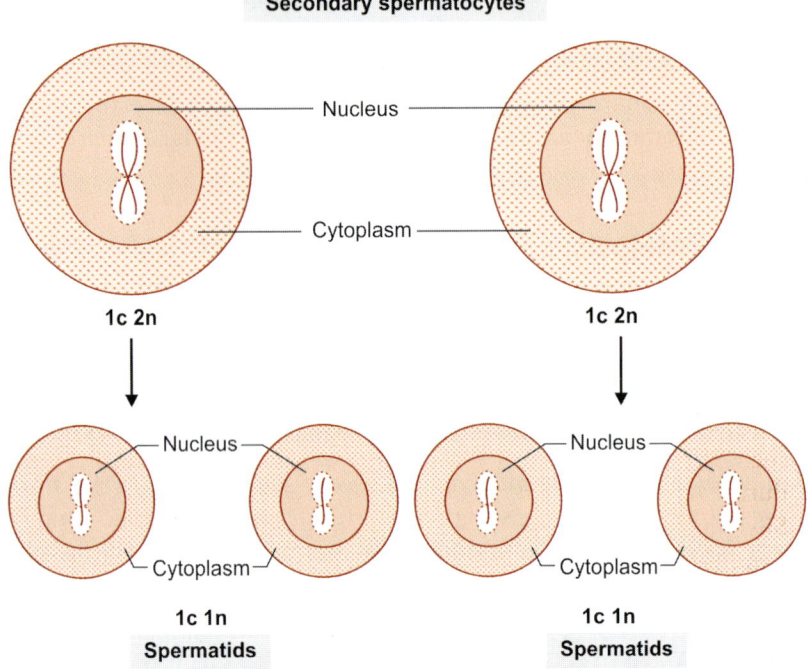

Fig. 7: Secondary meiotic division.

The diagrammatic representation of the entire process of spermatogenesis at molecular level is shown below.

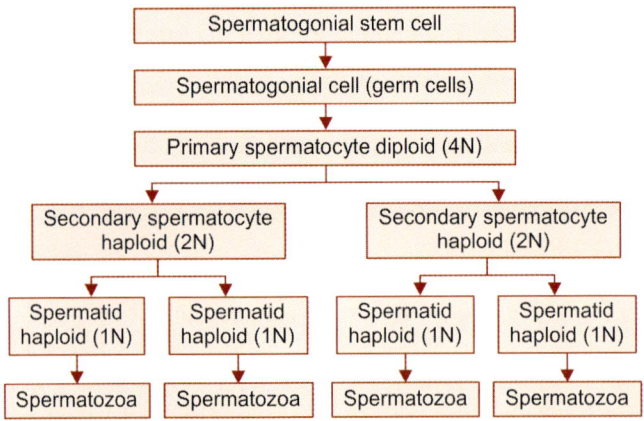

Possible Problems Arising during the Phase of Meiosis

For comprehensive meiotic division to occur, meiotic cell contains many novel proteins and enzymes. These are essential for chromosome and DNA alignment, DNA breakage, recombination and DNA repair. Occasionally DNA repair mechanism in the phase of meiosis may be defective; there may be anomalies in chromosomal segregation and pairing and crossing over of genetic material. These defects may lead to germ cell differentiation arrest at either primary or secondary spermatocyte level.

Phase of Spermiogenesis: Cytodifferentiation

During this phase, maturation of spermatozoa starts. From the stage of secondary spermatocyte a round-shaped spermatid forms followed by elongated spermatid and finally an adult spermatozoa develops.

During these transitional phases, the specific changes which occur consist of:
- Elongation of nucleus and nuclear condensation
- Appearance of acrosomal sac containing proteolytic enzymes
- Formation of neck and differentiation of the terminal part into three distinct segments—midpiece, principal piece, and end piece. These changes occur during six different stages; the stages have been designated as SA-1 and 2, SB-1 and 2 and SC-1 and 2
- Cytoplasmic reduction.

Specific and Remarkable Changes during Spermiogenesis

- Head nuclear protein consisting of histone is replaced by protamine, producing a tightly compacted nucleus. Protamine is a stronger DNA protein compared to histone. Unlike all other somatic cells of the body where histone is present with the DNA in the nucleus, spermatozoa is the only cell which contains protamine to offer compactness of the sperm head nuclear DNA.[5,6]
- Chromatin condensation during spermiogenesis results in DNA occupying nearly 70% of the total volume of sperm nucleus (somatic cell—only 5%).[7–10]
- The adverse effect of displacement of histone and replacement by protamine may result in haploid genome damage (after secondary spermatocyte, the sperm cell genome becomes haploid).
- Repair capabilities during spermiogenesis phase is limited (unlike those during meiosis phase).
- In addition to nuclear DNA structuring, axoneme, outer dense fiber and protein (dynein) in midpiece, principal piece and end piece develop.
- Mitochondria develops on the sheath of midpiece as germ cell differentiation by spermiogenesis continues.

As a consequence of massive changes during spermiogenesis there may be tremendous load on "haploid" spermatozoa, leading to germ cell arrest or blockage—thereby causing infertility in many individuals.

Defects in synthesis of midpiece and tail mitochondria may result in structurally abnormal spermatozoa with poor motility. Also mutation in protein essential for compaction of sperm nuclear DNA may result in spermatozoa with abnormal head.[11–17]

Minor genetic defects may not alter spermatozoa morphology but may lead to production of genetically defective spermatid. This will be a great concern for spermatid injection which is sometimes performed in the procedure of ICSI (ROSNI-round spermatid nuclear injection).

Difference of Initiation of Meiosis in the Male and Female Gamete

In female, meiosis starts at 12 weeks of intrauterine life, but remains arrested at meiosis-I. This is completed at puberty with onset of luteinizing hormone (LH) surge. In male, spermatogonial cells (the stem cells) remain at rest till puberty—meiosis and spermiogenesis start after puberty.

■ SPERMATOGENESIS—ANATOMICAL CONSIDERATION

Sperms develop and mature within seminiferous tubules. Seminiferous tubules consist of basement membrane and lumen (Fig. 8).

Basement Membrane

Basement membrane consist of two types of cells: Germ cells and Sertoli cells.

Sertoli cells are triangular-shaped cells with their apex projecting towards the lumen. The base of these triangular cells are situated peripherally. Apex of the Sertoli cells are interconnected by tight junction. This tightly interconnected apical junction forms "blood-testis barrier". Blood-testis barrier when intact does not allow seminal antigens to pass into the systemic circulation (reticuloendothelial system) to produce self antibodies.

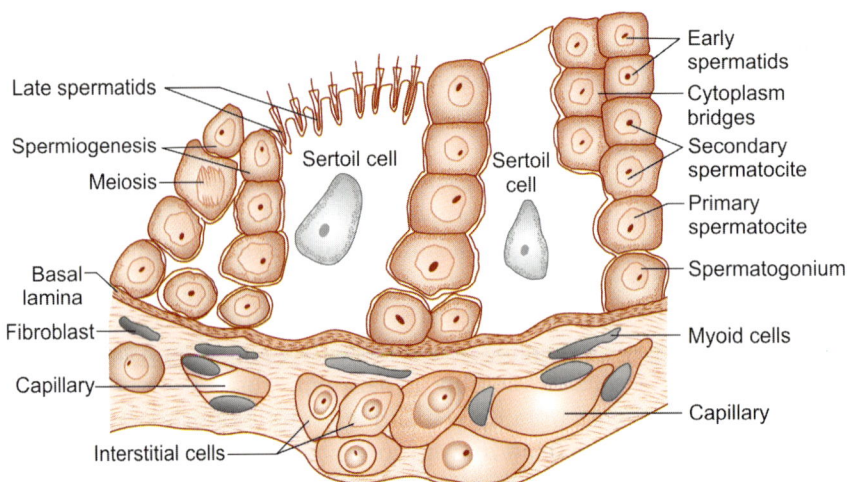

Fig. 8: Microscopic picture in spermatogenesis.

Germs cells lie in between the Sertoli cells, they are precursors of adult spermatozoa.

Lumen

Interconnected Sertoli cells divide the lumen of seminiferous tubules into two compartments:
1. Basal compartment
2. Adluminal compartment.

Significance of Two Compartments

- *Basal compartment*: In this compartment, maturation of early stages of spermatozoa occur. This compartment is in direct contact with interstitial cells containing Leydig cell, blood vessels, and lymphatics and therefore is directly exposed to immune phenomenon. But the tight interconnection of the apices of Sertoli cells, which forms the blood-testis barrier, prevents antigens to cross this barrier and prevents antibody formation. But when this blood-testis barrier is damaged as in infection, trauma, exposure to heat, and following vasectomy, antigens may crossover allowing antibodies to develop in reticuloendothelial system of the body. These antibodies then reenter the seminiferous tubules and damage the developing spermatozoa. Basement membrane contains myofibrils—which are under control of oxytocin. They help in forward sperm propulsion.
- *Adluminal compartment*: Within the adluminal compartment, late stages of spermatozoal maturation continues. This is a sealed compartment and therefore not exposed to external or environmental trauma.

Final Maturation and Acquisition of Motility of Spermatozoa

This occurs through exposure of spermatozoa to many biochemical components while the sperm travels through the seminal pathway. The principal sites where the sperm acquires significant motility are—rete testis, epididymis, seminal vesicles, and prostate. The important biochemical constituents which provide additional sources of sperm vitality, motility, and integrity are—carnitine, acid glycerophosphate from epididymis, fructose and coagulase (from seminal vesicle), liquefying enzymes and acid phosphatase from prostate.

Effect of Temperature on Spermatogenesis

Spermatogenesis requires a temperature considerably lower than that of the interior of the body. The testes are normally maintained at a temperature of about 32°C. They are kept cool by air circulating around the scrotum and probably by heat exchange in a countercurrent fashion between the spermatic arteries and veins. When the testes are retained in the abdomen or when, they are held close to the body by tight cloth binders, degeneration of the tubular walls and sterility result. Hot baths (43–45°C for 30 minutes per day) and insulated athletic supporters reduce the sperm count in humans, in some cases by 90%. In addition, evidence suggests a seasonal effect in men, with sperm counts being greater in the winter regardless of the temperature to which the scrotum is exposed.

Endocrine Control of Spermatogenesis (Flowchart 1)

Just like ovulatory control, spermatogenesis has also an endocrine control with feedback mechanism between hypothalamic pituitary control from one side and testicular control from the other side. Follicle-stimulating hormone (FSH) is secreted from the pituitary which stimulates Sertoli cell within the seminiferous tubules and Sertoli cells in turn produce two factors:
1. Inhibin which regulates the production of FSH from pituitary
2. Androgen binding globulin (ABG).[18]

Androgen binding globulin transports testosterone produced by Leydig cells which exist outside the seminiferous tubules into the lumen of the seminiferous tubules allowing maturation of germ cells. LH also produced by pituitary stimulates Leydig cells to produce testosterone (5–10 mg per day). Testosterone on one side helps maturation of germ cells and on the other hand regulates production of pituitary LH through negative feedback mechanism. The stages from spermatogonia to spermatids appear to be androgen-independent. However, the maturation from spermatids to spermatozoa depends on androgen acting on the Sertoli cells in which the developing spermatozoa are

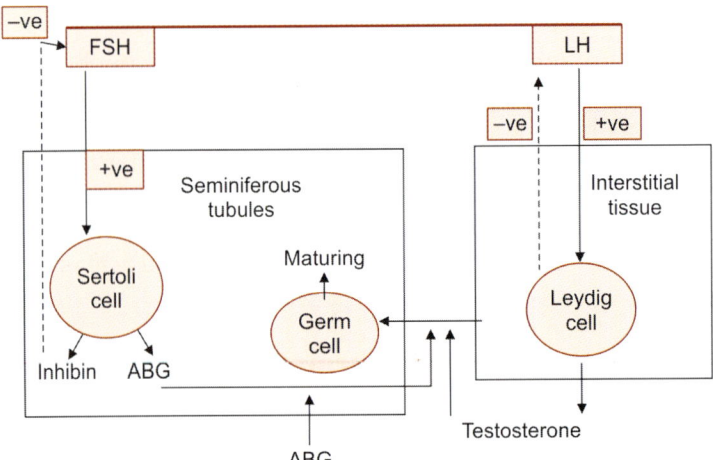

Flowchart 1: Endocrine control of spermatogenesis.

Growth factor, cytokine proteins, enzymes are the additional factors
(ABG: androgen binding globulin; FSH: follicle-stimulating hormone; LH: luteinizing hormone).

embedded. FSH acts on the Sertoli cells to facilitate the last stages of spermatid maturation. In addition, it promotes the production of androgen-binding protein (ABP).[18]

In addition to endocrine control there are other paracrine procedures which help in spermatogenesis. These paracrine factors consist of— IGF-1, cytokines, proteins, and enzymes.[19]

The estrogen content of the fluid in the rete testis is high, and the walls of the rete contain numerous estrogen receptors (ER). In this region, fluid is reabsorbed and the spermatozoa are concentrated. If this does not occur, the sperm entering the epididymis are diluted in a large volume of fluid, and infertility results.

After production in seminiferous tubules under tight hormonal control, sperm have to pass through a long pathway to act in its final destination. Spermatozoa leaving the testes are not fully mobile. They continue their maturation and acquire motility during their passage through the epididymis. During its journey, it gets matured, motility as well as sperm becomes susceptible to different type of damage by free radicals.

Following the morphological transformation of nucleus in the testis, as spermatozoa transit through the epididymis, there occurs a stabilization of the chromatin through establishment of disulfide bond between the thiol rich protamines.[20] Qualitative and quantitative modifications of the plasma membrane occurring in the lipidic composition[21] and the absorption of specific proteins secreted by the epididymal epithelium result in changes of its electric charges. The lack of all this changes is associated with a decreased ability of epididymal spermatozoa to bind and penetrate the oocyte.[22] Ejaculation of the spermatozoon involves contractions of the vas deferens mediated in part by P2X receptors for ATP and fertility is reduced in mice in which these receptors are knocked out.

KEY POINTS

- Spermatozoa is the male gamete which performs the function of reproduction. Each sperm is an intricate motile cell, rich in DNA, with a head that is made up mostly of chromosomal material. Covering the head like a cap is the acrosome, a lysosome-like organelle rich in enzymes involved in sperm penetration of the ovum and other events involved in fertilization. The motile tail of the sperm is wrapped in its proximal portion by a sheath holding numerous mitochondria.
- There are few unique characteristic of human spermatozoa; the important ones are: adult sperm cells do not grow or divide; unlike other somatic cells sperm head has a large nucleus and lacks large cytoplasm and the sperm cells are unique for the presence of plenty of abnormal forms in the ejaculate. This is because of frequency of aneuploidy due to specific chromosomal arrangements in the nucleus.
- There are four anatomical segments of adult spermatozoa, each with specific physiological function. The segments and their functions are: head, involved in the main biological function of fertilization; centriole, in the neck helping in the process of pronuclear apposition; while the midpiece and tail maintain sperm vitality metabolism respiration and locomotion.

- Spermotozoal developments occur within the testes from immature germ cells which are known as spermatogonial cells. There are three types of cells in our body; viz: somatic cell, stem cells, and germ cells. All cells are diploid except adult spermatozoa which is haploid. The entire process of adult sperm (haploid) formation from immature sperm (diploid) takes about 9–10 weeks and passes through several phases of divisions.
  Broadly, changes occur through three phases:
  1. Proliferation and differentiation of diploid spermatogonial germ cells.
  2. Phase of meiosis—chromosomal pairing and genetic recombination.
  3. Phase of spermiogenesis—series of changes occur, involving development of nuclear DNA, acrosomal cap, etc., ultimately developing into a haploid adult spermatozoa. This long period of spermatogenesis provides enormous opportunities for morphological and genetic abnormalities to occur in adult spermatozoa. This is one of the reasons for presence of large number of abnormal spermatozoa in the ejaculate.
- Anatomically, germ cells exist in the basal compartment of seminiferous tubules. Seminiferous tubule is divided into two compartments: basal and adluminal, by tight epical junction of Sertoli cells. Germ cells lie in between Sertoli cells.
- The primary development up to secondary spermatocyte occurs within basal compartment—whereas the final maturation occurs within the adluminal compartment. The biochemical environment for final maturation and acquisition of motility is provided by different molecular constituents available in the seminal pathway; epididymis, vas deferens seminal vesicles, prostate, and bulbourethral glands, etc.
- Like endocrine control of ovulation, spermatogenesis also has a similar mechanism of endocrine feedback regulation. The principle participants are: FSH, LH from pituitary and feedback control is provided through testosterone from Leydig cell and inhibin and androgen binding globulin (ABG) from Sertoli cells.

■ REFERENCES

1. Ward WS, Coffey DS. DNA packaging and organization in mammalian spermatozoa: comparison with somatic cells. Biol Reprod. 1991;44 (4):569-74.
2. Smith DJ. Human sperm accumulation near surfaces: a simulation study. Journal of Fluid Mechanics. 2009;621:289-320.
3. Ishijima S, Oshio S, Mohri H. Flagellar movement of human spermatozoa. Gamete Research. 1986; 13(3): 185-97.
4. Duijn CV. The structure of human spermatozoa. Journal of the Royal Microscopcial Society. 1952;72(4):189-98.
5. Zalenskaya IA, Brabdury EM, Zalensky AO. Chromatin Structure of Telomere: Domain in Human Sperm. Biochemical & Biophysical Research Communications. 2000;279(1):213-8.
6. Shettles LB. Nuclear Structure of Human Spermatozoa. Nature. 1960;186:648.
7. Fuentes-Mascorro G, Serrano H, Rosado A. Sperm Chromatin. Arch Androl. 2000; 45(3); 215-25.
8. Oliva R, Castillo J. Proteomics and the genetics of sperm chromatin condensation. Asian J Androl. 2011;13:24-30.

9. Gatewood JM, Cook GR, Balhorn R, et al. Sequence specific packaging of DNA in human sperm chromatin. Science. 1987; 236:962-4.
10. Bench GS, Friz AM, Corzett MH, et al. DNA and total protamine masses in individiual sperm from fertile mammalian subjects. Cytometry. 1996;23: 263-71.
11. Johnson GD, Lalancette G, Linnemann AK, et al. The sperm nucleus: chromatin, RNA, and the nuclear matrix. Reproduction. 2011;141:21-36.
12. Sakkas D, Mariethoz E, Manicardi G, et al. Origin of DNA damage in ejaculated human spermatozoa. Rev Reprod. 1999;4:31-7.
13. Ward WS. Deoxyribonucleic acid loop-domain tertiary structure in mammalian spermatozoa. Biol Reprod. 1993; 48:1193-201.
14. Zalensky AO, Allen MJ, Kobayashi A, et al. Well defined genome architecture in the human sperm nucleus. Chromosoma. 1995;103:577-90.
15. Solov'eva L, Svetlova M, Bodinski D, et al. Nature of telomere dimmers and chromosome looping in human spermatozoa. Chromosome Res. 2004;12:817-23.
16. Ward WS, Zalensky AO. The unique, complex organization of the transcriptionally silent sperm chromatin. Crit Rev Eukaryot Gene Expr. 1996; 6:139-47.
17. de Kretser DM, Loveland KL, Meinhardt A, et al. Spermatogenesis. HUM Reprod. 1998;13(Suppl 1):1-8.
18. McLachlan RI. The endocrine control of spermatogenesis. Best Practice and Research, Clinical Endocrinology and Metabolism. 2000;14(3):345-62.
19. McLachlan RI, Wreford NG, Robbertson DM, et al. Hormonal control of spermatogenesis. Trends in Endocrinology and Metabolism. 1995;6(3):95-101.
20. Calvin HI, Bedford JM. Formation of disulfide bonds in the nucleus and accessory structures of mammalian spermatozoa during maturation in the epididymis. J Reprod Fertil Suppl. 1971;13(suppl 13):65-75.
21. Neri QV, Hu J, Rosenwaks Z, et al. Understanding the spermatozoon. Methods Mol Biol. 2014;1154:91-119.
22. Kirchhoff C, Osterhoff C, Habben I, et al. Cloning and analysis of mRNAs expressed specially in the human epididymis. Int J Androl. 1990;13:155-67.

CHAPTER 2

Evaluation of Male Infertility

Shanti Roy

■ INTRODUCTION

Infertility is defined as failure to conceive after 1 year of regular and unprotected intercourse. In 50–60% of the couples presenting with infertility, a male factor either alone or as a cofactor is responsible. Evaluation for male factor follows a protocol similar to that for any other clinical condition:

- History
- General examination
- Local examination
- Investigations.

■ HISTORY

- Age, occupation, duration of married life and cohabitation, contraceptive use, any previous treatment for infertility, knowledge of fertile period and past fertility, if any, of either partner.
- Use of smoking, alcohol, tobacco, narcotics, regular hot/sauna baths and drugs as spironolactone.
- History of exposure to toxins such as DDT, polychlorinated biphenyl (plastic industry toxin), and BHC.
- Medical history of diabetes, tuberculosis, PUO, hypertension, vascular disease, DES exposure, measles, pubertal mumps orchitis, pneumonia, typhoid, sexually transmitted diseases and any other genitourinary infection.
- History of testicular torsion and testicular injury.
- Sexual history including frequency of intercourse and premature ejaculation, duration, frequency and effectiveness of sexual contact.
- History of general disease and current medications if any.
- Any surgery for descent of testes, bladder neck operation and vasectomy.

■ GENERAL EXAMINATION

It includes height, weight, gynecomastia, distribution of body hair, pattern of fat distribution, unusual length of extremities, general nutritional status, tests for anosmia and blood pressure, etc.

If androgen deficiency exists at the time of onset of puberty, the person is eunuchoid, tall, arm span exceeding the body length and the legs longer than the trunk. If androgen deficiency occurs after puberty there is no change in body proportions. Other features of hypogonadism are straight frontal hairline, a horizontal pubic hairline, sparse or no beard growth and gynecomastia.

■ LOCAL EXAMINATION

Size, shape and consistency of the testes, descent of both testes in scrotum, testicular torsion, urethral stricture, hypospadias, varicocele, hydrocele, lymphocele, urethral diverticulum, inguinal hernia, scrotal hernia, groin lymphadenopathy, any scarring or surgical scar.

Testicular volume is normally 12–30 mL per testis. Most of this volume is provided by the seminiferous tubules. Decreased testicular volume is a strong indicator of abnormal spermatogenesis. Extremely small but firm testes may be a sign of Klinefelter's syndrome whereas soft testes of normal or decreased size generally indicate a primary or secondary deterioration of spermatogenesis. Abnormalities of epididymis, pampiniform plexus and the vas deferens can be detected by palpation. Varicocele is a common finding which badly influences fertility. It means venous distension of pampiniform plexus and usually present on left side. According to the severity it is classified as Grade I, II and III.

Dystopic localization of the urethral orifice, phimosis or deviation of the penis during erections might lead to fertility problems.

■ INVESTIGATIONS

Semen Analysis

This is the most important single investigation for evaluation of male infertility. Further tests are decided depending upon its results. The semen should be analyzed after 2–3 days of abstinence. Long abstinence results in aging of sperms with decreasing motility. Shortened abstinence time might significantly reduce sperm concentration. Sperm output is not uniform in ejaculate and varies from time to time. Therefore, at least two semen samples at an interval of at least 2 weeks should be evaluated.

Collection of Specimen

The semen can be obtained in a jar by masturbation or after sexual intercourse with a specially designed silastic condom without lubricant. The sample should arrive in the laboratory within an hour of ejaculation for optimal analysis. Normally, semen liquefies within 30 minutes. If time for liquefaction taken is significantly reduced or prolonged it indicates a malfunction of the prostate or seminal vesicles. This should be further investigated with special tests.

Seminal Fluid Parameters

The main parameters assessed in the seminal fluid are:
- Ejaculate volume
- Liquefaction time
- Sperm concentration
- Sperm motility
- Sperm morphology
- Presence of leukocytes.

Reference Range

Data from World Health Organization (WHO) suggest a reference range for different parameters of seminal fluid, although it is still controversial what should be regarded as a normal semen profile (Table 1).

Volume: Normal range is 2–5 mL/ejaculate and less than 1.5 mL is considered to be low. A very low volume may be due to a poorly collected ejaculate, malfunction of accessory glands or genital tract obstruction. Semen volume of less than 1.5 mL is called hypospermia and more than 5.0 mL is hyperspermia. Hyperspermia may be due to prolonged sexual abstinence, infection or contamination with urine. Aspermia means absence of ejaculate during orgasm.

Count: A count of more than 15 million/mL is considered to be normal. When there is no sperm in the ejaculate it is called azoospermia while less than normal range of sperms is called oligozoospermia. When sperm count is less than 5 million/mL, it is unlikely that pregnancy will occur spontaneously. The prevalence of azoospermia is approximately 1% of all men. Azoospermia may result from outflow tract obstruction or testicular failure. Endocrine and genetic evaluation is indicated for men with abnormal sperm counts.

Motility: Motility is the single most important parameter of the semen analysis as far as fertility is concerned. More than 50% of sperms should be motile. WHO defines "normal motility", as at least 50% of total sperms to be motile in grade A + B (Progressive + Nonprogressive) or 25% of sperms in grade A (Progressive). Asthenozooserpmia is the term applied to less than 50% motile sperms in specimen. Circular or shaking motility is considered as abnormal.

Table 1: Reference range for different parameters of seminal fluid.

Parameter	Range
1. Volume	More than 1.5 mL
2. Count	More than 15 million/mL
3. Total Motility	More than 40%
4. Morphology	More than 4%
5. White blood cells	Less than 1 million/mL
6. Round cells	More than 5 million/mL

Asthenospermia has been attributed to prolonged abstinence, antisperm antibodies, genital tract infections or varicocele. To differentiate between the dead and nonmotile sperm, a hypo-osmotic swelling test can be performed. Unlike dead sperm, living sperm can maintain an ostotic gradient. Thus, when mixed with a hypo-osmotic solution, living, nonmotile sperm with normal membrane function swell and coil as fluid is absorbed.

Morphology: Evaluation of shape, length, width, volume, acrosome body and assessment of head and tail defects are done for morphological evaluation. It is an important predictor of male fertility and more than 4% should have normal morphology to have a pregnancy. Abnormal sperm morphology is termed teratospermia or teratozoospermia.

White blood cells (WBCs): Leukocytospermia is defined as greater than 1 million WBCs per milliliter of seminal fluid and may indicate chronic epididymitis or prostatitis.

■ RELEVANCE OF VARIOUS ABNORMALITIES IN SEMINAL FLUID

The relevance of various abnormalities in seminal fluid is given in Table 2.

Besides the above mentioned semen parameters, many other investigations can give a more detailed information of semen quality such as biochemical analysis or electron microscopic evaluation. But these methods have no special advantage as treatment is not influenced by their results. Various tests and treatment for antisperm antibodies were used in the past but is now obsolete as it has no definite role in improving male fertility. The same is true for other sperm function tests as hypo-osmotic swelling test, the eosin test and the zona binding test because no significant correlation between test results and outcome of these procedures have been demonstrated.

Hormone Analysis

The incidence of endocrine disorders as etiological factors for male infertility is extremely low. The following hormones are generally estimated for basic diagnosis.
- Serum testosterone
- Serum follicle stimulating hormone (FSH)
- Serum luteinizing hormone (LH).

Elevated FSH and low testosterone levels provide evidence of testicular failure and most men with oligospermia fall into this category. Low gonadotropin levels indicate a central cause (secondary hypogonadism). Low FSH and low testosterone levels are consistent with hypothalamic dysfunction, such as idiopathic hypogonadotropic hypogonadism or Kallman syndrome. In these patients, sperm production may be achieved with gonadotropin treatment.

Clinical symptoms of hyperprolactinemia, hyper- or hypothyroidism or dysfunction of the adrenal gland need to be assessed by respective analysis.

Table 2: Relevance of various abnormalities in seminal fluid.

Semen parameters	Cause
Low volume	Spillage No abstinence Vas aplasia Ejaculatory duct obstruction Partial retrograde ejaculation Chronic seminal vesiculitis Difficulty in masturbation
Increased volume	Prostatic infection, contamination with urine
Delayed liquefaction/Accessory gland dysfunction/increased viscosity	Some times due to unsuitable type of plastic container
Increased particulate debris pH acidic	Due to chronic infection Correlates with absence of fructose Obstruction of the ejaculatory ducts Bilateral congenital absence of vasa
pH >8	Acute prostatitis Vasculitis, epididymitis Sometimes because of delayed examination
Fructose absent	Vas aplasia, Ejaculatory duct obstruction, fibrosis of seminal vesicles
Sperm precursor cells absent	Rules out obstruction in cases of azoospermia
Sperm agglutination	Infection Antibodies Nonspecific
Pus cells increased	Infection in prostate/seminal vesicles. Possible laboratory error
Total azoospermia (with no premature cells)	Testicular failure, post-testicular obstruction
Oligoasthenozoospermia	Testicular dysfunction

Specific analysis of the testosterone receptors should be done if clinical symptoms of hypogonadism are present despite normal or elevated testosterone levels.

DNA Damage

Increased levels of DNA damage in sperms has been recently recognized as a cause of lowered fertility. This is associated with advanced paternal age and factors such as cigarette smoking, chemotherapy, radiation, environmental toxins, varicocele and genital tract infections. Numerous tests are currently available to analyze for DNA integrity. However till date, there is no sufficient evidence to recommend the routine use of these tests in infertile couples.

Antisperm Antibodies

Antisperm antibodies may be detected in as many as 10% of men with prevalence following vasectomy, testicular torsion, testicular biopsy or other conditions in which the blood-testis barrier is breached. However, it is not considered to be a routine component of infertility evaluation.

Genetic Testing

Approximately, 15% of azoospermic men and 5% of severely oligospermic men will have an abnormal karyotype. Karyotyping should be done in men with poor semen analysis results. A count between 3 and 10 million sperm per milliliter is considered poor.

Klinefelter syndrome (47 XXY) is observed in approximately 1 in 500 men in the general population and accounts for 1–2% of male infertility cases.

Autosomal abnormalities are also found in some men with severe oligospermia.

If a man with severely decreased sperm counts has a normal karyotype, testing for microdeletion of the Y chromosome should be done. Up to 15% of such persons will have small deletions in a region of the Y choromosome. These deletions are inherited by their offspring.

Obstructive azoospermia may be due to congenital bilateral absence of the vas deferens (CBAVD). Approximately 70–85% of men with CBAVD will have mutation found in the cystic *fibrosis transmembrane conductance regulator (CFTR) gene* although all of them will not have clinical cystic fibrosis.

Testicular Biopsy

Testicular biopsy is done for evaluation of severely oligospermic or azoospermic men to know whether viable sperms are present in the seminiferous tubules. Many azoospermic men even with raised FSH are found to have adequate sperms on biopsy which can be cryopreserved and used for IVF.

KEY POINTS

- Evolution of infertile male is an important issue as there is gradual rise in male infertility globally.
- Thorough history, extensive physical and laboratory investigation are required for proper evaluation for infertile male.
- There is no single global sperm test by which we can assess male fertilization potential, so we need a combination of test.
- Basic semen analysis is still the corner stone of laboratory investigation.
- Biochemical, functional semen analysis and endocrinal analysis of male partner are essential for proper management of infertile male.
- Recent advancement such as DNA fragmentation Index (DFI), ROS (Reactive oxygen Species /TAC (Total antioxidant capacity) estimation may further refine the evaluation process.

CHAPTER 3

Sperm Function Tests

Keshav Malhotra, Neharika Malhotra Bora, Jaideep Malhotra, Narendra Malhotra

■ INTRODUCTION

Since the advent of assisted reproductive techniques (ART), the use of semen function test as a modality for determining the prognosis of the couple has been questioned, but off late it has managed to gain acceptance both amongst patients and clinicians.[1] The new World Health Organization (WHO) manual for the examination and processing of human semen is a great improvement on the previous editions. The addition of sperm cryopreservation techniques, the expansion of the section on sperm preparation and the inclusion of new appendices have contributed to the production of a user-friendly laboratory manual. The most important change in the manual is the use of evidence-based publications as references to determine cutoff values for normality.[2] Owing to the constantly changing societal landscape today, the number of couples having difficulties conceiving has been exponentially increasing. Recent and past evidence have corroborated that approximately 25–50% of the couples deal with male infertility.[3] Moreover, it has also been documented that sperm of infertile men compared to that of fertile men has more functional impairment, which possibly has a detrimental effect on their fertility.[4,5] Therefore, it's paramount, to test the male partner adequately for favorable outcomes in natural or artificial fertilization.[6] Nonetheless, this is a controversial issue since present literature gives hardly any clue about it.

■ SPERM FUNCTION TESTING

These tests are usually best performed in a well-equipped laboratory with trained personnel. It is a well-documented fact that male infertility is on the rise and though many advances have been made in the field in the last decade or two, the knowledge about the molecular and biological basis of male infertility is still lacking.[2] A routine semen analysis does not give us enough evidence to distinguish a fertile population from an infertile one. Therefore, a battery of tests should be done in order to have a better understanding. Sadly these tests are expensive and result in many patients opting out of the cycle because these

Sperm Function Tests

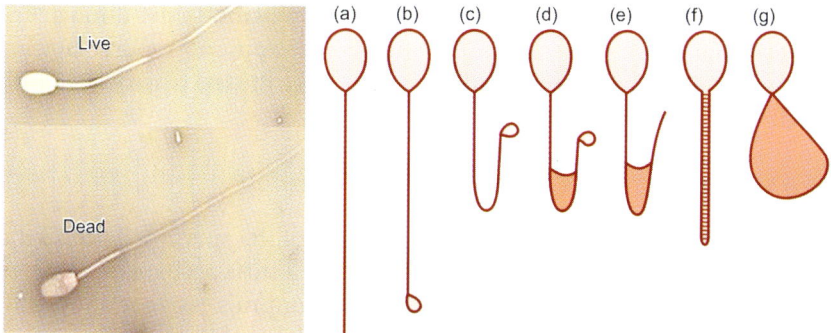

Fig. 1: Vitality testing by staining and hypoosmotic swelling test.
(a) Live; (b to g) Dead.

tests are prescribed. To understand these tests we must first understand the functions of the sperm (Fig. 1).

Spermatozoa must be capable of penetrating and passing through the cervical mucus, and through the uterus, undergo capacitation, acrosomal reaction, binding and penetration of the zona pellucida, and ultimately the ovum. Once the spermatozoon penetrates the ovum, it must then undergo nuclear decondensation to deliver the appropriate haploid chromosome complement. It then undergoes additional events required for fertilization and early embryonic development.

Based on these functions a variety of tests have been designed which are:
- Vitality tests
- Capacitation
- Acrosome reaction
- Zona binding assays
- Ovum penetration test
- DNA fragmentation
- Sperm aneuploidy.

Assessment of Vitality

Vitality or membrane integrity can be conducted on samples with a simple inexpensive dye- exclusion test. This is especially important for samples with poor motility or no motility at all. In such cases it becomes important for the embryologist to determine whether immotile spermatozoa are alive or dead, especially in cases where intracytoplasmic sperm injection (ICSI) is the considered therapy. A one-step staining technique using an eosin–nigrosin suspension is recommended. The WHO 2010 reference limit for vitality is 58%. The problem with staining the sample is that once stained these sperms cannot be used for ICSI, therefore a better test to do in such scenarios is a HOS or a hypoosmotic swelling test. Water permeability is a fundamental biophysical property of all living cells. It is known that one quality of the cell membrane is its ability to allow the selective transport of fluids and molecules through it.[2,7] This test might have some clinical use but there are opposing reports showing that the test does not have a prognostic value, since the test is associated with a high-level of false positive results.[8]

Capacitation

Capacitation is an important step in the ability of the sperm to fertilize the egg. During capacitation the sperm undergoes cell surface changes, achieves hyperactivated motility and attains vigorous nonprogressive motion with forceful amplitude bending, as shown in Figures 2A and B.

Capacitation can be tested in the following ways:

- Sperm wash and incubation in albumin-containing culture
  - Very simple
  - No need for oocyte or mucus
  - Identify changes in pattern of motility manually by microscopy or by using computer-assisted sperm analysis (CASA).
- Chlortetracycline-staining
  - Detection by fluorescence microscopy
  - Acrosome-reacted sperm show a staining pattern different from that of capacitated sperm with acrosomes still intact.

Acrosome Reaction

Over the last decade or so various researchers have demonstrated important parameters of sperm function, and acrosomal reaction is one of the most important ones. Liu and Baker, and Menkveld et al. have demonstrated that normal sperm acrosomal morphology (Fig. 3) correlates significantly with

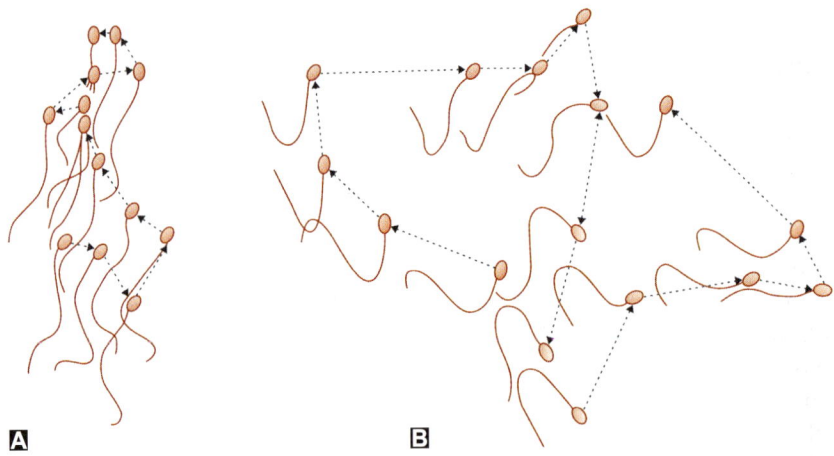

Figs. 2A and B: Change in pattern of motility during capacitation: (A) Non-hyperactivated; (B) Hyperactivated.

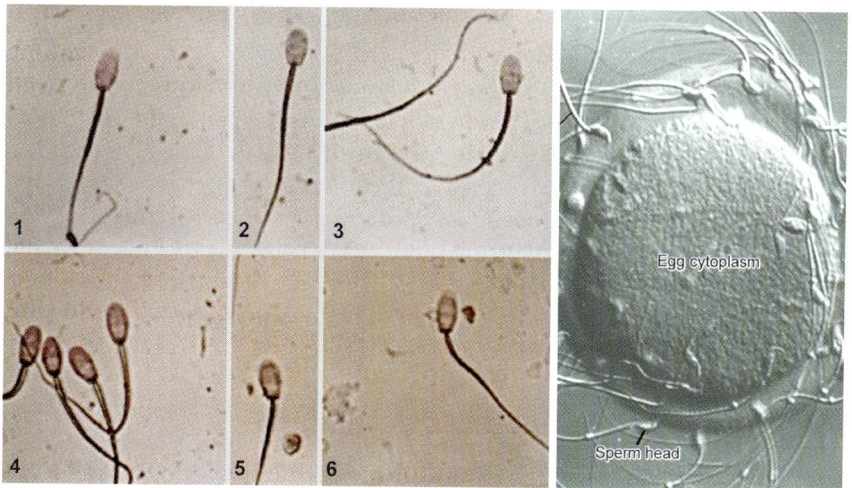

Fig. 3: Acrosomal staining and zone binding assay.

sperm binding to the zona pellucida, while Franken et al.[9] showed a strong relationship between normal sperm morphology and the inducibility of the acrosome reaction. Determining the ability of the acrosome to react is important in the diagnostic and therapeutic approach to couples undergoing conventional assisted reproductive technology treatment. Acrosomal reaction can be tested in a few ways, some of the now unconventional ways include: zona binding assays and the hemizona assay where the patient's zona or a donor zone pellucida is used to test for sperm attachment and penetration. However, the use of these tests is restricted as we waste precious oocytes on doing a diagnostic test. Acrosomal reaction can also be tested using stains like Trypan blue, triple stain, fluorescent lectins and antibody staining.

DNA Fragmentation[10]

In 1869, Frederich Miescher (German biochemist) observed for the first time, a molecule, whose significance was not known until 1953, when James Watson, Francis Crick, Maurice Wilkin, and Rosalind Franklin illustrated its structure as that of the deoxyribonucleic acid molecule (DNA). DNA is the genetic material that has all the instructions for an organism to develop, live and reproduce and is inherited by the children from their parents. Ovum and sperm from mother and father respectively are fused during fertilization to give rise to the zygote, which has half the set of chromosomes (genetic information) from both parents. Thus, the chemical and structural DNA integrity is imperative for development of embryo, and consequently fetus and child.[11] Owing to the constantly changing societal landscape today, the number of couples having difficulties conceiving has been exponentially increasing. Recent and past evidence have corroborated that approximately 25–50% of the couples deal with male infertility.[3] Moreover, it has also been documented that sperm of infertile men compared to that of fertile men has more DNA impairment, which possibly has a detrimental effect on their fertility.[4] Therefore, it is paramount, to test the stability of DNA for favorable outcomes in natural or artificial fertilization; failure to do so may or will affect the development of embryo, fetus, and child. Nonetheless, this is a controversial issue since literature also suggests that various tests to determine the integrity of DNA present no clue about the outcome of the procedure.[11] Moreover, routine DNA fragmentation testing shows no correlation with infertility, as has been stated by the American Society for Reproductive Medicine, since it provides information on seminal volume, pH, sperm concentration, motility, morphology, which is not the ultimate diagnosis of male infertility.[7]

Methods to Assess Sperm DNA Damage

Nowadays, there are batteries of diagnostic methods within easy reach to evaluate the DNA stability/integrity of the spermatocytes. Out of which three assays are popularly used among many laboratories, they are:
1. Sperm chromatin structure assay (SCSA)
2. Single-cell gel electrophoresis assay (COMET assay)
3. Terminal deoxynucleotidyl transferase-mediated dUTP nick end-labeling assay (TUNEL assay).

Besides the assays described above several other assays are used by some laboratories:

- Sperm chromatin dispersion tests (SCD) (Fig. 4)
- Acridine orange test (AOT)
- Toluidine blue test
- Aniline blue test.
  These are easy to perform and cheap but clinical effectiveness and relevance still remains to be established.

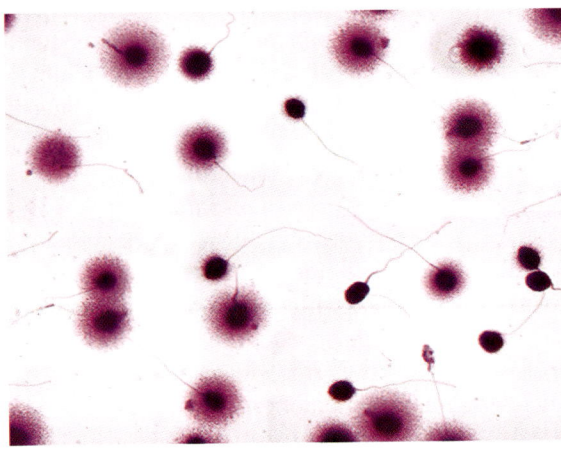

Fig. 4: Sperm DNA fragmentation staining by sperm chromatin dispersion method.

Sperm Function Tests

> **DFI %**
>
> <15% DFI = excellent fertility potential
> >15 to < 30% DFI = good fertility potential
> >30% DFI = fair to poor fertility potential
>
> The statistically significant DFI threshold for subfertility has been established at >30%
> Normal full-term pregnancies are possible with an elevated DFI, but the higher the level of fragmentation, the greater the incidence of reduced term pregnancies and miscarriage.

> **HDS %**
>
> <15% HDS = normal
> >15% HDS = above normal
>
> Immature chromatin can be measured by high DNA stainability (HDS) and is associated with asyngamy and poor IVF fertilization rates when it exceeds 15%

Fig. 5: Relevant values when using sperm chromatin dispersion.

All the above given tests calculate DNA fragmentation index % (DFI %) and/or high DNA stainability (HDS %); where DFI % is the percentage of sperm cells containing DNA damage and HDS % is the percentage of cells with immature chromatin. The depiction of their various percentages of DFI and HDS is illustrated in the Figure 5.

Sperm DNA integrity is imperative for precise conveyance of genetic information to the offspring. Therefore, it is paramount to test the stability of DNA, for a favorable outcome. There are numerous tests which are available to evaluate different aspects of DNA integrity and several clinical studies have failed to reach a consensus for the ideal technique to reliably and consistently describe clinical threshold levels to predict natural and artificial pregnancies. This may potentially be the case since most studies were comparatively small and the study aspects were unrelated and accuracy of various assays remains undetermined. Hence, additional studies are required with considerably larger sample sizes to investigate and elucidate the mechanisms leading up to the sperm DNA damage and subsequently improve clinical reproductive outcomes.

- Recurrent early pregnancy loss has a high association with high DFI/male factor, as paternal factor contributes to early embryonic development.
- Inadequate lifestyle is the most common etiological factor for high DFI.
- DNA fragmentation index greater than 30% is significant.
- High DNA fragmentation can also result in poor quality embryos or recurrent implantation failure.
- Antioxidant therapy should be given for at least 6 months so as to cover the spermatogenesis window.
- Antioxidants can help in reduction of DNA damage.
- Physiological intracytoplasmic sperm injection (PICSI) is a great tool for such cases as it selects the physiologically normal sperms for injection.

Testicular sperm aspiration can also be done in such cases as it is a known fact that most of the DNA damage occurs in the epididymis.
- Recurrent intrauterine insemination (IUI) failures or in cases of unexplained infertility, DNA fragmentation might be a probable cause and must be tested.
- Prevention is always better than cure and proper awareness about lifestyle can reduce occurrence.

Reactive Oxygen Species

When testing for reactive oxygen species (ROS) one has to figure out whether ROS has originated from external sources like leukocytes or it is present in the semen.[12] Henkel et al. data suggests that ROS that has been generated by leukocytes predominately affect the sperm plasma membrane and its related functions such as motility.[13] On the other hand, intrinsic ROS cause DNA damage as opposed to extrinsic ROS which cause plasma membrane damage.[14] There are several methods to measure seminal ROS in the clinical setting, most notably among them is the chemiluminescence assay. This technique measures the global ROS, i.e. both the intra- and extracellular ROS.

Sperm Aneuploidy Assay

Sperm aneuploidy screening has been used as a tool in diagnosis and determining treatment options for male factor infertility since the development of human sperm karyotyping by injection into hamster and mouse oocytes in the 1970s. From these studies and subsequent work with interphase chromosome analysis, at risk populations of men with teratozoospermia, oligozoospermia, and men with translocations, have since been identified. The current technique is an application of fluorescent in situ hybridization (FISH) on interphase sperm nuclei with careful enumeration of the labeled chromosomes to determine sperm ploidy.[15] Typically, five to seven chromosomes are evaluated in individual ejaculates to determine the percent of aneuploid sperm present. Sperm chromosomal abnormalities is associated with compromised motility and at times concentration. Aneuploidy does not affect fertilization rate but negatively influences pregnancy and delivery rates.[12]

■ CONCLUSION

Sperm function test practically evaluate the cellular processes of the spermatozoa from the time of ejaculation to fertilization and beyond. The standardization of these tests has been subjected to a lot of controversy and in most cases these tests are basically used as research tools in order to find out the cause of male infertility. As of now these tests are not recommended to be used as routine diagnostic tests but are gaining popularity among clinicians. The advent of ICSI has changed the rules and most ART specialists now ignore the need to test the sperm parameters, based on the thought that only one sperm is required to fertilize the egg and with ICSI we bypass the processes needed for the sperm to naturally fertilize the egg. However, it must be understood that when only one sperm is required to fertilize an egg that sperm has to be the best, functionally, and hence these tests are needed even more when using ICSI.[16]

REFERENCES

1. McDonough P. Editorial comment: has traditional sperm analysis lost its clinical relevance? Fertil Steril. 1997;67:585-7.
2. Franken DR and Oehninger S. Semen analysis and sperm function testing. Asian J Androl. 2012;14:6-13.
3. Safarinejad MR. Infertility among couples in a population-based study in Iran: prevalence and associated risk factors. Int J Androl. 2008;31:303-14.
4. Evenson DP, Jost LK, Marshall D, et al. Utility of the sperm chromatin structure assay as a diagnostic and prognostic tool in the human fertility clinic. Hum Reprod. 1999;14(4):1039-49.
5. Zini A, Bielecki R, Phang D, et al. Correlations between two markers of sperm DNA integrity, DNA denaturation and DNA fragmentation, in fertile and infertile men. Fertil Steril. 2001;75(4):674-7.
6. Ahmadi A, Ng SC. Developmental capacity of damaged spermatozoa. Hum Reprod. 1999;14(9):2279-85.
7. WHO. Laboratory manual of the WHO for the examination of human semen and sperm cervical mucus interaction. 2010.37(I-XII):1-123.
8. Barratt CL, Osborn R, Harrison PF, et al. The hypo-osmotic swelling test and the sperm mucus penetration test in determining the fertilisation of human oocytes. Hum Reprod. 1989; 4:430-4.
9. Franken DR, Bastiaan HS, Kidson A, et al. Zona pellucida mediated acrosome reaction and sperm morphology. Andrologia. 1997; 29:311-7.
10. Tavukçuoğlu Iş, Al-Azawi T1, Khaki AA, et al. Clinical value of DNA fragmentation evaluation tests under ART treatments. J Turk Ger Gynecol Assoc. 2012; 13(4): 270-4.
11. Avendaño C, Mata A, Sanchez Sarmiento CA, et al. Use of laptop computers connected to internet through Wi-Fi decreases human sperm motility and increases sperm DNA fragmentation. Fertil Steril. 2012;97(1):39-45.e2.
12. BRWolff H. The biologic significance of white blood cells in semen. Fertil Steril. 1995;63: 1143-57.
13. Henkel R, Kierspel E, Stalf T, et al. Effect of reactive oxygen species produced by spermatozoa and leukocytes on sperm functions in nonleukocytospermic patients. Fertil Steril. 2005;83:635-42.
14. Chance B, Sies H, Boveris H. Hydroperoxide metabolism in mammalian organs. Physiol Rev. 1979;59:527-605.
15. Emery BR. Sperm aneuploidy testing using fluorescence in situ hybridization. Methods Mol Biol. 2013;927:167-73.
16. ESHRE. Andrology Special Interest Group. Consensus Workshop on Advanced Diagnostic Andrology Techniques. Hum Reprod. 1996;11:1463-79.

CHAPTER
4

Screening of Male Partner before ART Procedure and its Recent Advancement

Swaminathan D, Sanketh Dhumal S

■ INTRODUCTION

Pregnancy rates by intercourse in normal couples are approximately 20–25% per month, 75% by 6 months and 90% by 1 year.[1] After one year of unprotected intercourse approximately 15% of couples of unknown fertility status are unable to conceive. In approximately 30% of these couples, infertility is due to a significant male factor alone, whereas combined male and female factors are present in an additional 20%.[2] Thus, a male factor is involved in approximately 50% of infertile relationships. The true incidence of male infertility is unknown due to great variability in the prevalence of infertility. However, in 30–50% of subfertile couples, the male partner has suboptimal semen quality, either because of low sperm count, poorly motile sperm or sperm with abnormal size and shape (morphology). In more than 50% of male infertility cases, the etiology remains unknown and the infertility is classified as idiopathic. *Male infertility evaluation must go far beyond a simple semen analysis which has to be complemented with a comprehensive history and physical examination as well as relevant endocrine, genetic, and other investigations.*

The primary goals of the evaluation of the male presenting with infertility are to identify:

1. Etiology conditions that may be reversed with resultant improvement in male's fertility status.
2. Irreversible conditions that may be best managed by the use of assisted reproductive techniques such as intrauterine insemination (IUI) or in vitro fertilization (IVF) using male partner's sperm.
3. Irreversible conditions not amenable to assisted reproductive techniques, and medically significant pathology underlying male infertility where donor insemination or adoption may be suggested.
4. Genetic consequence that have implications for the patient and/or his offspring.

■ HISTORY

A careful history should be obtained, including a detailed reproductive history and medical and surgical history, as well as review of pertinent lifestyle factors and potential gonadal toxic exposure. The male partner should be questioned about his erectile and ejaculatory function, as well as frequency of masturbation.

Childhood Illness and Conditions

History of specific childhood illness or conditions may be important in the evaluation of infertile male, such as bilateral cryptorchidism which results in the significant decline of spermatogenesis, while the effect of unilateral cryptorchidism appears to be much milder.[3] The timing of the pubertal development should be noted. Significantly delayed or incomplete development may suggest an endocrinopathy. Mumps does not appear to affect the testis when experienced prepubertally.

Systemic Diseases and Illnesses

Systemic diseases and illnesses such as diabetes and multiple sclerosis may affect erectile as well as ejaculatory function.[4] Myotonic dystrophy is associated with the development of testicular atrophy. Any generalized illness resulting in fever or viremia may cause impaired testicular function, the effects of which may not appear in the ejaculate for 1–3 months. The actual time lapse between the injurious event and the appearance of the abnormal cells in the ejaculate varies, depending on what stage of the spermatogenic process is affected. *For this reason, if a patient gives a history of acute medical problems in the 3 months before his first office visit, and if laboratory analysis shows subnormal semen quality, analyses should be repeated several months later before decision is made regarding the quality of the sperm production.*

Past Surgical History

Details of the past surgery should be obtained. Bladder neck surgery as well as prostate surgery may result in retrograde ejaculation, and patients will present with absent or low volume ejaculates and the presence of large numbers of sperms in the urine. Modifications of retroperitoneal lymph node dissection techniques utilizing a template method or a nerve-sparing approach preserve the sympathetic nerves and allow retention of the ejaculatory function in most patients.

■ CANCER AND CANCER TREATMENTS

Patients with testicular cancer may present with infertility either before or after the treatment of their cancer. Approximately 50% of testicular cancer patients have subnormal sperm densities prior to chemotherapy.[5] Radiation therapy given to patients with testicular seminoma results in impaired spermatogenesis 4–6 months after the completion of radiation, this may even occur with gonadal shedding. Patients with leukemia, lymphoma, and a variety of solid neoplasms often have subnormal parameters.[6] Most patients with Hodgkin's disease and leukemia become azoospermic after chemotherapy, however, some treatments may not result in permanent sterility. After bone morrow transplantation with a combination of chemotherapy and radiation therapy; permanent sterility usually results.

■ MEDICATIONS AND DRUG USE

A detailed history of medications including prescribed, over the counter, illicit, and nutraceuticals should be obtained. Exogenous androgens are well known to induce hypogonadotropic hypogonadism. This may be induced by testosterone directly or by synthetic anabolic steroids. The subsequent suppression of endogenous testosterone production usually results in azoospermia, which is frequently reversible over 3–6 months period of time. Of significance, some patients do not recover normal pituitary function. Alpha blockers may cause decreased ejaculate volume or anejaculation. This appears not to be due to retrograde ejaculation and appears to be more common with tamsulosin than with other alpha blockers.[7]

■ PHYSICAL EXAMINATION

The physical examination of the infertile male should focus on identifying abnormalities that may affect fertility. This includes the pattern of virilization, as well as patient's secondary sexual characteristics. Anatomical abnormalities of the penis can result in improper placement of the ejaculate in the vaginal vault. The scrotal contents should be carefully palpated, and testicular consistency should be noted as well as testicular size. It has been shown that a decrease in the size is often associated with impaired spermatogenesis. Testicular volume should be measured with an orchidometer, or length and width measured with calipers. Examination of the epididymis should be carefully performed, taking the note of the presence of the caput, corpus, and cauda as well as whether or not the epididymis feels indurated or full. Obstruction of the genital ductal system may be suggested by a fullness of the epididymis. Palpation of the spermatic cords should be performed with careful notation of the presence or absence of the vas deferens as well as any areas of vassal atrophy or nodularity. The patient should be examined in a standing position for the presence of a *varicocele* within the spermatic cord and surrounding the testicle.

■ INITIAL LABORATORY TESTING

The cornerstone of the evaluation remains the completion of at least 2–3 semen analyses. It is important for the clinician to understand the difference between average semen parameters and those threshold values below which fertility becomes statistically less likely.

SEMEN ANALYSIS

The laboratory techniques of semen analysis are defined by the WHO and the guidance was revised in 2010 (Table 1), including the publication of new references ranges. Historically, significant variation can exist in the data generated between laboratories that analyze aliquots of the same sample circulated for quality assurance purposes. It has been shown that the most precise measurements are made when semen analysis is performed in specialist embryology/andrology laboratories rather than general laboratories available in many hospitals. Clinicians should, therefore, be aware of such variability and make efforts to understand the robustness of the measures generated in the laboratories they use to undertake semen analysis on their patients.

In spite of the problems in performing semen analysis, follow-up studies of couples attempting to conceive show that where semen analysis is performed

Table 1: WHO reference values for human semen characteristics of fertile men (2010).

WHO (2010) reference values: The fertile ranges are a sperm concentration of ≥15 million/mL, vitality of 58%, progressive motility of ≥32% and morphological normal forms of ≥4%.

Parameter	Lower reference limit
Semen volume (mL)	1.5 (1.4–1.7)
Total sperm number (10^6 per ejaculate)	39 (33–46)
Sperm concentration (10^6 per mL)	15 (12–16)
Total motility (PR þ NP, %)	40 (38–42)
Progressive motility (PR, %)	32 (31–34)
Vitality (live spermatozoa, %)	58 (55–63)
Sperm morphology (normal forms, %)	4 (3.0–4.0)
Other consensus threshold values	
pH	≥7.2
Peroxidase-positive leukocytes (10^6 per mL)	<1.0
MAR test (motile spermatozoa with bound particles, %)	<50
Immunobead test (motile spermatozoa with bound beads, %)	<50
Seminal zinc (mmol/ejaculate)	≥2.4
Seminal fructose (mmol/ejaculate)	≥13
Seminal neutral glucosidase (mU/ejaculate)	≥20

robustly, there are good relationships between the individual measures of semen quality obtained (*concentration, motility and morphology*) and the probability of conception.

■ INTERPRETATION OF INITIAL EVALUATION

Following the history, physical examination, and initial semen analysis, a different diagnosis should be developed. Additional laboratory studies may then be employed to further refine the diagnosis and help determine management options.

Semen analysis results can be categorized into:
1. All parameters normal
2. Azoospermia
3. Diffuse abnormalities in sperm density, sperm morphology, and motility
4. Isolated problems restricted to one parameter of the semen evaluation such as seminal volume, sperm density, motility or morphology.

Variations in Semen Volume and Appearance

Low semen volume suggests incomplete collection, short duration of abstinence from ejaculation before the test, absence or obstruction of the seminal vesicles, or androgen deficiency. It may also occur in patients with retrograde ejaculation, and hence examination of a post-ejaculatory urine sample is of value. High semen volume (>8 mL) may be seen in association with oligospermia but is of little practical significance. Hemospermia is usually the result of minor bleeding from the urethra, but serious conditions, such as genital tract tumors, must be excluded. Discoloration of the semen may indicate inflammation of accessory sex organs. The semen may be yellow with jaundice or Salazopyrin (sulfasalazine) administration. Defects of liquefaction and viscosity are relatively common and presumably result from malfunction of the accessory sex organs. Although these may cause problems with semen analysis and preparation of sperm for assisted reproductive technology (ART), they are probably of little relevance to fertility. Sperm agglutination is common with sperm autoimmunity but can also occur for other reasons.

Azoospermia

The total absence of sperm from the semen needs to be confirmed in repeated tests with vigorous centrifugation of the semen and careful examination of the pellet.[8] Sperm may be found in apparently azoospermic samples using more sensitive sperm-counting methods by examining larger volumes with fluorescence microscopy. Rarely, an illness or difficulty with collection will cause transient azoospermia; however, this can also occur for unexplained reasons. With severe spermatogenic disorders and some obstructions, sperm may be present in the semen intermittently. If any live sperm can be found, these can be cryopreserved for intracytoplasmic sperm injection (ICSI).

Oligozoospermia

Sperm concentrations of less than 15 million/mL or preferably total counts less than 39 million/ejaculate are classified as oligospermic.[9] There is a correlation between sperm concentration and other aspects of semen quality. Both motility and morphology are usually poor with oligozoospermia.

Asthenozoospermia

Asthenozoospermia is defined as less than 40% sperm total motility or less than 32% with progressive motility.[10] Spurious asthenozoospermia caused by exposure of sperm to rubber (particularly condoms), spermicides, extremes of temperature, or long delays between collection and examination should be excluded. Low sperm motility is a frequent accompaniment of oligozoospermia and is often also associated with a mixed picture of morphologic defects suggesting defective spermiogenesis. Specific ultrastructural defects of the sperm can be evaluated by electron microscopy when there is zero sperm motility or extreme asthenozoospermia (<5% motile sperm). Such a test should also be performed if such patients have a history of chronic sinusitis, bronchiectasis, and dextrocardia, characteristics of immotile cilia syndrome. Absent dynein arms, other axonemal defects, mitochondrial abnormalities, disorganized fibrous sheath or outer dense fibers, or normal ultrastructure may be found. Standard semen analyses usually show normal sperm concentrations and morphology, but there may be tail abnormalities: short, straight, or thick tails or midpiece defects. Viability tests help to distinguish this group of patients from those with necrozoospermia. Patients with structural defects in the sperm may be able to be treated by ICSI. Asthenzooospermia may also be associated with sperm autoimmunity. The causes of other motility defects of moderate degree are unidentified.

Necrozoospermia

It is important to distinguish necrozoospermia from other types of severe asthenzooospermia, because some patients with necrozoospermia produce pregnancies despite low sperm motility.[11] Necrospermia is usually characterized by less than 20–30% total motility, less than 5% progressive motility, and a viability test of less than 30–40%, indicating a high proportion of dead sperm. Other causes of severe asthenozoospermia such as sperm autoimmunity and collection problems must be excluded. Necrozoospermia may fluctuate in severity, particularly with changes in coital frequency. Characteristic of necrozoospermia is an improvement of sperm motility with increased frequency of ejaculation. The condition may be caused by defective storage of sperm in the tails of the epididymides or stasis in the genital tract, and it also occurs with chronic spinal cord injury and with adult polycystic kidney disease associated with cysts in the region of the ejaculatory ducts. There are ultrastructural features of degeneration in the ejaculated sperm but normal structure of late spermatids in testicular biopsies. Treatment with antibiotics may have a beneficial effect, but this is not proved. The couple should have intercoursed once or twice every day for 3–4 days up to the time of ovulation.

Teratozoospermia

Teratozoospermia is a reduced percentage of sperm with normal morphology (4%) assessed by light microscopy.[12] It is important to distinguish mixed abnormalities of sperm morphology from those in which all or the majority of sperm show a single uniform defect, such as spherical heads with absence of the acrosomes (globozoospermia) and pinhead sperm. Pinhead sperm result when the centrioles from which the sperm tails develop are not correctly aligned opposite the developing acrosome. On spermiation, the sperm heads are disconnected from the tails and absorbed during epididymal transit so that there are only sperm tails in the ejaculate, the cytoplasmic droplet on the midpiece giving the pinhead appearance. Both conditions cause sterility but are extremely rare. In general, human spermatozoa are very variable in appearance, and the microscopic assessment of sperm morphology is highly subjective and difficult to standardize between laboratories. Only a small proportion (<25%) of the motile sperm from fertile men are capable of binding the zona pellucida (ZP) in vitro, and this zona-binding capacity is closely related to the morphology of the sperm head. The morphometric characteristics of the sperm that bind to the ZP may be useful as a standard for sperm morphology. Various histologic assessments of morphology have been used. The simplest is to record as normal only those sperm that have no shape defects in head, midpiece, or tail regions. In the strict morphology approach, although size measurements are set, the sperm are assessed by eye and those marginally abnormal are assigned abnormal. Automated methods involving image analysis by computer (like *CASA*) have been developed that could overcome the between-laboratory variability and greatly improve the predictive value of semen analysis for natural conception.

■ OTHER LABORATORY TESTS

In an attempt to improve the accuracy of laboratory tests, many researchers have developed more sophisticated tests designed to investigate specific aspects of sperm biology or to mimic in some way aspects of the journey sperm make to the site of fertilization. These are termed sperm function tests and include measuring the ability of sperm to:

- Enter and make progression in mid-cycle cervical mucus (sperm mucus penetration tests)
- Hyperactivate following capacitation
- Bind to the zona pellucida (ZP)
- Undergo the acrosome reaction
- Penetrate zona-free hamster eggs.

Although for each of these there is reasonable body of evidence to suggest correlations with outcome of IVF or unassisted conception, none of these tests has, to date, been universally incorporated into clinical practice. Perhaps the tests with most current promise are those that examine the integrity of sperm DNA. However, many studies have suggested correlations between the integrity of sperm DNA and the probability of spontaneous conception, the outcome of assisted conception treatment, embryo quality and the probability of miscarriage and early pregnancy loss. However, both the *American Society for Reproductive Medicine and the European Society for Human Reproduction and Embryology* have recently reviewed the evidence base for sperm DNA testing and have concluded, for the time being at least, that there is insufficient evidence for such tests to be offered on a routine basis. As such, patients should only be offered the option to have their DNA quality tested in the context of an appropriately designed clinical trial.

■ HORMONE ANALYSIS

If repeat semen analysis demonstrate severe oligozoospermia (<5 million spermatozoa/mL) or azoospermia, then *basal serum follicle-stimulating hormone (FSH), luteinizing hormone (LH), and testosterone* will be valuable. If serum concentrations of FSH, LH, and testosterone are normal and the man has azoospermia, a post-ejaculatory urine sample will provide evidence about retrograde ejaculation if sperms are seen in the urine. If spermatozoa are not present in the post-ejaculatory urine, the man has obstructive azoospermia or impaired spermatogenesis. Low serum FSH, LH, and testosterone warrants gonadotropin treatment (secondary hypogonadism). High serum FSH, LH, and low testosterone indicate primary hypogonadism (testicular failure). Men with low sperm counts and low LH (and FSH) who are well-androgenized should be suspected of anabolic steroid abuse (exogenous testosterone suppresses intratesticular testosterone production, which is an absolute prerequisite for normal spermatogenesis). The serum testosterone can be low, normal, or high depending upon the specific substance taken. Sperm production recovers in most men when they stop using anabolic steroids, however, this process can take months to years. Prolactin should be measured in men who complain of reduced libido and have low serum testosterone. Low serum inhibin B may be a more sensitive indicator of primary testicular dysfunction than high FSH.

■ GENETICS OF MALE INFERTILITY

Identifiable genetic abnormalities contribute to 15–20% of the most severe forms of male infertility (azoospermia), while the majority 30–60% are idiopathic and under investigation with a strong suspicion of genetic underpinnings.[13] Among known genetic causes of male infertility, chromosomal abnormalities, Y-microdeletions, X-linked and autosomal gene mutations have been previously described. In this chapter, we discuss known genetic etiologies of male infertility.

CHROMOSOMAL ANALYSIS

The incidence of chromosomal abnormalities is inversely proportional to sperm production. Less than 1% of men with normal sperm concentration are identified to have chromosomal abnormalities, while 5% of men with severe oligospermia defined as a sperm concentration less than 5 million sperm per milliliter, will have chromosomal abnormalities, and 10–15% of men with azoospermia will have chromosomal abnormalities.[14] Therefore, chromosomal analysis is not routinely performed, except for men with severe oligospermia or azoospermia, for recurrent pregnancy loss or unexplained repeat failures of assisted reproductive techniques. In such cases, a chromosomal analysis, i.e. karyotype, is obtained to evaluate men with insufficient spermatogenesis.

Chromosomal Abnormalities

Several forms of chromosomal abnormalities exist. Aneuploidies are defined by an abnormal number of chromosomes either more or less than the euploid state, i.e. 46, XY or 46, XX. This occurs because of nondisjunction of homologous chromosomes during meiosis I or chromatid pairs during mitosis or meiosis II; it may also be due to chromosomal lagging during anaphase resulting in loss (54). Most common aneuploidies involve the gonosomes (X and Y chromosomes), followed by autosomal disomies of chromosomes 13, 18, and 2. Examples include Klinefelter syndrome (KS) (47,XXY) and mixed gonadal dysgenesis (MGD) (45,XO/ 46,XY) with the latter being a mosaic of two different chromosomal numbers. Deletions of genetic material from the Y chromosome may result in a microdeletion within the Y chromosome that cannot be detected on karyotype (Y microdeletion) and are the cause of up to 10% of men with nonobstructive azoospermia.

Translocations may be balanced, i.e. reciprocal translocations or unbalanced, i.e. Robertsonian translocations (RTs). Reciprocal translocations involve an exchange of genetic material between two or more chromosomes. They are the most common chromosomal structural anomalies in humans and are 10 times more common among infertile men. RTs are the result of one portion of a chromosome translocating to another chromosome. RTs occur with an incidence of 0.9% of men with severe male factor infertility and occur because of the rearrangement of chromosomes with loss of genetic material resulting in a complement of 45 chromosomes. These occur among acrocentric chromosomes such as chromosomes 13, 14, 15, 21, and 22. Here, the long arms fuse, resulting in loss of genetic material among the chromosomal short arms. The most common translocations include t(13q;14q) and t(14q;21q) and carry an incidence of 0.9% or less. Here, "q" designates the long arm of the chromosome, and "t" designates a translocation of the chromosomes within the brackets. These men tend to be phenotypically normal; however, they may demonstrate impaired spermatogenesis with increased rates of sperm aneuploidy among those sperm produced. Autosomal inversions can be considered intrachromosomal reciprocal translocations and involve structural derangements without loss of genetic material. Inversions relevant to male infertility include that of chromosome 9. This inversion accounts for up to 3–5% of male infertility and results in a variable phenotype ranging from normospermia, oligospermia, azoospermia, and asthenospermia.

Y Chromosome Microdeletions

Ninety-five percent of the Y chromosome is contained in the male-specific region of the Y chromosome or MSY and contains unique genetic material for sex-specific embryogenesis such as the sex-determining region of the Y chromosome (SRY). However, the Y chromosome does not recombine in the same manner as autosomal chromosomes; it does contain approximately eight massive palindromic sequences that enable maintenance of the fidelity of the genetic material on the Y through intrapalindrome homologous arm-to-arm recombination. From an evolutionary standpoint, the Y chromosome is highly efficient, containing the entire male phenotypic developmental pathway in a minimum of DNA. However, unlike its autosomal counterparts, it does not have the luxury of having two copies of critical genetic material and the loss of any of its material has reproductive consequences for men. Any deviation from the intrapalindromic arm-to-arm recombination can lead to ectopic homologous recombination. Errors occur when two spatially separated palindromic segments of the Y chromosome are erroneously combined, deleting all the intervening genetic material. These losses are referred to as microdeletions because they are not visible on standard karyotype analysis.

Y chromosome microdeletions have been extensively studied because the recognition that Yq has factors important for spermatogenesis.[15] Y chromosome microdeletions are clinically important because they are associated with severe male infertility, and likelihood of treatment success can be determined by the location of the deletion. The azoospermia factor (AZF) loci harbor 14 protein coding genes critical for spermatogenesis. These genes are organized into three distinct locations: "a," "b," and "c." Each of these regions may be deleted independently or in combination and are implicated as the cause of defective spermatogenesis for 5% of men presenting with severe oligospermia and 10% of men with NOA (nonobstructive azoospermia). The six classic forms of AZF deletions and their corresponding phenotype, in order of decreasing severity include: AZFabc [Sertoli cell-only (SCO)], AZFa (SCO), AZFbc (SCO/maturation arrest), AZFb (maturation arrest), AZFc (severe oligospermia to azoospermia), and partial AZFc (normal spermatogenesis to azoospermia).

AZFb deletions account for 15% of Y microdeletions. Invariably, complete deletions result in azoospermia and SCO or early maturation arrest histology. AZFc deletions account for 60% of all clinically relevant Y microdeletions. Up to 70% of men with AZFc deletions have sperm in the ejaculate, typically less than 1 million sperm per milliliter for these cryptospermic men with AZFc deletions. In men with azoospermia and AZFc deletions, microdissection testicular sperm extraction (mTESE) can be used to harvest sperm from the testicle in 50–60%. Thus, fertility potential is present in some patients with AZFc deletions; however, Y microdeletions are passed to male offspring.[16,17]

KEY POINTS

- Much of idiopathic male infertility is likely to have a genetic cause.
- Male infertility evaluation must go far beyond a simple semen analysis which has to be complemented with a comprehensive history and physical examination as well as relevant endocrine, genetic, and other investigations.
- Men who have nonobstructive azoospermia or severe oligospermia with total motile count less than 5 million should have a karyotype and Y chromosome microdeletion.
- Klinefelter syndrome (47,XXY) is the most common chromosomal abnormality with a frequency of 1:600 males and has a wide spectrum of clinical presentation.
- Men with an AZFa, AZFb, AZFb/c microdeletion uniformly have complete absence of spermatogenesis.
- If a male has congenital bilateral absence of the vas deferens, it is critical to offer him and his partner genetic testing for cystic fibrosis mutations as well as genetic counseling.

REFERENCES

1. Spira A. Epidemology of human reproduction. Hum Reprod. 1986;1(2):111-15.
2. MacLeod J. Human male infertility. Obstet Gynecol Surv. 1971;26:335-51.
3. Mosher WD. Reproductive impairments in the united states 1965-1982. Demography. 1985;22:415-30.
4. Simmons FA. Human infertility. N Engl Med. 1956;255:1140-6.
5. Vine MF, Tse CK, Hu P, et al. Cigarette smoking and semen quality. Fertil Steril. 1996;65:835-42.
6. Aafjes JH, Van der Vijver JC, Schenck PE. The duration of infertility: an important datum for the fertility prognosis of men with semen abnormalities. Fertil Steril. 1978;30:423-5.
7. Wilcox AJ, Weinberg CR, Baird DD. Timing of sexual intercourse in relation to ovulation: effects on the probability of conception, survival of the pregnany, ans sex of the baby. N Engl J Med. 1995;333:1517-21.
8. Goldenberg RL, White R. The effect of vaginal lubricants on sperm motility in vitro. Fertil Steril. 1975;26:872-3.
9. Kutteh WH, Chao CH, Ritter JO, et al. Vaginal lubricants for the infertile couple: effect on sperm activity. Int J Fertil Menopausal Stud. 1996;41:400-4.
10. Tagatz GE, Okagaki T, Sciarra JJ. The effect of vaginal lubricants on sperm motility and viability in vitro. Am J Obstet Gynecol. 1972;113:88-90.
11. Tulandi T, Plouffe L, McInnes RA. Effect of saliva on sperm motility and activity. Fertil Steril. 1982;38:721-3.
12. Carroll PR, Whitemore WF, Herr HW, et al. Endocrine and exocrine profiles of men with testicular tumors before orchiectomy. J Urol. 1987;137:420-3.

13. Boyers SP, Corrales MD, Huszar G, et al. The effects of Lubrin on sperm motility in vitro. Fertil Steril. 1987;47:882-4.
14. Lee PA. Fertility after cryptorchidism: epidemiology and other outcome studies. Urology. 2005;66:427-31.
15. Lee PA. Fertility after cryptorchidism: does treatment make a difference? Endocrinol Metab Clin North Am 1993;22:479-90.
16. Graso M, Buonaguidi A, Lania C, et al. Postpubertal cryptorchidism: review and evaluation of the fertility. Eur Urol. 1991;20:126-8.
17. Ramalingam M, Kini S, Mohammed T. Male Fertility and Infertility. Obstetrics, Gynaecology and Reproductive Medicine. 2014;24(11):326-32.

CHAPTER
5

Role of Genetics in Clinical Evaluation of Male Infertility

Stacy Colaco, Deepak Modi

■ INTRODUCTION

Approximately 15% of couples in reproductive age experience involuntary childlessness that represents approximately 140 million people worldwide. Male factor, alone or in combination with female factors, is a cause of infertility in about half of the cases as determined by semen analysis. Amongst the risk factors that affect male fertility are lifestyles, diabetes, obesity, hormonal diseases, testicular trauma, cryptorchidism, varicocele, genitourinary infections, ejaculatory disorders, chemo/radio or surgical therapies. Despite proper diagnostic work-up, the cause of infertility in nearly half of these cases cannot be determined. In such cases genetic defects are involved as the cause of infertility in such men.

Assisted reproductive technology (ART) is overall successful regardless of the underlying infertility cause and is often the next step for many couples with unexplained infertility. However, the use of genetically compromised spermatozoa in ART is associated with a wide range of adverse outcomes including abnormal embryo development causing implantation failure, an increased risk of miscarriage and defects in the offspring. Therefore, it is imperative to determine the origin of the problem to allow appropriate counseling and management of infertile couples with male factor infertility.

■ GENETIC DEFECTS ASSOCIATED WITH MALE INFERTILITY AND THEIR INTERPRETATION

The major genetic defects observed in infertile are karyotypic abnormalities and Y chromosome microdeletions. The minor defects include gene copy number variations, gene mutations and polymorphisms. These genetic defects can interfere with the development of the male gonads and the urogenital tract, cause degeneration of the germ cells or arrest in spermatogenesis or lead to production of non-functional spermatozoa. The types of genetic testing done in infertile men are described below. Rather than comprehensive, we will focus on only those that are presently clinically relevant and aid in patient management.

A summary of the genetic alterations commonly found in infertile males and its effects on ART outcomes is given in Table 1. Flowcharts 1 and 2 give the algorithm for genetic testing to be followed while evaluation of infertile men.

Karyotype

Karyotyping is important in the work-up of infertile men because structural chromosomal aberrations are up to 10 times more common in infertile men than fertile controls. 3% of oligozoospermic men, 19% of men with non-obstructive azoospermia and 4% of men receiving ICSI for male subfertility harbor chromosomal abnormalities. Karyotyping is recommended by the American Urological Association (AUA) and the European Academy of Andrology (EAA) in all men with a total motile sperm count below 10 million and those who have nonobstructive azoospermia.[1] Identification of karyotype alterations is of vital importance for the following reasons:
1. Clarifying a probable cause of the infertility provides psychological relief
2. In the situation of clinical syndromes, it might predict future health issues which would otherwise go unnoticed in infertile and often young men
3. Genetic counseling would give an appraisal of the risk of transmission of the known genetic alteration to the offspring.

The common karyotypic abnormalities found in infertile males are mosaic or non-mosaic Klinefelter's syndrome (47, XXY karyotype). Phenotypically, males with 47, XXY have small testes (<10 cc) and elevated serum follicle stimulating hormone (FSH) and luteinizing hormone. Although men with 47,XXY can have adequate androgenic potential, many present to a pediatric endocrinologist or urologist with delayed virilization during puberty, it often is not diagnosed until men present to an andrologist with fertility concerns during their reproductive years.

The other genetic defect is detected in infertile men is 46**,** XX male. It is caused by the translocation of a portion of the Y chromosome that includes the sex-determining region (*SRY*), a gene that initiates the male phenotype. Male patients with 46, XX karyotype are always infertile since they lack the major portions of the Y chromosome. Other Y chromosome abnormalities, such as mosaicism, ring Y, truncated Y and isodicentric Y, are also observed in infertile males. The majority of these men are infertile had would not have complete spermatogenesis. Thus, testicular sperm aspiration (TESA) or any other attempts at having their own biological children through ART is not an option for 46, XX men or those having structural abnormalities of the Y chromosome.[2]

Balanced translocations are also reported in infertile couples. These translocation, usually do not result in net gain or loss of genetic material and hence usually will not manifest a phenotype. While some men may have abnormal seminogram, most will be normal in all phenotypic aspects. In these coupes the infertility is due to chromosomally abnormal embryos that will usually fail to implant or result in early miscarriage.

Table 1: Summary of the genetic defects observed in infertile males, their consequences on ART outcomes and key points for counseling and future action.

Diagnosis by semen analysis	Genetic defect	Diagnosed by	Testicular phenotype	TESA possible	Effects on fertilization and embryo development	Genetic abnormalities in embryo	Counseling
Azoospermia or oligozoospermia	47, XXY And other sex chromosome aneuploidies	Karyotyping	Normal to hypospermatogenesis progressing to azoospermia	Yes	Normal to low	Yes, higher than normal	Sperm cryopreservation PGS
Azoospermia	46XX male	Karyotyping and FISH or PCR for SRY gene	Sertoli cell only	No	Not possible	Not possible	Donor semen or adoption
Normozoospermia to azoospermia	Balanced translocation	Karyotyping	Variable	Variable	Variable	Variable	PGD for specific chromosome aneuploidy
Azoospermia to severe oligozoospermia	YCMD AZFa deletion	PCR	Sertoli cell only	No (95% cases)	Poor	100% transmission of deletion to male offspring	Poor ART outcomes, perpetuating infertility in future generation
Azoospermia to severe oligozoospermia	YCMD AZFb deletion	PCR	Sertoli cell only to maturation arrest	No (95% cases)	Poor	100% transmission of deletion to male offspring	Poor ART outcomes, perpetuating infertility in future generation

Role of Genetics in Clinical Evaluation of Male Infertility

Diagnosis by semen analysis	Genetic defect	Diagnosed by	Testicular phenotype	TESA possible	Effects on fertilization and embryo development	Genetic abnormalities in embryo	Counseling
Azoospermia to mild oligozoospermia	YCMD AZFc full and partial deletion	PCR	Variable, mostly maturation arrest to hypospermatogenesis progressive to azoospermia	Yes (70% cases)	Poor to normal	100% transmission of deletion to male offspring	Perpetuating infertility in future generation. Partial deletion may go to full deletion in next generation sperm cryopreservation
Obstructive azoospermia	CFTR gene mutation in both partners	PCR and sequencing	Normal	Yes	Normal	Same as general population	PGD for CFTR to asses cystic fibrosis
Obstructive azoospermia	CFTR gene mutation in only male partner	PCR and sequencing	Normal	Yes	Normal	Same as general population	No genetic testing required
Obstructive azoospermia	CFTR mutation not detected	PCR and sequencing	Normal	Yes	Normal	Same as general population	Extended CFTR gene analysis and appropriate counseling. If female partner normal no testing is essential

Flowchart 1: Algorithm for genetic testing in infertile males.

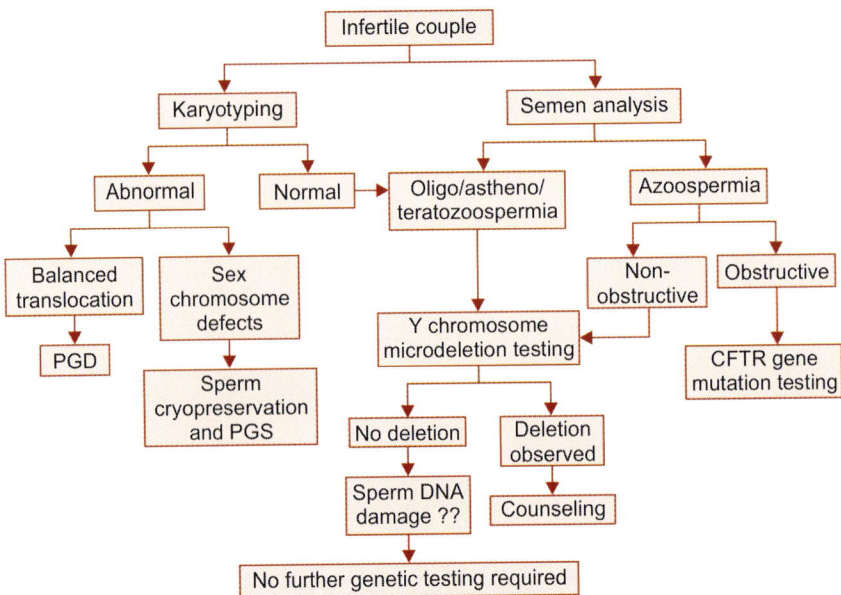

(PGD/PGS: preimplantation genetic screening/diagnosis)

Flowchart 2: Algorithm for genetic testing in men with obstructive azoospermia.

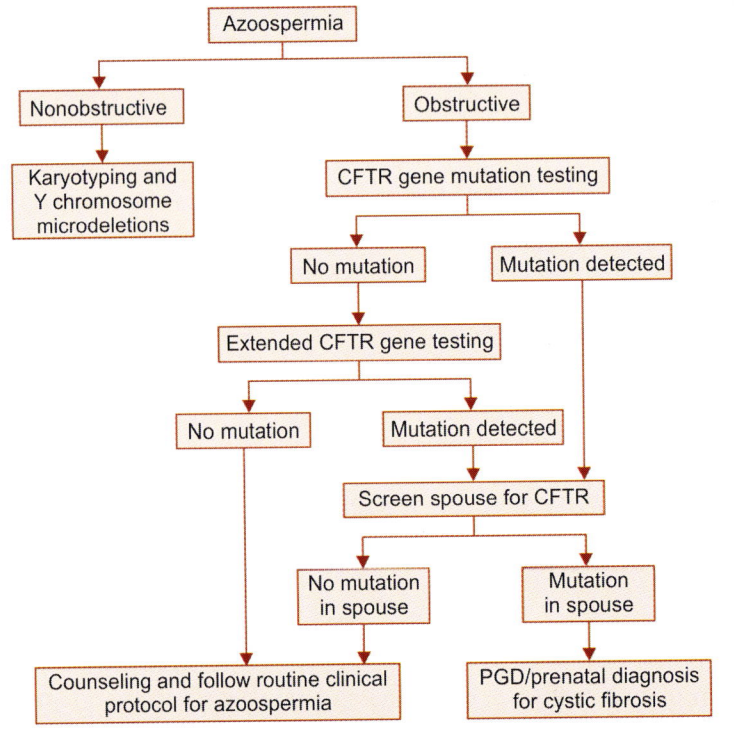

(PGD: preimplantation genetic diagnosis; CFTR: cystic fibrosis transmembrane conductance regulator)

Polymorphic variants, of certain chromosomes (commonly chromosome 1, 9, 16, Y) are often reported in karyotyping. While the frequency of the polymorphic variants is higher in infertile men, these are to be considered as normal variations and usually will have no pathogenic consequences.[2] According to general consensuses men with these variants should not be classified as genetically abnormal.

Y Chromosome Microdeletions

Y chromosome microdeletions (YCMD) are loss of one or more loci of Y chromosomes and these are not detected by standard karyotyping. YCMD testing is performed using a sequence-tagged sites polymerase chain reaction-based technique which determines the presence or absence of the three azoospermia factor region (AZF) regions (AZFa, AZFb and AZFc). Since these regions contain genes involved in spermatogenesis loss of one or more of these AZF loci would lead to arrest in spermatogenesis and hence male infertility.[3] Exclusively detected in infertile males, YCMD are observed in 5–10% of men with oligozoospermia and 10–20% of men with nonobstructive azoospermia.[3,4]

Y chromosome microdeletions are classified as AZFa, AZFb and AZFc deletions which can be either single or in combination. Deletions of AZFa lead to the complete depletion of germ cells and that of AZFb result in spermatogenic arrest and most of these men will manifest as azoospermia or severe oligozoospermia.[4] Deletions in the AZFc region are more frequent accounting for up to 90% of all Yq deletions with phenotypes varying from azoospermia to severe oligospermia.[4] Studies have revealed the presence of smaller deletions called as gr/gr, b1/b3, and b2/b3.[3] These sub-deletions are detected in some normozospermic men but its frequency is higher in infertile men.

Y chromosome microdeletions testing in all infertile men is recommended by the European Academy of Andrology (EAA) and American Society of Reproductive Medicine (ASRM) prior to performing intracytoplasmic sperm injection (ICSI). See Table 1 for the possible phenotypes observed in men with YCMD and the counseling points that need to be borne in mind while evaluating such patients.

■ CYSTIC FIBROSIS TRANSMEMBRANE CONDUCTANCE REGULATOR GENE MUTATION TESTING

Men with obstructive azoospermia (OA) have normal spermatogenesis but blocked flow in the male ductal system due to absence of vas deferens. This is a congenital defect and there could be absence of vas unilaterally or bilaterally and are called for congenital unilateral absence of vas deferens (CUAVD) or congenital bilateral absence of vas deferens (CBAVD). In men with low semen volume there is a strong suspicion of CUAVD or CBAVD and genetic testing for cystic fibrosis transmembrane conductance regulator (CFTR) gene mutation (chromosome 7q31.2) is recommended.[5]

Abnormalities in the CFTR gene result in cystic fibrosis which clinically has a progressive course adversely affecting lung, pancreas, and other parts of the gastrointestinal system. The vast majority of males with cystic fibrosis have CBAVD (more than 95%) with resultant OA. While patients with frank cystic fibrosis have two affected CFTR alleles with a strong mutation, in men with CAVBD without apparent cystic fibrosis there is most frequently one severe allele and one mild allele in 85% of patients.[5] Analysis of the CFTR gene is recommended for patients with CBAVD.[6]

In men with CBAVD with CFTR gene mutation, testicular biopsy will commonly shows active spermatogenesis and are suitable to be used in IVF/ ICSI and these men can father a child. However, since cystic fibrosis is autosomal recessive, the CFTR gene mutations can be inherited from the father to the offspring.[5] It is mandatory that the female partner testing for CFTR gene be carried out when the mutation is detected in the male partner. If the female partner is also identified to be CFTR gene mutation carrier (heterozygote) they should be counseled for possible occurrence of cystic fibrosis in the offspring.[5] See Flowchart 2 for the algorithm to be flowing while evaluating men with CBAVD and the points of counseling are given in Table 1.

These patients are offered prenatal testing in first trimester for determining the status of CFTR gene in the offspring. Alternately these are ideal candidates for preimplantation genetic diagnosis (PGD) for CFTR for selection of unaffected embryos and hence prevention of cystic fibrosis.[5] However, no prenatal diagnosis or PGD is essential if female partner has normal CFTR gene.

■ ALGORITHM FOR GENETIC TESTING IN INFERTILE MALES

Delineation between obstructive and nonobstructive causes of infertility is the most crucial factor in selection of appropriate genetic testing. A preliminary workup should include a comprehensive history and physical examination involving scrotal evaluation to quantitate testis volume and identify signs of hypogonadism combined with serum assays of several hormones such as FSH. Irrespective of the history, all men with azoospermia or oligozoospermia (including those with varicocele, history of mumps or smoking or alcohol consumption) must undergo genetic testing. Flowcharts 1 and 2 give the algorithm to be followed for genetic testing of infertile males.

When to Offer Karyotyping and What to Do When There is an Abnormal Karyotype

Irrespective of the sperm count, all infertile couples must be recommended karyotyping to rule out translocations as a potential cause of infertility. In the event one of the partner is found to have a chromosome abnormality a geneticist must be consulted to understand the prognosis and course of action. As mentioned above, do not consider variants to be pathogenic in nature and no action is essential. For a balanced translocation, ~25–50% of embryos will be chromosomally aneuploid and hence would not implant or result in miscarriage. Thus such patients will have low success rates even by conventional ART despite being clinically "normal" and having "good prognosis". In such patients, PGD with fluorescence in situ hybridization (FISH) with appropriate probes or comprehensive next generation Sequencing (NGS) is recommended to identify normal (euploid) embryos for embryo transfer. This should increase the chance of a successful pregnancy.

In the event the karyotype shows 47XXY (mosaic or non-mosaic type) or structural abnormalities of the Y chromosome, there will be progressive deterioration of spermatogenesis and these patients may progress from oligozoospermia to complete azoospermia.[2] Semen/TESA cryopreservation may be recommended in such cases. Studies have shown high incidence of chromosome abnormalities in sperm of such men and hence high risk of having abnormal embryos. PGS may be offered in such cases to increase chance of success. Table 1 summarizes the different manifestations observed in men with karyotypic abnormalities and the counseling points that must be taken care of during evaluation of an infertile male.

Who to Offer YCMD Testing and What to Expect When There is an Abnormality

Traditionally YCMD testing was offered to men with nonobstructive azoospermia or oligozoospermia when no cause was known. However, studies have shown that YCMD may be been found in men with varicocele, cryptorchidism and Klinefelter's mosaics.[4] Thus YCMD must be offered to all men with nonobstructive azoospermia or oligozoospermia. Table 1 summarizes the manifestations observed in men with different YCMDs and the counseling points that must be taken care of during evaluation of an infertile male.

We recommend YCMD testing in routine clinical practice for the following seven reasons:

1. *Identifying the cause of infertility*: YCMD testing will determine the underlying etiology of male factor infertility. Knowledge regarding these deletions will aid to provide more effective solutions to problems. For example, low sperm count and motility can be treated with hormones, anti-oxidants and lifestyle changes to improve the seminogram. However, these strategies of treatment will fail in men with YCMD. Also deletion carriers will most likely not benefit from the varicocelesurgical procedure.[5] Therefore, men with YCMD can directly be offered ART and not subjected to medical treatments to improve sperm count and motility.
2. *Predicting the prognosis of infertile males*: Oligozoospermic men with YCMD have progressive decline in sperm counts and can progress to azoospermia over time.[3] Thus males with mild or moderate oligozoospermia and YCMD would require a multiple follow-up for their possible progression to

azoospermia and provide an option of sperm cryopreservation for biological parenthood in future.

3. *Predicting outcome of testicular sperm aspiration (TESA)*: The occurrence and type of Yq microdeletion has correlate with testicular phenotype and chance of sperm retrieval. In general men with AZFa and AZFb deletions will rarely have sperm in their testis while AZFc deleted men would have hypospermatogenesis.[5] Thus YCMD testing can aid in decision making and predicting outcomes of procedures like TESA.[3,4]

4. *Predicting the success of ART*: Men with YCMD have low fertilization rate, poor embryo quality, impaired blastocyst rate and lower overall success of ART in men.[3] Hence, Yq microdeletion screening would also help in determining the probability of success rates after taking up ART.

5. *Prevention of vertical transmission of the genetic defects*: While men with YCMD (especially AZFc deletion) can technically father a child via ICSI, the defect is passed down to all the 100% of male offspring who will also infertile.[3] Thus the couple and the clinician must make an informed choice of having biological parenthood at the risk of perpetuating infertility in the family.

6. *Risk of testicular cancers*: Men with gonadal dysgenesis that bear a full or even partial fragments of Y chromosome have a high risk of developing gonadal tumors specifically gonadoblastoma.[7,8] While these are limited observational studies, it appears that that beyond infertility, the knowledge of YCMD would be a predictor occurrence of cancers in men and they should be appropriately counseled for further routine check-ups with andrologist/oncologist.

7. *Neuropsychiatric disorders*: A subset of men with YCMD are reported to have higher prevalence mild to severe neuropsychiatric disorders[9] indicating that the occurrence of other health risks beyond infertility in such men. While these reports are preliminary, it is better to be cautious and appropriately counsel the men for follow-up with neurologist.

Testing for Cystic Fibrosis Transmembrane Conductance Regulator Gene Mutations

By rule CFTR gene testing is only recommended in men with CAVBD or with low semen volume and is not otherwise indicated. As discussed above, in case there is a mutation detected, the female partner must be tested for a carrier status. In the event the female partner is identified to be CFTR gene heterozygote they must be offered prenatal testing in first trimester for determining the status of CFTR gene in the offspring and risk of cystic fibrosis. Alternately PGD for CFTR gene can also be offered. However, no further action is essential if female partner has normal CFTR gene. Flowchart 2 gives the algorithm for genetic testing of men with obstructive azoospermia.

CFTR gene mutations are expected in most men with CAVBD, however, in the event the results return as negative is a matter of concern. In such men detailed analysis of the entire CFTR gene is recommended. But clinician and the patient must be informed that a negative result does not mean the gene is normal, it only means our inability to detect the mutation. The family must be informed about the increased risk of cystic fibrosis in the offspring in case of CAVBD. Table 1 summarizes the counseling points that must be taken care of during evaluation of men with obstructive azoospermia.

What Care Should be Taken While Genetic Testing

It is of utmost importance that the clinician appropriately counsels the patient regarding the role of genetic testing and the prognostic and psychological effects of these genetic tests. Also testing should be done from certified laboratories where there are adequate quality control measures.[10] The clinician must also be aware of the limitation of the testing. For example, normal karyotype will not always mean absence of genetic abnormality. Small deletions and duplications that are observed by molecular testing in various parts of the genome and these might cause infertility.[11] In case of YCMD testing, it is presently offered using the genetic markers recommended by EAA/EMQN or by using the commercially available kits.[5,10] However, it must be noted that not all these markers are sufficient or essential for Indian population. It is reported that and almost 50% of patients can be missed if the EAA markers are used.[5] Thus the clinicians must insist on laboratories to provide testing using more appropriate markers for the population.

The Future of Genetics and Male Infertility

Genetic Testing of Spermatozoa

Genetic testing of spermatozoa like DNA fragmentation analysis is routinely employed in some clinics but the differences in the assays utilized, as well as by methodological variations for each individual assay have contributed to the controversial nature of this test. DNA fragmentation analysis is useful in certain patients such as those with unexplained poor IVF outcome and individuals with DNA fragmentation of index above 30 have poor outcomes in ART.[12] These men may be treated with antioxidants as it seems to improve the number of good quality sperm.[12,13] Although not all clinics agree to this consensus and hence presently sperm DNA fragmentation assay must be considered at best experimental. Sperm chromosome aneuploidy analysis involves tests to assess the presence of aberrant numbers of chromosomes in spermatozoa using FISH. Elevated aneuploidy has been associated to oligozoospermia, asthenozoospermia and teratozoospermia but the testing has limited clinical value. Although may be useful in cases of unexplained recurrent pregnancy loss or repeated IVF failure.

Sperm Epigenetics

One of the newest areas of future progress in unraveling the basis of male infertility is the area of epigenetics.[14] Epigenetic changes are non-coding changes to the genome brought about by methylation of cytosine bases of DNA and different chemical modifications to histones, which in turn, either increase or inhibit gene expression. Differences in sperm epigenetic profiles are noted in infertile males. Because the epigenome is transient and is subject to be influenced by a plethora of environmental factors such as age, diet, exposures, medicines and supplements and is thought to serve as an important link between environmental influences and altered fertility. Although the clinical implementation of epigenetic testing seems promising, essential validation studies are yet underway. Epigenetic profiling of spermatozoa from infertile men may help to assess the potential of the spermatozoa to contribute to normal embryogenesis and in assessing risks associated with environmental exposures.[14]

CONCLUSION

Male infertility is a complex multifactorial condition that presents with highly heterogeneous phenotypes. With clear-cut cause—effect relationship with severely impaired spermatogenesis, karyotyping and YCMD testing are now almost mandatory in clinical practice. These tests will not only allow determining cause of male infertility but also aid in predicting the success rates of ART. Further as YCMD has 100% transmission rate to male offspring, the couple needs to be aware that the males in the future generation will also be infertile. Beyond these immediate applications, there are some clinically relevant issues with YCMD testing needing urgent attention. These include the higher risk of testicular cancers and the occurrence of neurological dysfunctions. It is imperative that we carry out detailed analysis of men with YCMD with an outlook beyond infertility. CFTR investigations are limited to patients with CAVBD and there is an important role of genetic counseling for prevention of frank cystic fibrosis in future generations. The role of sperm DNA testing (DNA fragmentation, aneuploidy and epigenetics) is yet in experimental phase and has limited clinical utility. We believe that careful clinical assessment of male factor together with appropriate genetic analysis will offer important insights on the cause and consequences of male infertility and aid the clinicians to make the best use of the new field of androgenetics in future.

KEY POINTS

- Genetic testing is essential component of clinical evaluation for infertile male.
- Karyotyping and Y chromosome microdeletion testing are basic test that must be performed in all cases with abnormal spermiogram.
- These tests will aid in rational decision making for success of ART.
- 100% transmission rate of Y chromosome microdeletions from father to son after ART would perpetuate infertility and the associated risk in the family for generations.

ACKNOWLEDGEMENTS

SC is thankful to ICMR for the postdoctoral fellowship and DM laboratory is supported by grants from ICMR. The manuscript bears the NIRRH ID: OTH/613/02-2018.

REFERENCES

1. Ventimiglia E, Capogrosso P, Boeri L, et al. When to Perform Karyotype Analysis in Infertile Men? Validation of the European Association of Urology Guidelines with the Proposal of a New Predictive Model. Eur Urol. 2016;70(6):920-3.
2. Wosnitzer MS. Genetic evaluation of male infertility. Translational andrology and urology. 2014;3(1):17.
3. Colaco S, Lakdawala A, Modi D. Role of Y chromosome microdeletions in the clinical evaluation of infertile males. MGM J Med Sci. 2017;4:79-88.
4. Hotaling J, Carrell DT. Clinical genetic testing for male factor infertility: current applications and future directions. Andrology. 2014;2(3):339-50.
5. Sen S, Pasi AR, Dada R, et al. Y chromosome microdeletions in infertile men: prevalence, phenotypes and screening markers for the Indian population. J Assist Reproduct Genet. 2013;30(3):413-22.
6. de Souza DAS, Faucz FR, Pereira-Ferrari L, et al. Congenital bilateral absence of the vas deferens as an atypical form of cystic fibrosis: reproductive implications and genetic counseling. Andrology. 2018;6(1):127-35.
7. Machiela MJ, Dagnall CL, Pathak A, et al. Mosaic chromosome Y loss and testicular germ cell tumor risk. J Hum Genet. 2017;62(6):637-40.
8. Kido T, Lau YF. Roles of the Y chromosome genes in human cancers. Asian J Androl. 2015;17(3):373.
9. Castro A, Rodríguez F, Flórez M, et al. Pseudoautosomal abnormalities in terminal AZFb+ c deletions are associated with isochromosomes Yp and may lead to abnormal growth and neuropsychiatric function. Hum Reprod. 2017;32:465-75.
10. Krausz C, Hoefsloot L, Simoni M, et al. EAA/EMQN best practice guidelines for molecular diagnosis of Y chromosomal microdeletions: state of the art 2013. Andrology. 2014;2(1):5-19.
11. Halder A, Kumar P, Jain M, et al. Copy number variations in testicular maturation arrest. Andrology. 2017;5(3):460-72.
12. Agarwal A, Cho CL, Majzoub A, et al. The Society for Translational Medicine: clinical practice guidelines for sperm DNA fragmentation testing in male infertility. Transl Androl Urol. 2017;6(Suppl 4):S720-33.
13. Cho CL, Agarwal A, Majzoub A, et al. Transl Androl Urol. Clinical utility of sperm DNA fragmentation testing: concise practice recommendations. 2017;6(Suppl 4):S366-73.
14. Jenkins TG, Aston KI, James ER, et al. Sperm epigenetics in the study of male fertility, offspring health, and potential clinical applications. Syst Biol Reprod Med. 2017;63(2):69-76.

CHAPTER 6

Sperm Preparation Techniques and its Modification According to Different Sperm Seminopathy

Charudutt Joshi

■ INTRODUCTION

In modern era with development modifications in life style, infertility is also becoming a major problem increasing day by day. This leads to development of science of assisted reproduction techniques (ART). The best technique was selected on basis of indications and prognosis of infertility.

Intrauterine Insemination

Intrauterine insemination (IUUI) is first line treatment offered to a infertile couple. First time this technique was reported by John Hunter in 1970's, since than it has undergone many developments and changes. Before performing intrauterine insemination procedure first semen sample has to be processed to get highly motile fraction of sperm.

■ SEMEN

It is natural nutritious medium formed by secretion of prostrate (1/3rd), secretions of seminal vesicles (2/3rd) portion having tiny motile haploid cells called sperm.

Sperm is a courier by which delivers paternal parcel to the egg. This parcel contains 50% genetic material of future human being.

Semen Analysis (According to WHO 2010 Manual)

Liquefaction	: 30-45 minutes after collection at room temperature
Appearance	: Homogenous, gray opalescent
Odor	: Fresh and characteristic
Consistency	: Leaves pipette as discrete droplets
Volume	: In between 2 mL and 6 mL
pH	: 7.2–7.8
Sperm concentration	: More than 20 million spermatozoa/mL

Sperm Preparation Techniques and its Modification

Total Count : More than 40 million spermatozoa per ejaculate sample
Motility : More than 50% forward progression
Morphology : More than 4% normal sperms (strict criteria)
Vitality : More than 705 live spermatozoa
WBC : Less than 1 million cells per mL.

Sperm Preparation Laboratory

Ideal laboratory should be able to perform 100% sterile conditions for processing sperm sample. It should be in accordance with the guidelines from competent authority. Basic instrumentation include (Fig. 1):
- Binocular compound phase contrast microscope
- Laminar flow
- Test tube warmers
- Bacteriological incubator
- CO_2 incubator (optional)
- Centrifuge with timer and RPM meter
- Sperm counting chamber
- Cryocans for storage of sperm samples.

Sperm Preparation Procedure

All semen samples looks same in appearance but actually all of them are different from each other. It depends upon various parameters like count, motility, morphology amount of debris, anti-sperm anti-bodies, etc. Hence, the procedure also varies according to type of sample.

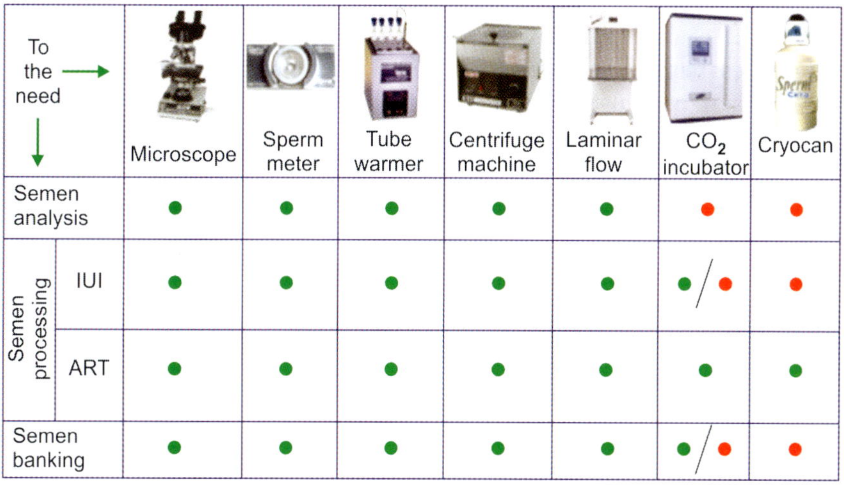

To the need	Microscope	Sperm meter	Tube warmer	Centrifuge machine	Laminar flow	CO_2 incubator	Cryocan
Semen analysis	●	●	●	●	●	●	●
Semen processing — IUI	●	●	●	●	●	●/●	●
Semen processing — ART	●	●	●	●	●	●	●
Semen banking	●	●	●	●	●	●/●	●

Fig. 1: Instruments required for andrology laboratory set up.
(*Note*: Green color (●), used in the process; Red color (●), not used in the process)

Semen is mixture of tiny cells called sperms, seminal plasma constitute of secretions from prostrate gland, seminal vesicles and epididymis. It also has cellular components like leukocytes and micro-organisms.

The ultimate aim of all procedures applied for sperm preparation is to separate out fraction of high quality functional motile sperm from seminal fluid without causing damage to sperms.

Advantages

- Removal of seminal plasma helps in reducing pelvic infections caused by microorganisms present
- It helps in removing prostaglandins which can cause uterine contraction after coming in contact with uterine wall
- It helps in reducing viral load from samples which are positive for HbSAg and HIV
- Very effective method for removing antisperm antibodies
- It helps in removing cellular debris and other unwanted material from the sample
- In some selected cases of low progression of sperm energy enhancing substances can be added during preparation.

Sperm Preparation Techniques

Over the years sperm preparation technique for intrauterine insemination (IUI) has undergone many changes according to the need. Many methods has been developed considering parameter involved like (a) Count, (b) Motility, (c) Volume, (d) Viscosity, (e) Presence of cellular debris.

The most important factor to be considered for sperm preparation by any technique is viscosity. Normal semen liquefies in 30 minute. There are some samples which coagulate or highly viscous in nature, takes more time to liquefy. Sometimes they do not liquefy at all. Such semen samples need to be treated differently. If previously reported than these patients can be given container for sample collection containing 2 mL of sperm washing media, so that sample directly collected in media. Clear instructions should be given to tight cap the container after collection as when it comes in contact with air it gets coagulate and become more viscous. In extreme cases when it does not liquefy at all than proteolyses enzymes can be added in the sample. The parameter to consider complete liquefaction is there should be free fall of sample in form of drops without leaving a mucus thread.

Centrifuging sperm at a definite speed can cause generation of ROS (reactive oxygen species) due to presence of debris, pus cell, and other cells, etc. which react with cell membrane of sperm resulting oxidative stress to damage the sperm.

All kind of sperm preparations need a basic physiological culture media like (a) EBSS (Earle's Balanced salt solution), (b) HAM's F10 media, (c) PBS

Sperm Preparation Techniques and its Modification

(Phosphate buffer saline), (d) Ringer's Lactate (e) HTF media (Human Tubal Fluid), etc. with pH adjusted to 7.2–7.4.

All available techniques can be categorized into three types:
a. Swim up with centrifugation
b. Swim up without centrifugation
c. Density gradient centrifugation

Swim Up with Centrifugation (Fig. 2)

Most common method used for sperm preparation. This is easy to perform and applied for normal samples. It helps in recovery of motile sperms leaving behind seminal plasma with cellular debris. It does not help in selecting morphologically normal sperms.

Steps:
1. Take liquefied sample in a well labeled graduated conical bottom tube.
2. Add double volume of media and mix well with pipette.
3. Centrifuge at 1500 rpm for 10 minutes.
4. You will see a compact pallet at bottom. Remove complete supernatant.
5. Loose the pallet by gently tapping it and slowly layer the pallet with 1 mL of media.
6. Keep it at 37°C in slanting position to increase surface area for 30–45 minutes.

Sometimes we see high amount of cellular debris in sample in such cases one more wash and spin can be given.
1. Take liquefied sample in a well labeled graduated conical bottom tube
2. Add double volume of media and mix well with pipette.
3. Centrifuge at 1500 rpm for 10 minutes.
4. You will see a compact pallet at bottom. Remove complete supernatant.
5. Add another 2 mL of media and mix well.
6. Again centrifuge at 1500 rpm for 10 minutes.
7. Remove complete supernatant.
8. Loose the pallet by gently tapping it and slowly layer the pallet with 1 mL of media.
9. Keep it at 37°C in slanting position to increase surface area for 30-45 minutes.

You will see turbid cloudy upper layer. Remove around 7 mL of this supernatant and keep it in another fresh tube till insemination.

Swim Up without Centrifugation

This method is also known as layering. Useful method for normal sperm sample (count more than 20 million/mL) with normal viscosity.

Steps:
1. Take 2 mL of sperm washing media in a 10 mL round bottom tube.
2. Now with help of transfer pipette add 2 mL of liquefied semen sample to the bottom gently without disturbing the interphase.
3. Keep it at 37°C for 60–90 minutes vertically.

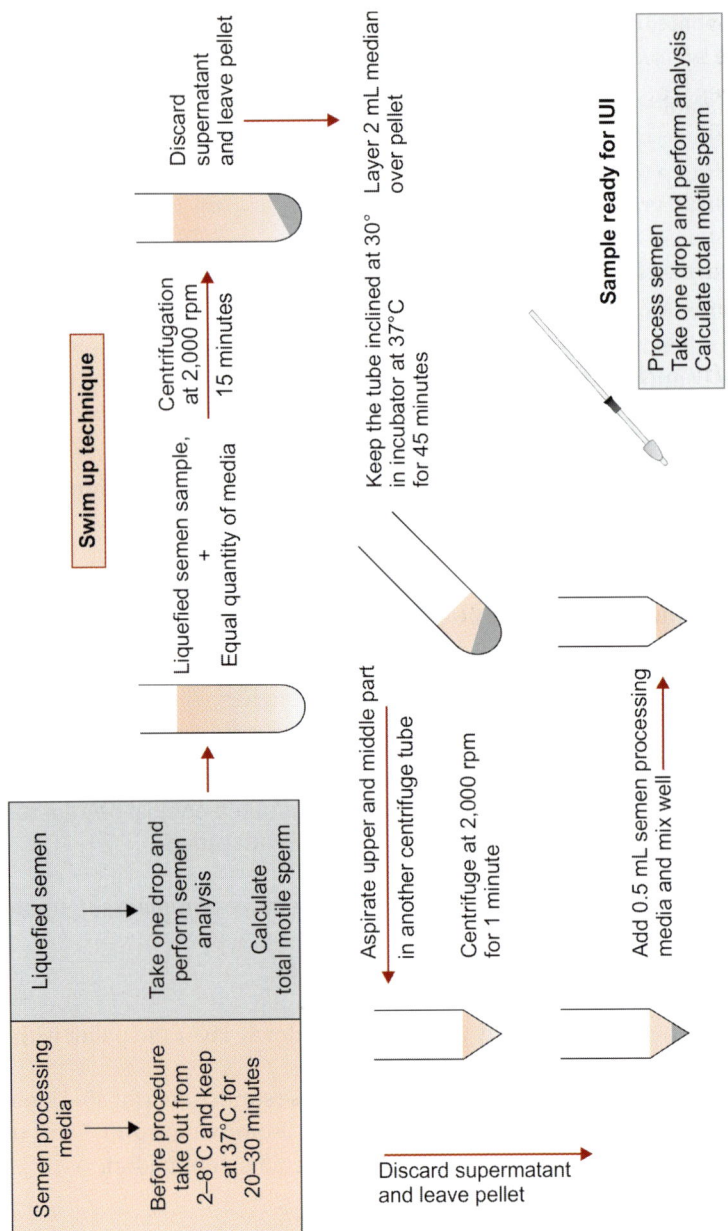

Fig. 2 : Illustration of normal sperm wash by swim up technique.

4. Remove top 0.5 to 0.7 mL cloudy layer in separate tube till insemination.
5. Use it for insemination.

Sometimes this upper layer is too cloudy that means high concentration of sperm; in such cases this method is slightly modified. It is combination of layering and swim up method.

1. Take 2 mL of sperm washing media in a 10 mL round bottom tube.

2. Now with help of transfer pipette add 2 mL of liquefied semen sample to the bottom gently without disturbing the interphase.
3. Keep it at 37°C for 60–90 minutes vertically.
4. Remove top 0.5 to 0.7 mL cloudy layer in separate tube till insemination.
5. Add another 1 mL media, mix it well.
6. Centrifuge at 1,000 rpm for 5 minutes.
7. Remove supernatant completely.
8. Add 0.5 mL media gently on pallet and incubate at 37°C for 30–45 minutes.
9. Remove supernatant and use it for insemination.

Density Gradient (Fig. 3)

Earlier percoll gradient were used. It is silica particle. Coated with polyvinylpyrrolidone. There was some reports published about carcinogenic effect of percoll and hence it is banned. Now in place we use colloidal silica particle solution in saline. It is available as 100% stock solution from which we can make different gradient solutions. Commonly used gradients are 40% and 80%, 45% and 90% and 90%, 70% and 40%. This technique is very effective when a sample has high amount of cellular debris, pus cells, abnormal sperms, oligospermia, and asthenozoospermia conditions.

Steps:
1. Make a gradient column in conical bottom centrifuge tube keeping highest concentration at bottom and lowest on the top.
2. Different gradient solutions should be layered very slowly taking care not to disturb the interphase between them.
3. Gently layer liquefied sample on top of the column.
4. Centrifuge it at 2000 rpm for 20 minutes with proper balance.

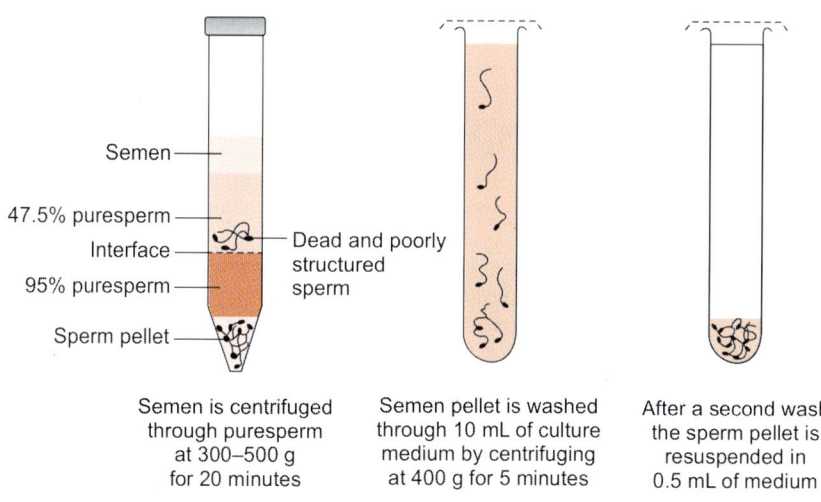

Fig. 3: Illustration of density gradient technique.

5. Remove upper layers of semen and top layers of gradient solutions leaving behind 50% of the bottom 90% gradient layer.
6. Transfer this layer to another fresh tube and add 2 mL washing medium to it. Mix well.
7. Again centrifuge it at 1,500 rpm for 5 minutes.
8. Remove supernatant leaving behind pallet.
9. Mix it gently with 0.5 mL of media and is ready to use for insemination.

There are different kinds of semen sample and method of preparation depends upon the type and specific characters of the sample. Various papers published till date comparing different techniques available; however, no conclusive evidence or report state that one method is better than other. Nowadays most commonly used method is density gradient.

KEY POINTS

- Some semen samples are highly viscous and do not liquefy completely in time or some time does not liquefy at all. To get good motile sperm fraction its complete liquefaction is important. In such cases sample can be given with media added in it so that sample directly collected in media.
- If a sample is not liquefies in time than it can be added with media mix it and again keep it for 15 minutes, it will liquefy.
- Still some samples does not liquefy than entire sample is taken in 5 mL syringe without putting needle than needle 22 G is fixed on it and entire sample is passed through it along side wall of container. It will liquefy. It is called needle processing. However, it is not recommended as it causes sperm damage.
- Nowadays photolytic enzymes are used to break mucus fibers in semen sample to liquefy.
- To confirm whether sample is liquefied, aspirate semen in the pasture pipette hold vertically and see free fall of sample drop wise. If completely liquefy than there will be free fall of drops without mucus thread.
- Samples containing excessive amount of pus cells and cellular debris is strong indication of infection. It should be send for culture and after treating with proper antibiotic than only this sample should be prepared.
- Some sample collected with very low volume (less than 0.5 mL) which does not contain sperms or very less sperm. Than such patient should be counseled and asked for it. It is quite possible that sample is not collected properly or there may be spillage. In such conditions he should be asked to produce one more sample after some time. If sample has good count but quantity is very low than it should be added with washing media (1–2 mL) in it to avoid drying of the sample.
- In cases of oligospermia, asthenospermia, terratozoospermia, etc. density gradient technique is best to get good yield of motile sperm friction.
- Some samples shows agglutination or clumping of sperms. It should be carefully observed that this clump is due to mucus fiber or it is actual binding of sperm to each other. In case of actual binding it may be a case of antisperm antibody positive. In such cases container should be given for collection with 2 mL of media and during preparation it should be washed twice.
- In cases of HIV or HbSAg positive it should be prepared with density gradient followed by washing it twice significantly reduces viral load.

FURTHER READING

1. Aitken RJ, Clarckson JS. Significance of reactive oxygen species in defining efficiency of sperm preparation technique. J Androl. 1988;9:367-76.
2. Amelar RD. Coagulation, Liquefaction and viscosity of human semen. J Urol 1962;87:187-90.
3. Chocrane database syst. Rev. 2007;17(4):CD004507.
4. Drevius LO. The spermrise test. J Reprod Fertil. 1971;24(3):427-9.
5. Jaquier AM, Crich JP. Semen analysis; A practical guide. Blackwell Scientific Publication, Oxford; 1986.
6. Marshburn PB, Kutteh WH. The role of antisperm antibodies in Infertility. Fertil Sterli. 1994;61(5):799-811.
7. Mencaglia L, Falcon P, Lentini GM, et al. ICSI for treatment of HIV virus serodiscordant couples with infected male partner. Human Reprod. 2005;20:2246-6.
8. Nayar KD, Sehgal P, Tiwari A. P-994 Comparative study of various sperm preparation techniques in IUI and their effects on pregnancy rates. Fertil Sterl. 2006;86:S502-3.
9. Pandian N (Ed): Handbook of Andrology, TR Publications, Chennai; 1999.
10. Prakash P, Leykin L, Chen Z, et al. Preparation by differential gradient centrifugation is better than swim up in selecting sperm with normal morphology Fertil Steril. 1998;69(4):722-6.
11. Savasi V, Ferrazzi E, Lanzani C, et al. Safety of sperm washing and ART outcome 741 HIV-I discordant couples. Hum Reprod. 2007;22:772-7.
12. Soliman S, goyal A. RCT comparing two different method of sperm preparation. Fertil Steril. 2005; 84(suppl 1):S156.
13. The infertility manual Edited by Kamini Rao.
14. WHO manual on Semen Analysis; 2010.
15. Zimmerman ER, Robertson KR, Kim H, et al. Semen preparation with sperm select system verses washing technique. Fertil Steril. 1994;61(2):269-75.
16. Zini A, Mak V, Phang D, et al. Potential adverse effect of semen processing on human DNA and its integrity. Fertil Sterl. 1999;72:496-9.

CHAPTER

7

Advanced Sperm Selection Technique for ART

G Manjula

■ INTRODUCTION

Selection of sperm is a crucial part in assisted reproductive treatment (ART). Sperm preparation methods do mainly differentiate according to sperm motility and are indispensable for therapies like intrauterine insemination, in vitro fertilization (IVF) and intracytoplasmic sperm injection (ICSI). Although in the beginning of the era of ICSI andrology was thought to play a minor role, ICSI has offered new options by correlating the treatment outcome to parameters of the individual applied spermatozoon. Hence the possibility for selecting spermatozoa has shifted from parameters which characterize the entire sperm cohort to a single-sperm specific assessment technology. Consequently, sperm selection is a topic which is intensively discussed nowadays. This article gives a comprehensive overview of the technologies which can be applied today and give a prospective on future techniques.

In vitro fertilization is a form of assisted reproductive technology used for treating infertility, a condition affecting an estimated 15% of the population. IVF usually involves controlled ovarian hyperstimulation, surgical oocyte retrieval, in vitro fertilization and embryo transfer. Intracytoplasmic sperm injection is a form of ART where instead of relying on spontaneous entry of the sperm into the oocyte, a single sperm is injected into the cytoplasm of each oocyte to achieve fertilization. ICSI is commonly used as a treatment for male factor infertility where semen parameters are poor, when sperm has been surgically retrieved or following repeated failed fertilization with standard IVF (Palermo 1992).

Successful embryo development and subsequent pregnancy outcome are likely to be impacted by the quality of the sperm which fertilizes an oocyte (Sakkas 2000). Ideally only sperm with a high chance of successful fertilization and subsequent embryo growth would be used for ART. These sperm would be viable, mature, have high DNA integrity and be structurally sound. Sperm preparation and selection in IVF is limited to semen washing, density gradient centrifugation and the use of the swim-up techniques (Boomsma 2007). In

ICSI, routine sperm selection is based on motility and gross morphology (sperm are examined under a microscope at 200–400x magnification) after one or more of the above methods of semen preparation. Advanced sperm selection techniques based on alternative characteristics might enable further selection of the most appropriate sperm for use in ART.

Through the use of advanced sperm selection techniques a structurally intact and mature sperm with high DNA integrity may be selected for fertilization. Each modality utilizes differing characteristics of sperm structure, physiology or function to allow selection of the most normal sperm. Advanced sperm selection protocols aim to improve ART outcomes and may limit the possible deleterious effects on offspring of using sperm with defective DNA (Aitken 2007). Advanced sperm selection techniques have developed as a means of improving ART outcomes in certain clinical scenarios. Techniques can be categorized as follows.

■ ADVANCED SPERM SELECTION TECHNIQUES

Based on the main criteria used to select a sperm subpopulation, these procedures can be classified as:

Selection by Differential Sperm Surface Charge

There are two different approaches to select sperm based on the differential net electric charge on the sperm plasma membrane:
1. *Electrophoretic system* (SpermSep® CS-10, NuSep Ltd., Frenchs Forest, Australia) (Ainsworth et al. 2005)
2. *Zeta potential method* (Chan et al. 2006).

Electrophoretic System (Fig. 1 and Table 1)

The electrophoresis-based technology was developed at Dr. Aitken's laboratory in Australia (Ainsworth et al. 2005) and later commercialized by NuSep Ltd. as Microflow® CS-10 (renamed to SpermSep® CS-10). This device uses an electric field to separate sperm cells based on size and electronegative charge. It is composed of four chambers: two outer chambers and two inner chambers (incubation and collection). The semen specimen is loaded into the incubation chamber and allowed to equilibrate for 5 minutes before applying a current of 75 mA and variable voltage (18–21 V). The selected sperm subpopulation is recovered from the collection chamber after 5 minutes of application of the electric field and it is ready for ARTs. There is evidence that the electronegativity on the sperm surface indicates normal differentiation and is associated with CD52 expression on sperm membrane (Schroter et al. 1999) and other glycoproteins (Ainsworth et al. 2011). These observations and the fact that CD52 is correlated with normal sperm morphology and capacitation (Giuliani et al. 2004), may account for the ability of the electrophoresis separation method to select sperm with significantly improved morphology with low levels

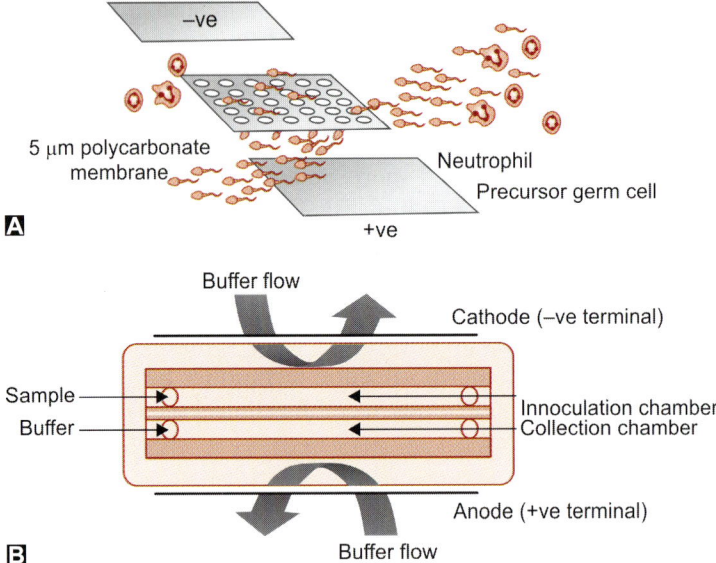

Figs. 1A and B: The electrophoretic system used for sperm selection. (A) Competent spermatozoa move in the applied electric field, and cell contaminants are excluded based on size; (B) Graphic representation of the system configuration including restriction and separation membranes, buffer flows and sample inoculation and collection locations.

Table 1: The electrophoretic system used for sperm selection.	
Advantages	Disadvantages
Relatively fast as it requires only 5 minutes of current application	Complexity of the separation apparatus used may be the limiting factor
No centrifugation steps thus it avoids ROS production	
Can be employed for oligozoospermic samples, testicular samples and frozen spermatozoa	

of DNA damage (Ainsworth et al. 2005). Key features of the electrophoresis system that make it attractive for ART laboratories are: the whole process of selection can take only a few minutes and the generation of ROS is minimized because of lack of centrifugation steps. On the other hand, the cost associated with acquisition of the electrophoresis separation device may be prohibitive for andrology laboratories with limited resources.

The first live birth from an embryo conceived with a spermatozoon selected by the novel electrophoretic approach was reported in 2007 (Ainsworth et al. 2007). The study involved a couple with long-term infertility associated with extensive sperm DNA damage. Later, a prospective controlled trial was performed to demonstrate that the membrane-based electrophoresis system is as effective as and considerably faster than the DGC to prepare spermatozoa for both IVF and ICSI (Fleming et al. 2008).

Zeta Potential Method (Fig. 2 and Table 2)

Sperm cells can be selected based on their negative zeta electrokinetic potential (Chan et al. 2006) which is the overall charge a particle, in this particular case a spermatozoon, acquires in a specific medium. A mature sperm cell has a negative zeta potential of 16–20 mV (differential potential between the sperm membrane and its surroundings) (Ishijima et al. 1991). The zeta potential method is very simple to perform and it does not require special equipment, therefore, it is inexpensive. Briefly, washed sperm in serum-free medium is introduced in a conical tube which has been positively charged by rubbing or rotating the tube on a latex glove.

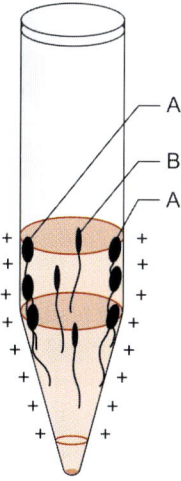

Fig. 2: Sperm selection using zeta potential method. Diagram for sperm selection using zeta potential. Sperm suspension is pipette into a positively charged tube. Negatively charged mature sperm (A) will adhere to the tube, while non-mature sperm (B) will not adhere and are discarded.

Table 2: Sperm selection using zeta potential method.

Advantages	Disadvantages
Easy to perform and inexpensive	Low recovery of processed sperm limits their use in oligozoospermic samples
Permits rapid recovery of sperm with improved sperm parameters	Not useful in testicular and epididymal sperms aspirates as they lack sufficient net electrical charge on sperm surface membrane
Sperm progressive motility and hyper-activation is improved	Not tested in humid environment that is known to neutralize electrical charges
High voltage electricity is not applied	

Electronegatively charged sperm (mature) attach to the walls of the tube by electrostatic forces and the non-adherent sperm fraction and other contaminants are removed by inverting the tube. Selected adherent sperm cells are recovered by rinsing the tube with serum-supplemented medium. Regarding the morphology and functional characteristics of sperm selected by zeta potential, experimental data indicated that this method advantages the conventional DGC in terms of percentage of morphologically normal sperm, hyperactivation, DNA integrity and maturity, but not motility (Chan et al. 2006).

Results from a randomized prospective study with sperm selected with a combination of DGC/zeta potential or DGC alone previous to ICSI indicated that the combination may increase fertilization rates and possibly pregnancy rates in infertile couples associated with male factor infertility (Kheirollahi-Kouhestani et al. 2009). However, definitive data that demonstrate the benefits of applying the zeta potential approach to select sperm for human assisted conception is still missing.

Selection of Non-apoptotic Spermatozoa from Apoptotic

- Magnetic cell sorting
- Annexin V glass wool filtration

Magnetic Cell Sorting (Fig. 3 and Table 3)

The externalization of the phospholipid phosphatidylserine (PS) to the sperm plasma membrane is a characteristic feature of the apoptotic phenomenon that occurs early during the process of sperm cell death. This basic knowledge has prompted investigators to develop a magnetic-based selection system for sperm cells that can separate early apoptotic from non-apoptotic germ cells (MACS, Miltenyi Biotec GmbH, Bergisch Gladbach, Germany). Since externalized PS has high affinity to Annexin V, apoptotic sperm cells bind to Annexin V-conjugated paramagnetic microbeads. The magnetically labeled sample is passed through a magnetic column where magnetically labeled apoptotic or dead spermatozoa are retained in the column while the unlabeled non-apoptotic spermatozoa are collected in the flow-through for further processing for ARTs (Grunewald et al. 2001; Manz et al. 1995).

Magnetic activated cell sorting (MACS) separates apoptotic spermatozoa from non-apoptotic spermatozoa. 100 µL of sperm sample is mixed with 100 µL of MACS microbeads and incubated at room temperature for 15 minutes. The mixture is loaded on top of separation column which is placed in magnetic field. Apoptotic sperm with Annexin V beads (magnetic) are retained in the column while the non-apoptotic sperm are eluted out and collected in a tube below the collection device. Annexin V-negative sperm cells show significantly higher motility and survival rates following cryopreservation than annexin V-positive sperm cells. Magnetic activated cell sorting improves the acrosome reaction in couples with unexplained fertility.

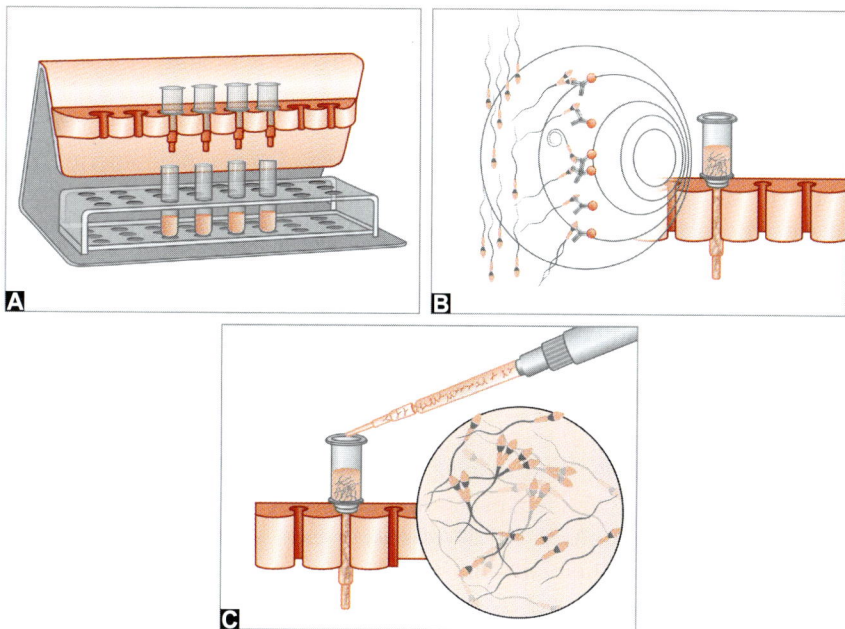

Figs. 3A to C: Magnetic cell sorting: Magnetic activated cell sorting: (A) The Octatet magnetic collection device can be used for loading up to a maximum of 8 samples. The tubes are placed between each open slot surrounded by the magnetic field; (B) The apoptotic and the nonapoptotic cells are labeled with the Annexin V antibody beads (magnetic). These attach to the outer surface of the sperm that are apoptotic. Annexin V beads (magnetic) do not bind to the sperm that are nonapoptotic and have intact membranes; (C) Apoptotic sperm with Annexin V beads (magnetic) are retained in the column while the nonapoptotic sperm are eluted out and collected in a tube below the collection device.

Table 3: Magnetic cell sorting.

Advantages	Disadvantages
MACS acts at molecular level	MACS which removes apoptotic sperms needs to be used in conjunction with other techniques such as density gradient to remove other substances
It is the only known technique which separates apoptotic sperms from non-apoptotic sperms	
Rapid, convenient and noninvasive	
Bead detachment after MACS is not necessary	
MACS can be used to optimize the cryopreservation thawing outcome	

Annexin V Glass Wool Filtration

In order to avoid the problems associated with freely floating microbeads, another system for selection of non-apoptotic spermatozoa has been recently described. The system is based on modifying commercially available glass wool separation columns to add the ability of retaining apoptotic sperm. This was achieved by coating the glass wool with Annexin V that binds to apoptotic sperm. The technique referred to as Annexin V glass wool (Annexin V-GW) or molecular glass wool is easy to use on both fresh and cryopreserved semen samples; AnnexinV glass wool has an ability to select spermatozoa with lower caspase activation and higher mitochondrial membrane potential.

Glass Wool Filtration (Table 4)

Glass wool filtration separates motile sperm cells from other contents of semen by filtration through densely packed glass wool fibers. The filtration separates out immotile sperm cells, leukocytes and debris. Henkel et al. reported that glass wool filtration eliminates 87.5% of leukocytes in semen. This is important since leukocytes are the main source of ROS in semen. After filtration, the semen is centrifuged to remove seminal plasma from viable sperm cells. The fact that centrifugation is carried out without leukocytes and non-viable spermatozoa are important since the absence of these populations limits the production of ROS.

Selection of Highly Motile Sperms from Immotile Sperms

Micro-fluidic sperm cell sorter (MACS, Miltenyi Biotec GmbH, Bergisch Gladbach, Germany).

Microfluidic Sperm Cell Sorter (Fig. 4 and Table 5)

Semen sample added in inlet A and MEDIUM is added into inlet B. Spermatozoa are sorted depending on their ability to swim across the semen stream into the medium stream. Only motile sperms swim towards outlet C. In contrast, immotile sperms keep flowing to outlet D. During the separation method, spermatozoa do not undergo added physical stress due to centrifuge.

Table 4: Glass wool filtration.

Advantages	Disadvantages
Easy to perform	Relatively expensive
Recovers sperms with good motility and normal chromatin condensation	Debris and immotile sperms may pass through the mesh and be present in the sample even after filtration
Eliminates leukocytes	
Low ROS	

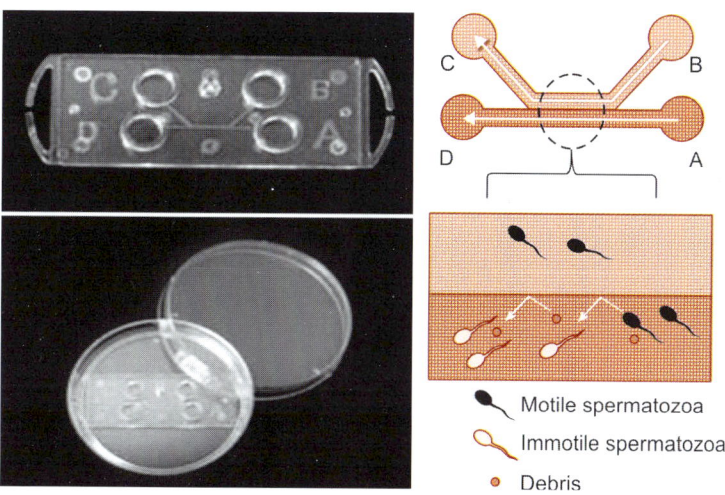

Fig. 4: Microfluidic sperm cell sorter.

Table 5: Microfluidic sperm cell sorter.	
Advantages	*Disadvantages*
Simple and safe method of obtaining motile sperm of enriched normal morphology	Expensive
Because no centrifugation, there is reduced opportunity to cause DNA damage to sperm	Not capable of processing an entire sample due to its small capacity

Selection Based on the Sperm Membrane Maturity

Hyaluronic acid sperm binding test (physiological intracytoplasmic sperm injection—PICSI).

Hyaluronic Acid Sperm Binding Test (Fig. 5)

The presence of hyaluronic acid (HA) binding sites on sperm outer membrane is regarded as a sign of sperm maturity, and constitutes the basic principle for a sperm binding assay (Jakab et al. 2005). In this assay, HA is immobilized on a solid surface (polystyrene culture dish) and the washed sperm sample is allowed to interact with the HA coated surface for 15 minutes. An individual sperm attached to the dish is picked up with the ICSI pipette and used for oocyte injection.

As HA is a natural occurring compound present in cervical mucus, cumulus cells and follicular fluid, the binding method is considered to have minimal biosafety risks for both the embryo and the patient. The device called PICSI® (preselected intracytoplasmatical sperm injection), commercialized by ORIGIO MidAtlantic Devices Inc. (Mt Laurel, NJ, USA), uses a conventional polystyrene culture dish enhanced with tree microdots of hyaluronan where

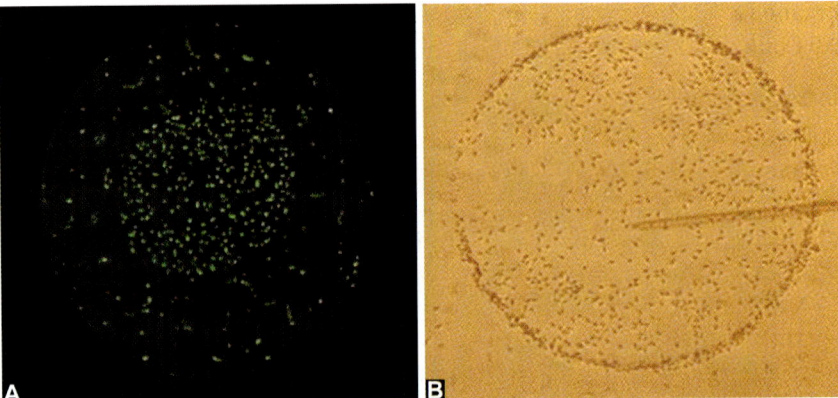

Figs. 5A and B: Sperm selection using PICSI dishes: (A) Sperm drop is placed at the periphery of a HA drop, mature sperm binds to the HA-spot, while immature sperm moves freely; (B) Bound sperm could be picked up with the ICSI pipette.

the sperm suspension is added. Sperm maturity has been associated with certain desirable sperm traits such as: improved viability and motility, intact acrosomes, lower caspase-3 activation and lower frequency of chromosomal aneuploidy (Huszar et al. 2007; Huszar et al. 2003). Studies documenting the use of sperm selected by HA method in the clinical ART setting is still scarce and somehow contradictory.

While one study reported significantly increased fertilization rate of oocytes injected with HA-selected sperm and only a marginal effect on pregnancy rate (Nasr-Esfahani et al. 2008), in other studies by Permegiani et al. (2010a; 2010b) oocytes injected with sperm selected by the binding method originated better quality embryos but no effect was detected on fertilization and pregnancy rates.

Selection Based on Ultra Morphology

- Real-time motile sperm organelle morphology examination (MSOME)
- Intracytoplasmic morphologically selected sperm injection (IMSI)
- Sperm birefringence using polarization microscopy.

Real-time Motile Sperm Organelle Morphology Examination

A new sperm selection method has been developed based on the inclusion of only normal sperm assessed using real-time motile sperm organelle morphology examination (MSOME) at a magnification of ×6300 (Bartoov et al. 2002). During MSOME, a micro-droplet of motile sperm suspension prepared by a routine sperm preparation technique is examined under oil immersion, with an inverted light microscope fitted with high-power Nomarski optics with digital enhancement. MSOME assesses five sperm organelles (acrosome, postacrosomal lamina, neck, tail and mitochondria) that can be classified as either normal or abnormal. The sixth organelle (the nucleus) is evaluated for both shape and chromatin content (vacuolar area) (Fig. 5). Among the six organelles, the sperm nucleus appears to be the most important in influencing ART outcome (Bartoov et al. 2002).

Intracytoplasmic Morphologically Selected Sperm Injection (Figs 6A and B)

Subsequently, a modification of ICSI termed intracytoplasmic morphologically selected sperm injection (IMSI) has been developed (Bartoov et al. 2003). This approach is of particular benefit when used in situations where identification of specific sperm organelles is required, such as the acrosomal components in cases of globozoospermia (Check et al. 2007).

MSOME followed by IMSI is an elaborate procedure that involves prolonged sperm manipulation, adding significantly to the routine ICSI processing times. It was reported that it could take up to 5 hours to perform (Berkovitz et al. 2005). It also requires special instrumentation with considerable expense. The subjectivity of the sperm ultra morphology assessment may be another limiting factor that prevents its widespread use.

Sperm Birefringence by Using Polarization Microscopy

A different optical system has been developed to identify the sperm birefringence, which occurs in mature forms due to the presence of subacrosomal protein filaments that are longitudinally oriented (Baccetti, 2004). Sperm birefringence can be evaluated using an inverted microscope equipped with polarizing and analyzing lenses, which allows the selection of birefringent, acrosome-reacted spermatozoa during ICSI without negatively impacting sperm motility or viability (Gianaroli et al. 2008). Birefringent spermatozoa can be selected for microinjection and these are thought to present with higher quality as the proportion of birefringent sperm has a significant positive correlation with other sperm parameters such as

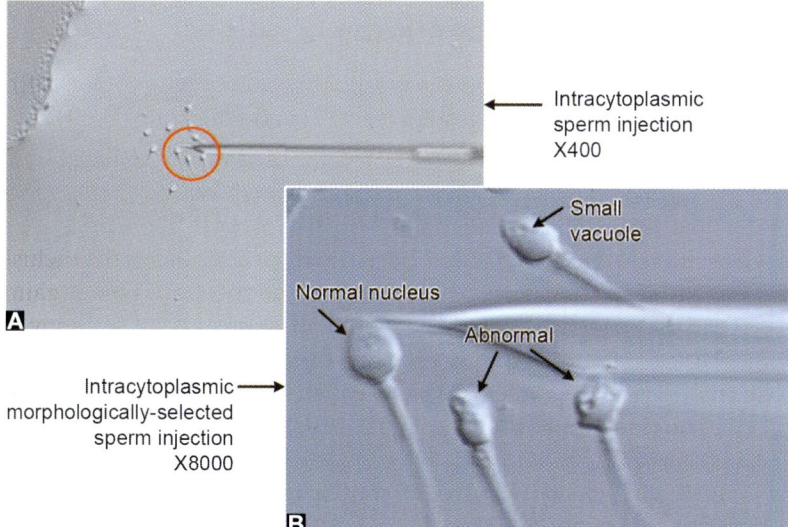

Figs 6A and B: Intracytoplasmic morphologically selected sperm injection

concentration, motility and viability (Gianaroli et al. 2008). As for MSOME and IMSI, the selection of spermatozoa using polarizing microscopy will require additional instrumentation, time and technical expertise.

■ CONCLUSION

Even if the best quality spermatozoa are used in ICSI, no more than 55% of the selected sperm have normal DNA (Ramos et al. 2004). Sperm selection methods currently used prior to ART are inadequate and that other methods need to be considered to ensure that only spermatozoa with optimum quality are included. Several advanced sperm selection methods have been described based on different approaches for targeting functionally competent and intact spermatozoa. More research is needed to identify which infertility cases, if not all, will benefit from the application of these selection methods. Care should be taken to investigate safety and efficacy aspects of advanced sperm selection methods before their widespread implementation in ART.

■ KEY POINTS

- Advanced sperm selection protocols aim to improve ART outcomes by isolate mature, motile, structurally intact and non-apoptotic spermatozoa and may limit the possible deleterious effects on offspring of using sperm with defective DNA.
- MACS is the only known technique which separates apoptotic spermatozoa from non-apoptotic spermatozoa.
- Key futures of the electrophoresis system that make it attractive for ART laboratories are: the whole process of selection can take only a few minutes and the generation of ROS is minimized because of lack of centrifugation steps.
- The zeta method can be carried out immediately as sperm cells loose the charge with the onset of capacitation.
- Interestingly, sperm birefringence was found to be linked to the acrosomal status where the more beneficial birefringence patterns were characteristic for spermatozoa which had undergone the acrosome reaction.

■ FURTHER READING

1. Ainsworth C, Nixon B, Aitken RJ. Development of a novel electrophoretic system for the isolation of human spermatozoa. Hum Reprod. 2005;20(8):2261-70, ISSN 0268-1161 (Print) 0268-1161 (Linking).
2. Ainsworth C, Nixon B, Jansen RP, et al. First recorded pregnancy and normal birth after ICSI using electrophoretically isolated spermatozoa. Hum Reprod. 2007;22(1): 197-200, ISSN 0268-1161 (Print) 0268-1161 (Linking).
3. Ainsworth CJ, Nixon B, Aitken RJ. The electrophoretic separation of spermatozoa: an analysis of genotype, surface carbohydrate composition and potential for capacitation. Int J Androl. 2011;34(5):e422-34, ISSN 1365-2605 (Electronic) 0105-6263 (Linking), 2011.
4. Alvarez Sedo C, Uriondo H, Lavolpe M, et al. Clinical outcome using non-apoptotic sperm selection for ICSI procedures: report of 1 year experience. Fertil Steril. 2010;94:S232.

5. Bartoov B, Berkovitz A, Eltes F, et al. Real-time fine morphology of motile human sperm cells is associated with IVF-ICSI outcome. Journal of Andrology. 2002; 23(1):1-8.
6. Beydola T, Sharma RK, Agarwal A. Sperm Preparation and Selection Technique, Chapter 29, RK-2013.
7. Castillo-Baso J, Garcia-Villafaña G, et al. Embryo quality and reproductive outcomes of spermatozoa selected by physiologic-icsi or conventional icsi in patients with kruger <4% and >4% normo-morphology. Fertil Steril. 2011;96(3):S159.
8. Chan PJ, Jacobson JD, Corselli JU, et al. A simple zeta method for sperm selection based on membrane charge. Fertil Steril. 2006;85(2):481-6,ISSN 1556-5653 (Electronic) 0015-0282 (Linking).
9. Dirican EK, Ozgun OD, Akarsu S, et al. Clinical outcome of magnetic activated cell sorting of non-apoptotic spermatozoa before density gradient centrifugation for assisted reproduction. J Assist Reprod Genet. 2008;25(8):375-81, ISSN 1058-0468 (Print) 1058-0468 (Linking).
10. Ebner T, Filicori M, Tews G, et al. A plea for a more physiological ICSI. Andrologia. 2012;44(1):2-19.
11. Gianaroli L, Magli MC, Collodel G, et al. Sperm head's birefringence: a new criterion for sperm selection. Fertil Steril. 2008;90(1):104-12, ISSN 1556-5653 (Electronic) 0015-0282 (Linking).
12. Junca AM, Dumont M, Cornet D, et al. Is intracytoplasmic morphologically sperm injection (IMSI) detrimental for pregnancy outcome? Fertil Steril. 2010;94:S31.
13. Lee TH, Liu CH, Shih YT, et al. Magnetic-activated cell sorting for sperm preparation reduces spermatozoa with apoptotic markers and improves the acrosome reaction in couples with unexplained infertility. Hum Reprod. 2010;25:839-46.
14. McDowell S, Kroon B, Ford E, et al. Advanced sperm selection techniques for assisted reproduction (Protocol). The Cochrane Collaboration and published in The Cochrane Library 2013, Issue 3.
15. Montag M, Toth B, Strowitzki T. Sperm Selection in ART. Journal of Reproductive Medicine and Endocrinology, 2012;9(6):485-9.
16. Ortega NM, Bosch P. Methods for Sperm Selection for In Vitro Fertilization. In Vitro Fertilization—Innovative Clinical and Laboratory Aspects Edited by Professor Shevach Friedler Published in print edition April, 2012.
17. Poenicke K, Grunewald S, Glander H, et al. Sperm Selection in Assisted Reproductive Techniques. In: Rao KA, Agarwal A, Srinivas MS (Eds). Andrology Laboratory Manual. 1st edition India: Jaypee Brothers Pvt Ltd; 2010.pp.173-87.
18. Razavi SH, Nasr-Esfahani MH, Deemeh MR, et al. Evaluation of zeta and HA-binding methods for selection of spermatozoa with normal morphology, protamine content and DNA integrity. Andrologia. 2010;42(1):13-9.
19. Said T, Land JA. Effects of advanced selection methods on sperm quality and ART outcome: a systematic review. Human Reproduction Update. 2007;17(6):719-33.
20. Said TM, Land JA. Effects of advanced selection methods on sperm quality and ART outcome: a systematic review. Human Reproduction Update. 2011;17(6):719-33.

CHAPTER

8

Effects of Oxidative Stress on Different Sperm Functions: How to Evaluate and Manage

Sulagna Dutta, Ahmad Majzoub, Ashok Agarwal

■ INTRODUCTION

Reactive oxygen species, the unavoidable byproducts obtained from oxygen metabolism, are exclusively toxic metabolites that may also exert beneficial effects through regulating vital cell signaling cascades. Intracellular reactive oxygen species (ROS) concentrations are determined by the balance between the rates of ROS production and their rates of clearance by various antioxidant defense mechanisms. Under normal physiologic levels, ROS regulate intracellular signaling cascades thus mediating essential physiological mechanisms such as sperm maturation, hyperactivation, capacitation, acrosome reaction (AR) as well as fertilization.[1] However, when ROS concentration exceeds the physiologic limit, adversities occur. Antioxidants are capable of negating such adversities, however, when ROS generation overwhelms the antioxidants' threshold of ROS clearance, or when antioxidant production is diminished, a state of oxidative stress (OS) ensues.[2] This imbalance in the redox potential carries significant negative effects on various cellular components such as carbohydrates, nucleic acids, proteins, and lipids.[3] The spermatozoa are exceptionally susceptible to OS owing to their inadequate cell repair systems as well as insufficient antioxidant defenses due to very little cytoplasmic content. They are susceptible to lipid peroxidation (LPO) due to high content of polyunsaturated fatty acids (PUFA) in their plasma membrane resulting in disruption of membrane permeability, and thus efflux of adenosine triphosphate (ATP) impairing flagellar movement.[4] Sperm viability, motility, and fertilization potential are disrupted by OS in the reproductive tissues evidenced by the presence of significantly higher levels of ROS in the semen of infertile men when compared to fertile controls.[5]

This chapter aims to provide a concise perception regarding the generation of ROS in the male reproductive system along with their ameliorating and deleterious effects on male reproductive functions. It also explores the evaluation methods of ROS in order to assess the progression of OS in male reproductive tissues which is vital to understand the clinical corrections of ROS induced male infertility.

■ REACTIVE OXYGEN SPECIES GENERATION IN MALE REPRODUCTIVE TISSUES

Spermatozoa can generate ROS mostly via two methods:
1. At the sperm plasma membrane, ROS may be produced by the nicotinamide adenine dinucleotide phosphate (NADP) oxidase system and/or
2. At the mitochondrial level, ROS is generated via the nicotinamide adenine dinucleotide dependent redox reaction, which is the most predominant mechanism. Spermatozoa are mitochondria rich cells owing to their constant requirement of energy for their motility.[6] Increase in the number of dysfunctional spermatozoa in semen significantly induces higher ROS production, affecting its mitochondrial function and motility. The prime ROS in human spermatozoa is superoxide (O_2^-) which reacts with itself through dismutation reactions to yield hydrogen peroxide (H_2O_2). If transition metals such as iron and copper are present, H_2O_2 and O_2^- can generate the most destructive and extremely reactive hydroxyl radical (OH^-) via the Haber-Weiss reaction (Fig. 1) which can initiate a LPO cascade disrupting membrane fluidity and impairing sperm functions.[7]

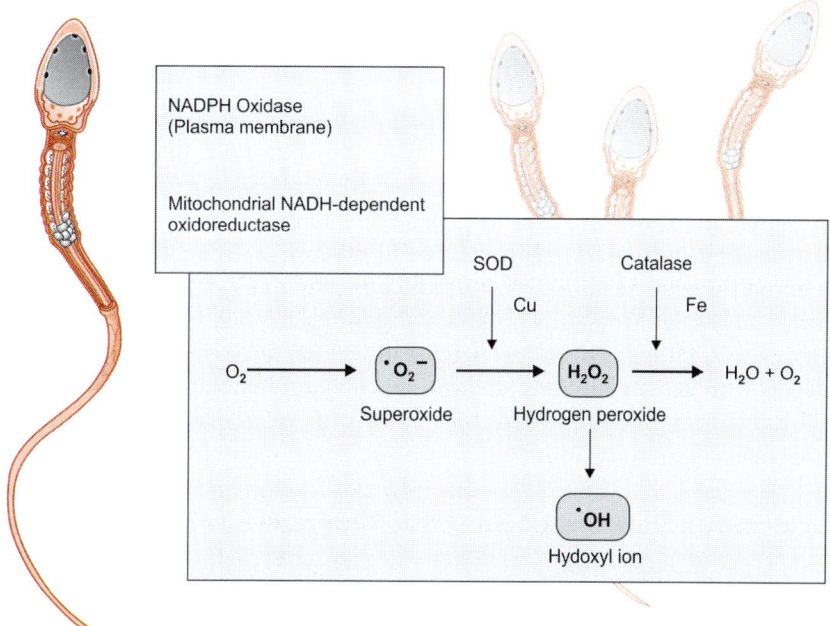

Fig. 1: Reactive oxygen species generation in spermatozoa.[14]
(NADPH: nicotinamide adenine dinucleotide phosphate, NADH: nicotinamide adenine dinucleotide, SOD: superoxide dismutase, Cu: copper, Fe: Iron).

Endogenous Sources of Reactive Oxygen Species in Seminal Plasma

Leukocytes

Peroxidase-positive leukocytes [polymorphonuclear leukocytes (50%~60%) and macrophages (20%~30%)] originate from the male prostate and seminal vesicles. Infectious or inflammatory responses can trigger these cells which in turn can produce 100 times more ROS than normal as part of the defense mechanisms and also elevate NADPH production through the hexose monophosphate shunt.[3] Also, the elevation of proinflammatory mediators and reduction of antioxidants seen in inflammatory reactions can induce a respiratory burst resulting in OS. Leukocytospermia is a sperm disrupting disorder characterized by the presence of greater than one million peroxidase-positive leukocytes per milliliter of semen.[8]

Immature Spermatozoa

Under normal circumstances, the cytoplasm gets extruded from the developing spermatozoa to prepare itself for fertilization. However, an arrest to spermiogenesis may result in retention of excess cytoplasm around the midpiece of the damaged spermatozoon [excess residual cytoplasm (ERC)]. ERC is capable of activating the NADPH system via the hexose-monophosphate shunt, which is a source of electrons for ROS production and potentially, OS.[9]

Varicocele

Varicocele, characterized by an abnormal venous dilation in the pampiniform plexus around the spermatic cord, is detected in about 40% of male partners of all infertile couples and is thought to be the leading cause of male factor infertility.[10] Many mechanisms have been postulated in the pathophysiology of varicocele. Testicular hyperthermia and hypoxia are the most commonly accepted theories resulting in OS induced testicular dysfunction.[10,11] One meta-analysis confirmed the presence of significantly higher oxidative stress parameters such as ROS and lipid peroxidation in semen samples from infertile patients with varicocele compared with normal fertile donors.[10] The seminal ROS levels have been reported to be directly associated with the grade of varicocele.[12]

Exogenous Sources of Reactive Oxygen Species

Radiation from mobile phones can induce ROS in human semen impairing semen quality and inducing sperm DNA damage, thus affecting sperm count, motility and vitality.[13] The radiofrequency electromagnetic waves can impair the intracellular electron flow along the internal membranes due to numerous cytosolic charged molecules, thus disrupting normal functioning of the germ cells.[14]

Toxins from domestic or industrial products may intrude into the body and induce ROS production in the testes, impairing sperm structure and function. Phthalates (in plastic objects) as well as metals such as cadmium, chromium, lead, manganese, and mercury have been found to impair spermatogenesis, sperm quality and count.[14]

Smoking causes an imbalance between ROS and antioxidants in the semen of smokers. Smoking may increase seminal leukocyte concentrations by 48% and seminal ROS levels by 107%, decrease seminal plasma antioxidants and increase 8-hydroxy-2'-deoxyguanosine (8-OHdG) concentrations (a biomarker of oxidative damage).[14] Furthermore, smoking induces increased blood and semen cadmium and lead concentrations which may exaggerate ROS production and impair sperm motility.[14] Increased sperm DNA damage and apoptosis are commonly identified in smokers and carry detrimental effects on male infertility.[15]

Alcohol is a promoter of ROS generation and also affects antioxidant defense mechanism. Acetaldehyde, a by-product of ethanol metabolism, can produce ROS by interacting with proteins and lipids, thus, damaging cellular components decreasing percentage of normal spermatozoa.[16]

■ EFFECTS OF REACTIVE OXYGEN SPECIES ON DIFFERENT SPERM FUNCTIONS

Physiological Functions

As mentioned previously, higher concentrations of ROS can inflict detrimental effects on semen quality ultimately resulting in infertility. Nonetheless, low and regulated concentrations of ROS play vital physiologic roles on male reproduction, such as sperm capacitation, hyperactivation, acrosome reaction, as well as sperm-oocyte fusion (Fig. 2).[1]

Maturation

Spermatozoal maturation occurs in the epididymis and is characterized by alteration of cell membrane, rearrangement of surface proteins together with nuclear and enzymatic remodeling.[1] This vital step in sperm development is regulated by cellular signal transduction machineries which are influenced by ROS levels. Chromosomal DNA in the mammalian spermatozoon is densely packed as its histones are replaced by the smaller sized protamines. Inter- and intra-molecular disulfide bonds are established between cysteine residues of protamines to convey chromatin stability. ROS may assist the disulfide bond formation ensuring chromatin stability and protecting DNA from damage. Peroxides may also aid proper formation of the *mitochondrial capsule*, which is composed of a protein network rich in disulfide bonds to secure mitochondria from proteolytic degradation.[1]

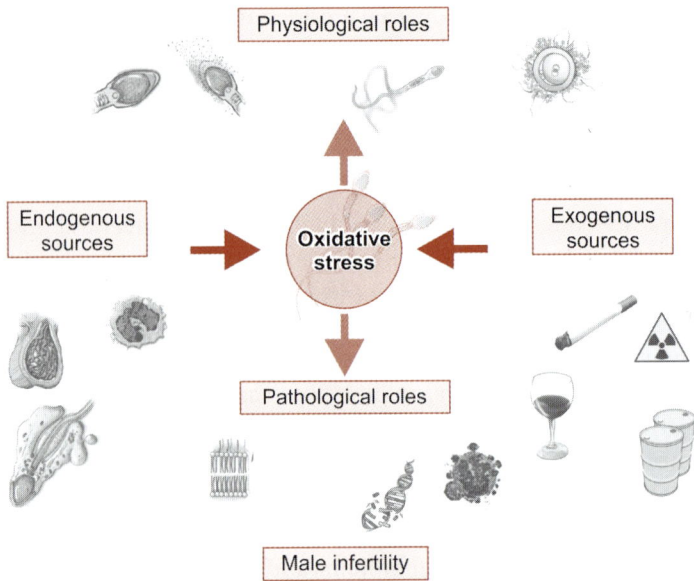

Fig. 2: Oxidative stress in male reproduction.[14]

Reactive Oxygen Species as Signal Transducers

Reactive oxygen species, owing to their small size, ubiquitous nature and short half-life, aid sperm functions at different physiological phases such as maturation, activation, capacitation and acrosome reaction. The underlying mechanism of action may be via the redox regulation of cysteine residues. The redox states of the thiol groups determine enzymatic activity. ROS activates adenyl cyclase (AC) inducing intracellular cyclic adenosine monophosphate (cAMP) production which in turn activates protein kinase A (PKA) molecules. PKA mediates the activation of various downstream pathways according to the spermatozoa maturational state.[1]

Motility and Hyperactivation

Hyperactivation is a particular state of sperm motility characterized by high amplitude, increased and asymmetric flagellar movement, elevated side-to-side sperm head displacement, along with nonlinear motility.[17] It is considered to be part of capacitation and is required for successful sperm penetration of the zona pellucida and fertilization. ROS has positive impacts on the hyperactivation processes in spermatozoa. The initiation process of capacitation and hyperactivation is induced by the influx of Ca^{2+} and HCO_3^-, probably by the inactivation of an ATP-dependent Ca^{2+} regulatory channel (PMCA) and alkalization of the cytosol. Calcium ions and ROS, specifically O_2^-, lead to the activation of AC, generating cAMP. cAMP via PKA activation triggers NADPH oxidase and thereby stimulate greater ROS generation. PKA also phosphorylates Ser and Tyr residues which can also activate protein tyrosine kinase (PTK). Consequently, PTK triggers phosphorylation of tyrosine residues in the fibrous sheath around the axoneme and the cytoskeleton of the sperm flagellum. ROS, especially H_2O_2, elevates tyrosine phosphorylation by inducing PTK and inhibiting phosphotyrosine phosphatase (PTPase), which lead to dephosphorylation of Tyr residues. The final step in the process of hyperactivation is presumably the increased tyrosine phosphorylation.[1] Superoxide anion (O_2^-) has been observed to be the major ROS contributor to this ameliorating effect.[14]

Capacitation

The ultimate functional process in spermatozoal maturation needed for making the sperm competent to fertilize an ovum is capacitation. The established molecular pathway by which ROS facilitates capacitation is by triggering intracellular cAMP levels inducing downstream PKA which in turn phosphorylates mitogen-activated protein kinase (MEK, extracellular signal regulated kinase)-like proteins, threonine-glutamate-tyrosine, and fibrous sheath proteins. These signaling cascades bring about final capacitation of the sperm rendering it totally prepared for the acrosome reactions.[14]

Acrosome Reaction

To ensure fertilization, the hyperactivated spermatozoon must pass across the cumulus oophorous, bind to the zona pellucida of the oocyte and create a pore in its extracellular matrix via exocytotic release of proteolytic enzymes. These acrosome reactions are mediated through phosphorylation of tyrosine proteins, Ca^{2+} influx resulting in intracellular rise in cAMP and PKA thereby enabling the spermatozoon to penetrate and fuse with oocyte. ROS has been observed to facilitate actions on the zona pellucida of the spermatozoon by various means including phosphorylation of three relevant plasma membrane proteins.[1]

Sperm-Oocyte Fusion

Reactive oxygen species may increase the membrane fluidity required for successful sperm-oocyte fusion after aiding the biochemical cascades of spermatozoa capacitation and acrosome reaction. Throughout capacitation, ROS prevents deactivation of phospholipase A2 (PLA2) by inhibiting protein tyrosine phosphatase activity so that PLA2 can cleave the secondary fatty acid from the membrane phospholipid triglycerols to increase fluidity of the membrane.[18]

Pathological Functions

When the highly reactive ROS overpowers the antioxidant defense systems and disturbs the homeostatic balance between ROS generation and antioxidants activities, pathological defects arise in vital biomolecules such as proteins, nucleic acids, lipids, and sugars (Fig. 2).[16]

Lipid Peroxidation

The sperm cell is characterized by having high levels of lipids in its plasma membrane mostly in the form of PUFAs having unconjugated double bonds between its methylene groups. The double bond near to the methylene group declines the strength of methyl carbon-hydrogen bond, rendering hydrogen exceedingly susceptible to oxidative damage. As the intracellular levels of ROS rise uncontrollably, they initiate a cascade of reactions ultimately resulting in LPO [11] in which almost 60% of the membrane fatty acids are lost, diminishing its fluidity, enhancing non-specific permeability to ions, and also inhibiting the actions of membrane receptors and enzymes. LPO is thus an autocatalytic self-propagating chemical reaction leading to abnormal fertilization, and the mechanism of this oxidative damage may propagate through three major steps, namely, initiation, propagation, and termination.[14]

Initiation includes hydrogen atoms abstraction from the carbon-carbon double bonds thus propelling free radicals which in turn generate lipid radicals, and the later react with oxygen forming the peroxyl radicals. These peroxyl radicals may again abstract hydrogen atom from the lipids, especially when metals like copper and iron are present, progressing the chain of autocatalytic reaction. The propagation stage of oxidative damage continues with the formed radicals reacting with successive lipids, generating cytotoxic aldehydes owing to degradation of hydroperoxide. The formation of peroxyl and alkyl radicals proceed in a cyclical manner in this propagation step until a stable end product is formed which is malondialdehyde (MDA) and the reaction chain reaches its termination. Thus, MDA is an essential biochemical marker to analyze and monitor the level of peroxidative damage affecting the spermatozoa. 4-hydroxynonenal, another product of LPO, is hydrophilic and can lead to severe spermatozoa dysfunction at both proteomic as well as genomic levels.[14]

DNA Damage

Several deleterious effects of ROS on sperm nuclear DNA are evident owing to increased DNA fragmentation, chromatin cross-linking, base-pair modifications, and chromosomal microdeletions.[14] ROS is also responsible for reduced sperm motility by inhibiting energy generation, via LPO and importantly mitochondrial DNA (mtDNA) mutations. Damage to at least one of the 13 genes coding for the electron transport system (ETC) transporter system in the mitochondria will reduce ATP production and induce intracellular ROS production.[14] ROS may reduce sperm motility also by oxidation of a thiol group in glyceraldehydes-3- phosphate dehydrogenase (GAPDH) which is a glycolytic enzyme, or deletion of adenine and pyridine nucleotides by LPO.[14]

Apoptosis

Reactive oxygen species is capable of disrupting the inner and outer mitochondrial membranes releasing cytochrome C. This cytochrome C in turn activates the apoptotic caspases.[14] This mechanism of induction of apoptosis in the spermatozoa by ROS is evident in infertile men as high levels of cytochrome C was observed in the seminal plasma of infertile men which is an indicator of severe mitochondrial damage.[14]

■ EVALUATION OF SEMINAL OXIDATIVE STRESS

Reactive oxygen species-mediated damage to sperm is evidently a major contributing pathology in 30–80% of unexplained infertile male patients.[19] Therefore, analysis of elevated ROS levels in the infertile men is quite reasonable. Factors, such as inconvenience of ROS screening, its high cost and lack of overall accepted efficient analysis method, hinder consideration of ROS measurement as an integral part of male infertility assessments, despite its immense importance. At present, more than 30 different assays are in practice by which ROS is measured and OS is analyzed in the semen of infertile men.[14]

Routine Semen Analysis

The routine analysis of semen parameters (sperm count, morphology and motility) allows clinicians to make almost perfect diagnosis of OS, where asthenozoospermia is perhaps the best marker for OS.[20] The hyperviscosity of seminal plasma marks a rise in seminal plasma MDA and a decrease in seminal plasma antioxidant status.[20] Moreover, *Ureaplasma urealyticum* infection in the semen is also associated with high viscosity of seminal plasma and high ROS production.[20] The detection of a considerable number of round cells may signify the presence of leukocytospermia which is a well-known source of exaggerated ROS production as stated previously. However, to ensure that the round cells are not immature spermatozoa, ancillary tests such as the peroxidase test, seminal elastase measurement or CD45 (transmembrane glycoprotein expressed on the cell surface) antibody staining, should be done. Disrupted sperm morphology and cytoplasmic droplets are prime features of anomalous spermatozoa leading to uncontrolled production of ROS. Lastly, poor sperm membrane integrity, which may be assessed by the hypo-osmotic swelling test (HOST), has been linked to the presence of OS.[14]

Reactive Oxygen Species by Chemiluminescence

Seminal ROS measurement is mostly assessed by the chemiluminescence assays. The procedure involve a luminometer and a chemiluminescent probe such as luminol (5-amino-2,3,-dihydro-1,4-phthalazinedione; Sigma-Aldrich, St. Louis, MO, USA). Aliquots of liquefied semen are subjected to centrifuge at 300×*g* for 7 minutes followed by freezing the aliquoted seminal plasma at −20°C for measurement of the total antioxidant levels. The pellet is then washed using phosphate buffered saline (PBS, pH 7.4) and 400 μL aliquots of 2×10^6 sperm/mL concentration are resuspended in the washing medium and used for the assessment of basal ROS levels. The negative control contains 10 mL of 5 mM luminol in 400 mL of PBS. Luminol (5 mM stock in dimethyl sulfoxide) is added to the mixture to serve as a probe and the test tubes are loaded in the luminometer for 15 minutes for measuring the level of ROS levels. Luminol measures both extracellular and intracellular ROS. The free radicals contained in the semen sample, produce a light signal reacting with luminal, which is converted by the luminometer to an electric signal (photon). The measurement of the number of free radicals generated is done as relative light units/s/10^6 sperm. The range of normal ROS levels in washed sperm suspensions is 0.10–1.03×10^6cpm *per* 20×10^6 sperm.[21]

Total Antioxidant Capacity

Luminol is also used for the measurement of the total antioxidant capacity (TAC) within the seminal plasma, which is quantified against a vitamin E analog *Trolox* (a water-soluble tocopherol analog). The results are articulated as an ROS-TAC score indicating the combined antioxidant activities evoked by all the constituents, including vitamins, lipids and proteins.[21]

Lipid Peroxidation Markers

Lipid peroxides accumulation in the spermatozoa produces a variety of decay end-products such as MDA, 2-propenal (acrolein), hydroxynonenal, and isoprostanes, which can be measured as indicators of OS. MDA measurement, the most commonly utilized method, is mediated by thiobarbituric acid (TBA) assay where MDA combines with TBA producing a 1:2 adduct, a colored substance measured by fluorometry or spectrophotometry.[14,21]

Seminal Oxidation-Reduction Potential

Oxidation-reduction potential, also known as the redox potential, is a measure of the potential for electrons to move from one chemical species to another.[22] Oxidation-reduction potential (ORP) is a measure of this relationship between oxidants and antioxidants, providing a comprehensive measure of OS. Recently, a novel technology based on a galvanostatic measure of electrons has been developed, and it has been used to assess changes in OS in trauma patients and as a function of extreme exercise.[23,24] ORP in the semen has been easily and comprehensively measured using the MiOXSYS System (AytuBioScience, USA) that enables wider application of OS analysis in clinical and research settings.[25] ORP results provided by the MiOXSYS system are standardized, reliable and reproducible compared to previously used ROS assays.[25,26]

PREVENTION AND MANAGEMENT OF MALE REPRODUCTIVE OXIDATIVE STRESS

The first step in the management of OS should be to verify the underlying cause(s) of the imbalance between the ROS load and antioxidant level in order to deliver effective treatment strategies. Some important management factors are discussed below:

Lifestyle Modifications

Increased professional and personal stresses mostly owing to developed society lead to bad habits such as, substance abuse, smoking, and an unbalanced diet which are all recognized as potential causes for OS. Therefore, minimizing such behaviours should aid in OS alleviation. In addition, exposure to pollution, heat, toxins, heavy metals, etc. contribute largely in the development of OS. Apart from these, any other activities raising the scrotum's temperature such as saunas, hot baths, long period of driving, and long sedentary office hours should be monitored. There should be adequate aeration and protection at work places to limit exposure to any noxious chemicals or vapors that may potentiate OS.[19]

Antioxidants

Antioxidants eliminate ROS or reduce its formation to halt the oxidative chain reaction. Preventive antioxidants (metal chelators or binding proteins), such as lactoferrin and transferrin, inhibit the formation of ROS; whereas scavenging antioxidants, such as vitamins C and E, eliminate ROS. Antioxidants can also be enzymatic and nonenzymatic. Enzymatic antioxidants include natural antioxidants such as glutathione reductase (GSH), superoxide dismutase (SOD), and catalase, while some important nonenzymatic antioxidants include vitamins C, E, and B; carnitines; cysteines, carotenoids; pentoxifylline, taurine, metals, hypotaurine, and albumin. The nonenzymatic antioxidants can be acquired from vegetables or fruits containing the supplements.[14]

Surgery

Varicocele is marked by abnormal elongation and dilation of the pampiniform plexus of veins surrounding the spermatic cord. Corrective surgery occludes these dilated veins in subfertile males or male patients suffering from testicular pain. This technique has been observed to reduce seminal ROS levels protecting the sperm from oxidative damage.[19] Surgical repair also ameliorates other major biomarkers of infertility, including sperm parameters as well as successful pregnancy rates.[14,27]

CONCLUSION

Oxidative stress results from disturbances in the intricate balance between ROS generation and elimination. While physiologic levels of ROS are vital for optimal sperm function, when present in exaggerated levels, ROS may incite detrimental effects on sperm quality and function and ultimately result in infertility. Several markers and measurement methods for OS have been described and their assessment should provide valuable information during the evaluation of infertile men. Effective prevention and treatment of OS is mandatory in order to improve the reproductive potential of infertile men.

KEY POINTS

- Reactive oxygen species (ROS) are vital for normal physiological processes of sperm such as maturation, capacitation, acrosome reaction and sperm-oocyte fusion required to undergo proper fertilization.
- Oxidative stress (OS) incurs male infertility if the intricate balance between ROS generation and mitigation via antioxidants, is disturbed.
- High levels of seminal ROS lead to pathological defects by damaging the biomolecules such as proteins, nucleic acids, lipids, sugars and inducing the apoptosis of germ cells.
- Evaluation of seminal ROS may provide vital information during the evaluation of male infertility.
- Several methods for assessment of OS exist. The most commonly utilized ones include: chemiluminescence assessment of ROS or total antioxidant capacity (TAC) and measurement of lipid peroxidation markers or seminal oxidation-reduction potential (ORP).
- OS can be prevented by adopting a healthy life style and may be managed by either antioxidants supplementation or correction of varicocele.

REFERENCES

1. Thompson A, Agarwal A, du Plessis SS. Physiological role of reactive oxygen species in sperm function: A review. In: Parekattil, SJ, Agarwal, A (Eds.) Antioxidants in male infertility. New York: Springer Science; 2013. pp. 69-89.
2. Halliwell B, Cross CE. Oxygen-derived species: their relation to human disease and environmental stress. Environ Health Perspect. 1994;102 Suppl 10:5-12.
3. Agarwal A, Saleh RA, Bedaiwy MA. Role of reactive oxygen species in the pathophysiology of human reproduction. Fertil Steril. 2003;79(4):829-43.
4. Alvarez JG, Storey BT. Assessment of cell damage caused by spontaneous lipid peroxidation in rabbit spermatozoa. Biol Reprod. 1984;30(2):323-31.
5. Agarwal A, Sharma RK, Nallella KP, et al. Reactive oxygen species as an independent marker of male factor infertility. Fertil Steril. 2006;86(4):878-85.
6. Henkel RR. Leukocytes and oxidative stress: dilemma for sperm function and male fertility. Asian J Androl. 2011;13(1):43-52.

7. Chen SJ, Allam JP, Duan YG, et al. Influence of reactive oxygen species on human sperm functions and fertilizing capacity including therapeutical approaches. Arch Gynecol Obstet. 2013;288(1):191-9.
8. WHO Laboratory manual for the examination and processing of human semen. Geneva: World Health Organization; 2010. pp. 7-113.
9. Rengan AK, Agarwal A, van der Linde M, et al. An investigation of excess residual cytoplasm in human spermatozoa and its distinction from the cytoplasmic droplet. Reprod Biol Endocrinol. 2012;10:92.
10. Agarwal A, Prabakaran S, Allamaneni SS. Relationship between oxidative stress, varicocele and infertility: a meta-analysis. Reprod Biomed Online. 2006;12(5): 630-3.
11. Makker K, Agarwal A, Sharma R. Oxidative stress and male infertility. Indian J Med Res. 2009;129(4):357-67.
12. Will MA, Swain J, Fode M, et al. The great debate: varicocele treatment and impact on fertility. Fertil Sterility. 2011;95(3):841-52.
13. Agarwal A, Deepinder F, Sharma RK, et al. Effect of cell phone usage on semen analysis in men attending infertility clinic: an observational study. Fertil Steril. 2008;89(1):124-8.
14. Agarwal A, Virk G, Ong C, et al. Effect of oxidative stress on male reproduction. World J Mens Health. 2014;32(1):1-17.
15. Saleh RA, Agarwal A, Sharma RK, et al. Effect of cigarette smoking on levels of seminal oxidative stress in infertile men: a prospective study. Fertil Steril. 2002;78(3):491-9.
16. Agarwal A, Prabakaran SA. Mechanism, measurement, and prevention of oxidative stress in male reproductive physiology. Indian J Exp Biology. 2005;43(11):963-74.
17. Suarez SS. Control of hyperactivation in sperm. Hum Reprod Update. 2008;14(6):647-57.
18. Khosrowbeygi A, Zarghami N. Fatty acid composition of human spermatozoa and seminal plasma levels of oxidative stress biomarkers in subfertile males. Prostaglandins, Leukot Essent Fatty Acids. 2007;77(2):117-21.
19. Tremellen K. Oxidative stress and male infertility: A clinical perspective. Hum Reprod Update. 2008;14(3):243-58.
20. Aydemir B, Onaran I, Kiziler AR, et al. The influence of oxidative damage on viscosity of seminal fluid in infertile men. J Androl. 2008;29(1):41-6.
21. Agarwal A, Majzoub A. Laboratory tests for oxidative stress. Indian J Urol. 2017;33(3):199.
22. McCord JM. The evolution of free radicals and oxidative stress. Am J Med. 2000;108(8):652-9.
23. Rael LT, Bar-Or R, Aumann RM, et al. Oxidation-reduction potential and paraoxonase-arylesterase activity in trauma patients. Biochem Biophys Res Commun. 2007;361(2):561-5.
24. Rael LT, Bar-Or R, Mains CW, et al. Plasma oxidation-reduction potential and protein oxidation in traumatic brain injury. J Neurotrauma. 2009;26(8):1203-11.

25. Agarwal A, Sharma R, Roychoudhury S, et al. MiOXSYS: a novel method of measuring oxidation reduction potential in semen and seminal plasma. Fertil Steril. 2016;106(3):566-73.
26. Agarwal A, Roychoudhury S, Sharma R, et al. Diagnostic application of oxidation-reduction potential assay for measurement of oxidative stress: clinical utility in male factor infertility. Reprod Biomed Online. 2017;34(1):48-57.
27. Hamada A, Esteves SC, Agarwal A. Insight into oxidative stress in varicocele-associated male infertility: part 2. Nat Rev Urol. 2013;10(1):26-37.

CHAPTER
9

Sperm DNA Fragmentation and its Clinical Implication

Niladitya Sanyal, Subir Chatterjee, Gautam Khastgir

INTRODUCTION

Traditionally, the assessment and diagnosis of male infertility or subfertility is based upon the analysis of semen volume, sperm concentration, motility and morphology and although there is a direct relationship between semen quality and pregnancy rates both in natural conception and medically assisted reproduction (MAR), there is no predictive threshold for success of conventional semen parameters.

Conventional semen analysis does not assess all aspects of the functions of the testis and sperm quality therefore, newer tests for predicting the chance of pregnancy needs to be clinically useful and relevant. Under such circumstances sperm DNA fragmentation holds promise to be a capable marker for assessment of male reproductive capability.[5,6]

The integrity of our genome is continuously challenged by endogenous metabolic by-products and exogenous factors. Depending on variable like cell type, cell cycle, stage and type of DNA damage, a cell has several ways to repair damaged DNA and inaccurate repair can have different and often undesirable consequences. While our somatic cells die of old age/disease, the germ line cells (gametes) have to maintain sufficient DNA integrity to pass on our DNA to forthcoming generations (these cells survive longer due to higher telomerase activity).

The process of spermatogenesis induces double stranded DNA breaks (ds-DNA breaks) first during meiosis (to allow meiotic cross-over) and second during spermiogenesis, when the chromatin of the haploid round spermatids is compacted by the replacement of histones by protamines. Furthermore the sperm DNA may accumulate damage/fragmentation during maturation and storage in the epididymis. In addition to the above DNA fragmentation can be caused due to defective apoptosis, excessive reactive oxygen species (ROS) production and decreased seminal antioxidants. Also, toxic effects of drugs, cigarette smoking, pollution and other factors like high testicular temperature (fever, varicocele) and advanced age have been associated with increased sperm DNA fragmentation or damage.[7-12]

Recent studies have highlighted the significance of sperm DNA integrity as an important factor that affects the functional competence of the sperm cells. Therefore the assessment of SDF could be a clinically useful tool/test for male fertility prediction in MAR or ART. For this process of DNA assessment or measurement several techniques are available and have been evaluated in separate studies.

In this review we shall discuss the different factors behind sperm DNA damage/fragmentation, the approaches or tests to determine, assess and measure DNA fragmentation and its clinical implications and a general consensus with regards to its efficacy in MAR.[2]

■ FACTORS CONTRIBUTING TO SPERM DNA FRAGMENTATION

Biological Factors Contributing to Sperm DNA Fragmentation

Although the mechanism causing DNA damage of sperm has been partially identified the origin and precise mechanism of DNA damage in mature sperm cells is difficult to elucidate. Three main hypotheses have been proposed to explain the phenomenon of DNA fragmentation in sperm cells (Fig. 1).[13]

The 1st hypothesis suggests that the presence of DNA breakage is related to replacement of histones with protamine during the process of spermatogenesis. The histone-protamine transition occurs during spermatogenesis facilitates better compaction of the DNA molecule as compared to somatic cells. During this process nicking of DNA occurs by topoisomerase II to prevent forced twisting of DNA molecule. This is a highly specialized mechanism controlled thoroughly by the genetic dictate of the cell. Under these circumstances, any mechanism affecting the process of protamination is detected and then deleted in the process of sperm maturation using check point like mechanisms and apoptosis is triggered. In fact protamine deficiency correlates with morphological sperm alteration or increased DNA damage.

The 2nd hypothesis suggests that DNA fragmentation results due to excessive oxidative stress in the male reproductive tract. The process of oxidative stress occurs when high quantities of ROS is released by leukocytes and macrophages in a similar process such as inflammation followed subsequently by redox

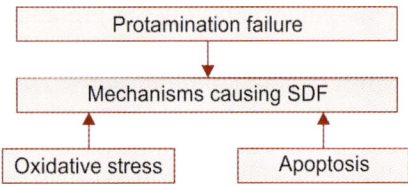

Fig 1: Primary mechanisms producing SDF.
(SDF: Sperm DNA fragmentation).[13]

process on the cells membranes and later on the sperm DNA. The presence of immature sperm cells with residual cytoplasm in the ejaculate contributes an abnormally elevated oxidation level that induces endogenous redox reaction.

In general the process of oxidative stress is initiated when ROS production exceeds the activity of seminal plasma antioxidants, such as superoxide dismutase, glutathione peroxidase, catalase etc. that block the redox reaction cascade. The oxidative stress this produces contributes mainly towards single stranded DNA breaks but lipidic peroxidation and protein alterations are also possible.

The 3rd hypothesis implicates apoptotic events during sperm cell maturation within the epididymis similar to somatic cells, DNAses get activated which cause double stranded DNA breaks and degrade the DNA molecule. The presence of caspases 1, 8 and 3 in the acrosomal region and caspases 9 in the equatorial region has been implicated in DNA degradation. Presence of apoptotic factors in the mature sperm cells like Fas, Bcl-X, P^{53} and Annexin V all support apoptosis in cells with ds-DB.

Finally it may be considered that all aforementioned reasons could damage sperm DNA in combination with each other.[13]

External Factors Contributing to Increased DNA Fragmentation

A lot of studies have shown that over the last couple of decades there has been a progressive decrease in the quality of human semen resulting from environmental toxicants and lifestyle changes.

Sherry et al. in 2000 showed that sperm motility and concentration is markedly reduced due to air pollution, also, specific mutations occur due to air pollution under experimental conditions.

Additionally, in developed countries obesity is occurring in epidemic proportions. It has been established that overweight men tend to produce high concentration of fragmented sperm cells. Similarly, tobacco smoking has been implicated as one of the main causes of male infertility and sperm DNA fragmentation.

Finally ageing, stress, exposure to pollutants and high temperature may adversely affect levels of reproductive hormones, pregnancy outcome, genital development and semen quality.[13]

Types of Lesions Associated with Sperm DNA Fragmentation

The main type of DNA breaks, ss-DB and ds-DB affects DNA in both somatic cells and gametes (sperm or egg) (Figs. 2A to C).

The factors for such DNA damage has been already been discussed under the aforementioned headings.

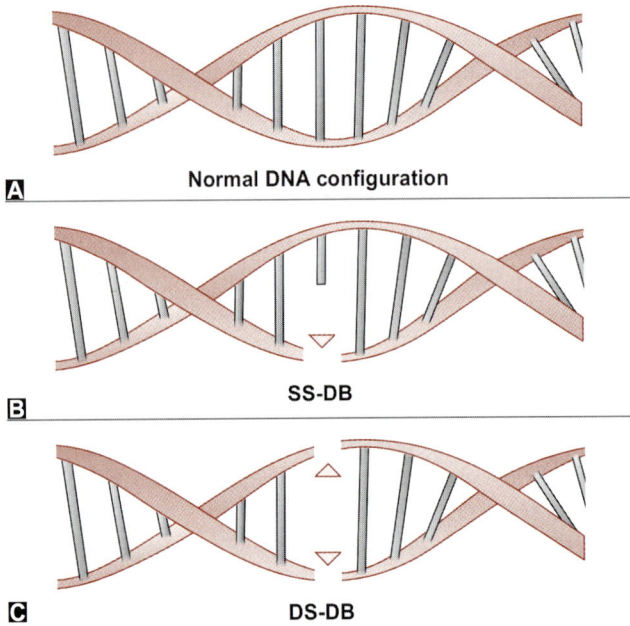

Figs. 2A to C: (A) Normal DNA configuration, (B) Single stranded DNA break (SS-DB), (C) Double stranded DNA break (DS-DB).[13]

The end result of these breaks is apoptosis or degradation of sperm DNA. However in some cases certain enzymes may repair the DNA of the sperm however structural and functional integrity of the sperms may be lost due to that.[13]

However, one important contradiction still remains to be discussed. We are all aware of approximately 1.5% of the total DNA can produce proteins the rest of the genome (introns) that cannot be transcribed have been implicated in secondary genetic functions. Therefore, any ss-DB and ds-DB breakages may not completely spoil or damage the sperm DNA.[13]

Nunez-Calonge. et. al. (2012) and Zini et. al. (2005) suggest that embryo development may be significantly altered in intracytoplasmic sperm injection (ICSI) compared to IVF cycles, as some form of natural selection occur in the latter.[13-15]

Also, the ability of the oocyte to repair the sperm DNA and the extent to which it can be repaired needs to be kept in mind before coming to a conclusion on SDF measure and treatment procedures. However, this is a gray zone and cohort studies have not been performed to get to a unanimous decision on this.

■ TESTS AVAILABLE FOR SPERM DNA DAMAGE/ FRAGMENTATION

The most important factor for a clinically useful sperm DNA fragment assessment is strong predictive capacity for pregnancy with least possible overlap between fertile and infertile samples.[1]

The four tests most often used today are:
1. Sperm chromatin structure assay
2. Sperm chromatin dispersion (HALO) test
3. Terminal deoxynucleotidyl transferase mediated deoxyuridine triphosphate nick end labeling assay
4. Single cell gel electrophoresis assay.

Sperm Chromatin Structure Assay

The SCSA is a fluorescent cell sorter test which measures the susceptibility of sperm DNA to denaturation after exposure to heat or acid conditions. The strength of this test is to measure a large number of sperm cells rapidly. This gives it robust statistical power. It measures only single stranded fragments. In terms of sensitivity it can detect sperm DNA damage in approximately 20% of unexplained couples.[1]

Sperm Chromatin Dispersion/HALO Test

The SCD or HALO test is a cheap and convenient kit based assay for sperm DNA damage testing. The test is simple and available in fertility labs for in house use. The test is based on the principle that sperm cells with fragmented DNA fail to produce a characteristic halo of dispersed DNA loops that is observed in sperm with non-fragmented DNA, following staining after acid denaturation and removal of nuclear proteins. However, one limitation of this test is that its low density nucleoids are relatively faint with less contrasting images. Recent studies suggest that this has better sensitivity than the TUNEL assay.[1,16]

Terminal Deoxynucleotidyl Transferase Mediated Deoxyuridine Triphosphate Nick End Labeling Assay

This assay detects *nicks* (free ends of DNA) by incorporating fluorescent stained nucleotides. This allows detection of single and double stranded DNA damage. The cells can be assessed either microscopically or by flow cytometric analysis. The downside to this test is that this assay has many protocols and the absence of a standard protocol makes it difficult to be compared. Recently in 2011 Aitken's group has improved the TUNEL assay.[1]

Single Cell Gel Electrophoresis Assay

This is a second generation sperm DNA test. COMET assay actually quantifies the actual amount of DNA damage per sperm. As the mass of DNA fragments stream out from the head of unbroken DNA, they resemble a *heavenly COMET* tail hence the name of the assay. One advantage of this assay is that it uses only 5000 sperms so it is suitable for measuring small quantities of sperm cells. This test can identify both single and double stranded DNA breaks and with an additional step can also measure altered bases. This is useful as we do not know yet which types of DNA damage are most deleterious to male fertility. The COMET assay is sensitive, repeatable and able to detect damage in every single sperm cell (even fertile ones). Since 2010, clinical thresholds for the diagnosis of male infertility and prediction of successful IVF have been established for COMET assay for sperm.[1]

CLINICAL PARAMETERS AND IMPLICATIONS

Role of Sperm DNA in Fertility

Several tests are applied to evaluate the relationship between the degree of DNA damage and the fertilization rate, embryo cleavage rate, implantation rate, pregnancy rate and live birth rate of offsprings.[17]

When 30% or more of a sperm sample DNA is damaged, the female has difficulty conceiving. In patients with DNA fragmentation index (DFI) of less than 25% the chances of pregnancy is comparatively higher.[9,18]

However, sperm DNA fragmentation does not correlate with fertilization and embryo fragmentation rates.[4]

Pregnancy loss may occur with an increase in the degree of sperm DNA damage and this could be the cause of unexplained pregnancy loss in some patients.[10]

If sperm DNA is unable to decondense after entering the ooplasm, fertilization may fail or a post fertilization failure could occur due to defective sperm DNA, e.g. poor embryo quality.[19]

Pregnancy Rate After In Vitro Fertilization/Intracytoplasmic Sperm Injection/Intrauterine Insemination

Patients undergoing intrauterine insemination (IUI) are approximately 7.3 times more likely achieve a pregnancy if DFI was greater than 30% or approximately 3 times more likely to achieve a pregnancy in case of IVF procedure if DFI is greater than 30% as compared to when DFI is less than 30% (as shown in a couple of cohort studies). Patients undergoing IVF or ICSI tend to show more spontaneous abortions with DFI values greater than 30%.[4]

FUTURE RESEARCH AND TOPICS TO ADDRESS

Future research is needed to answer the following questions:
- Is sperm DNA fragmentation of clinical importance in ART?
- If so, what are the criteria for clinically acceptable tests including the SCD assay?
- What is the mode of action of the quality and quantity and location of DNA defect on reproductive process?
- If any of the available tests can specifically detect important fertility related DNA defects?

- Can current and (or) new techniques measure the DNA status of whole cell population, not excluding the presence of a sub population with no significant DNA damage?
- What is the best technique to identify the type of DNA defects that affect fertility regardless of quantity of damaged DNA and to identify and isolate spermatozoa with intact DNA for use in ART?[4]

Finally, we feel that in case of sperm DNA damage or DFI over 30% we recommend opting for a sperm donor.

REFERENCES

1. Sharif K. Sperm DNA fragmentation testing: To do or not to do? Middle East Fertil Soc J. 2013;18:78-83.
2. Cissen M, Wely MV, Scholten I, et al. Measuring sperm DNA fragmentation and clinical outcomes of medically assisted reproduction: A systematic review and meta-analysis. Plos One. 2016;11(11):e0165125.
3. DeJong C. The clinical value of sperm nuclear DNA assessment. Hum Fertil. 2002;5:51-3.
4. Shafik A, Shafik A, Shafik I, et al. Sperm DNA fragmentation. Arch Androl. 2006;52:197-208.
5. Adams C, Anderson L, Wood S. High, but not moderate, levels of sperm DNA fragmentation are predictive of poor outcome in egg donation cycles (abstract no. 0-110). J Am Soc Reprod Med. 2004;82(Suppl 2):S44.
6. Agarwal A, Saleh RA, Bedaiwy M A. Role of sperm chromatin abnormalities and DNA damage in male infertility. Fertil Steril. 2003;79:829-43.
7. Belen-Hererero M, Gagnon C. Nitric oxide: a novel mediator of sperm function. J Androl. 2001;22:349-56.
8. Belokopytova IA, Kostyleva EI, Tomilin AN, et. al. Human male infertility may be due to a decrease of the protamine P2 content in sperm chromatin. Mol Reprod Dev. 1993;34:53-7.
9. Bungum M, Humaidan P, Spano M, et al. The predictive value of sperm chromatin structure assay (SCSA) parameters for the outcome of intrauterine insemination, IVF and ICSI. Hum Reprod. 2004;19:1401-8.
10. Carrel D, Liu L, Peterson CM, et al. Sperm DNA fragmentation is increased in couples with unexplained recurrent pregnancy loss. Arch Androl. 2003;49:49-55.
11. Chohan KR, Griffin JT, Lafromboise M, et al. (2004): Sperm DNA damage relationship with embryo quality and pregnancy outcome in IVF patients (Abstract no. 0-137). J Am Soc Reprod Med. 2004;82(Suppl 2):S55.
12. Dadoune JP (1995): The nuclear status of human sperm cells. Micron. 1995;26:323-45.
13. Gosalvez J, Lopez-Fernandez, C, Fernandez JL, et al. Unpacking the mysteries of sperm DNA fragmentation: Ten frequently asked questions. J Reprod Biotech Fertil. 2015;4:1-16.
14. Nunez-Calogne R, Caballero P, Lopez-Fernandez, C et al. (2012). An improved experimental model for understanding the impact of sperm DNA fragmentation on human pregnancy following ICSI. Reprod Sci. 2012;19(11):1163-8.

15. Zini A, Meriano J, Kader K, et al. (2005). Potential adverse effects of sperm DNA damage on embryo quality after ICSI. Human Reprod. 2005;20(12):3476-80.
16. Fernández JL, Muriel L, Rivero MT, et al. The sperm chromatin dispersion test: a simple test for the determination of sperm DNA fragmentation. J Androl. 2003;24(1):59-66.
17. Agarwal A, Allemande SS. Sperm DNA damage assessment: a test whose time has come. Fertil Steril. 2005;84:850-85.
18. Evenson DP, Jost LK, Marshall D, et al. Utility of the sperm chromatin structure assay as a diagnostic and prognostic tool in the human fertility clinic. Hum Reprod. 1999;14:1039-49.
19. Tomsu M, Sharma V, Miller D. Embryo quality and IVF treatment outcomes may correlate with different sperm comet assay parameters. Hum Reprod. 2002;17:1856-62.

CHAPTER
10

DNA Fragmentation Index and Magnetic Activated Cell Sorting: A Practical Approach

Rishina Bansal, Ritu Hinduja, Navin Desai

■ INTRODUCTION

In the clinical practice of assisted reproduction, usually, a conventional sperminogram comprising of basic parameters such as motility, count, and morphology of the sperms is the only work up of males that is advised.[1] We classify male fertility attending to these parameters only, but sometimes the conventional semen analysis is not enough to predict male fertility or the likelihood of pregnancy after infertility treatment. Any type of DNA damage from the maternal or paternal origin can lead to hampering of the reproductive process. In male gametes, it can be recognized as chromosomal aberrations, epigenetic modifications, mutations, base oxidation and sperm DNA fragmentation. In fact, sperm DNA fragmentation might be the most frequent cause of paternal DNA anomaly transmission to progeny, especially in subfertile and infertile men. A sperm containing fragmented DNA can be alive, motile, morphologically normal and capable to fertilize an oocyte. There are evidences that the oocyte can have the ability to repair DNA damage depending on the type of DNA damage as well as oocyte quality and age, but in assisted reproduction techniques an important number of female patients have advanced age or have an ovarian cause of infertility than can difficult the natural capacity of DNA reparation.

The sperm DNA fragmentation test in assisted reproduction detects late apoptosis in sperm as high levels of DNA fragmentation is linked with increased sperm apoptosis. One of the early markers of apoptosis is the loss of membrane integrity, which leads to externalization of phospholipid phosphatidylserine (a molecule with a high affinity for annexin V).[2]

Using this affinity of the phosphatidylserine to annexin V a novel sperm preparation technique has been devised where annexin V (used as an apoptotic sperm marker) conjugated with magnetic microspheres get attached to the externalized phosphatidylserine, which are then exposed to a magnetic field in an affinity column. This helps separate apoptotic from non-apoptotic sperm. This procedure is called magnetic activated cell sorting (MACS). This technique was used in 1995 by Pesce and De Felici to isolate and purify the primordial germ cells (PGCs) from mouse embryos (MiniMACS magnetic separation system).[3]

Many studies have recently evaluated the use of MACS as a method to reduce apoptotic sperm and improve sperm and embryo quality. Based on the findings from these studies, other groups studied MACS as a sperm selection method for ART. Recent studies have recommended MACS selection regardless of DNA fragmentation results because apoptotic sperm is not exclusively associated with sperm DNA fragmentation.[4]

■ SPERM DNA FRAGMENTATION

Paternal contribution to the fertilization and to the development of healthy offspring is of vital importance. There have been reports of an increased risk of autism, leukemia and cancer in offspring from fathers with increasing age or fathers with increased level of DNA fragmentation due to smoking. Furthermore, some spontaneous dominant genetic diseases, epilepsy and some birth defects are linked to paternal contribution.[5] A number of studies involving DNA fragmentation of spermatozoa have reported an association between an increase in DNA fragmentation in the spermatozoa and subfertility. Comparing studies of fertile and infertile males have shown that the amount of DNA damage is significantly higher in the infertile group.[6] An abnormal chromatin packing is more recurrent in men with normospermia undergoing ART treatment than in fertile men.[7] If the man has increased DNA fragmentation in the spermatozoa, a prolonged time to pregnancy (TTP), an increased risk of a missed abortion,[8] and a significantly reduced chance of in vivo fertilization of the partner have been suggested.[9]

When seeking fertility treatment, DNA fragmentation in the spermatozoa also seems to be of vital importance when planning the course of treatment. Until now, no clear association between increased amount of DNA fragmentation and fertilization rate after in vitro fertilization (IVF) or intracytoplasmic sperm injection (ICSI) has been established.[9] However, it may affect the clinical pregnancy rate. It thus seems that an increase of DNA fragmentation primarily affects in vivo fertility, either by reducing natural conception or by a significant reduction in successful intrauterine inseminations (IUIs). It is estimated that up to 20% of males with semen parameters otherwise suitable for IUI treatment present with a DNA fragmentation index (DFI) greater than 30%, and on this basis the authors behind this study recommend that IVF or ICSI being the first choice of treatment if the amount of DNA fragmentation exceeds 30%.[10] Together, these studies provide important insight into the significance of DNA fragmentation in the spermatozoa when treating couples for infertility.

Origin of Sperm DNA Fragmentation

Varicocele

Varicocele is defined as abnormally dilated scrotal veins and is present in almost 15% of the normal male population and in about 40% of infertile men.

There is an adverse effect of varicocele on spermatogenesis due to the venous reflux and testicular elevation of temperature. It is proved that the presence of varicocele can cause a decrease in sperm motility, concentration, and morphology, but also can cause an increase in sperm DNA fragmentation as well as an increase in mitochondrial inactivation. This fact suggests that in cases of males with varicocele, determination of DNA fragmentation could be an important factor in deciding the treatment option.

Obesity

There is clear evidence based on epidemiological studies that obesity in men has a clear negative impact on fertility. It is associated with hypogonadism and became consistent the fact that also is linked with impaired spermatogenesis and sperm function, including DNA fragmentation. Analysis of chromatin integrity suggests that overweight and obese men show increased chromatin damage. Sperm from obese men that is used in in vitro fertilization is correlated with a higher rate of pregnancy loss and less likely to result in live births.[11] It is also a fact that in obese male there is an increased presence of reactive oxygen species (ROS) that is an indicator of perturbed mitochondrial function and seems that is originated from macrophages. Experimental and epidemiological data show that male fertility and offspring health may improve by weight loss in obese and overweight men, especially if is achieved by exercise and a healthy diet.

Age

There is an increasing population that wants to parent at older ages. It is well known that female fecundity declines with increasing age. Increasing age in men seems to decline their fecundity but the risks of abnormal pregnancies and heritable effects associated with advancing paternal age are still poorly understood. The effects of male aging on semen quality, DNA fragmentation and chromosomal abnormalities in infertile patients and fertile donors are being reported since 1970 but results are conflicting. It is known that the activities of antioxidant enzymes within the seminal plasma and spermatozoa from older men may be reduced and spermatozoa are more vulnerable to mutational changes than spermatozoa from younger men, and this is a fact to take into consideration because late spermatids and immature and mature spermatozoa do not have DNA repair system. In addition, apoptotic functions of spermatogenesis may be less effective in older men and who delay fatherhood may have an increased risk of unsuccessful and abnormal pregnancy as a consequence of fertilization with damaged sperm.[12] Age may not only impact semen quality, but also the genetic integrity of the sperm and sperm DNA damage can be attributed to a variety of intra- and extra-testicular factors.

Cancer, Chemotherapy, and Radiotherapy

Assessment of sperm DNA integrity has been proposed as a method to determine the impact of cancer and cancer therapy on sperm function. In a study conducted by Meseguer et al, fragmented DNA was determined from cancer patients before surgery, chemotherapy or radiotherapy treatments and compared with a group of infertile men and a control group of sperm donors of proven fertility. The sperm DNA fragmentation was statistically lower in the control group of donors, not statistically different with the infertile group and no statistically differences were found in the levels of DNA fragmentation when comparing cancer types, including those of testicular origin.

One conservative attitude can be the use of sperm cryopreservation before treatment that does not constitute a risk of transmitting defect DNA and use it in a reproduction technique in case of no spontaneous pregnancy after treatment.

Cigarette Smoking

There are abundant works that point the cigarette smoking habit as a cause of fertility descends. Nicotine is proved to be a potent pro-oxidant to the biological samples like spermatozoa and is able to alter men fertility potential by inducing membrane impairments, altering the Glutathione metabolism cycle, changing the sperm morphology and motility, and inducing DNA fragmentation. DNA integrity is significantly affected in smoker patients related to nonsmokers.[13] Cigarette smoking may have deleterious effects on sperm nuclear quality that affects the prognosis in a treatment of infertility.

Alcohol

Alcohol consumption is found to have a deleterious effect on sperm parameters and DNA fragmentation suggesting that can contribute to infertility.[13]

Days of Abstinency

Sperm DNA fragmentation varies as a function of ejaculatory abstinence and it is recommended to the male being overcoming a reproduction technique not to have ejaculatory abstinence or a short (1 day) abstinence.[14] This can be due to epididymal stasis that is kept at a minimum by short abstinence and decreasing the exposition to oxidative stress. It is proved the improvement in sperm DNA fragmentation index when short abstinence and repeated ejaculated samples are collected especially in oligospermic men.

Measuring Sperm DNA Fragmentation Index

There are four techniques to measure sperm DNA fragmentation index (DFI) (Fig. 1):
1. Sperm chromatin structure assay
2. Comet assay
3. Terminal deoxynucleotidyl transferase mediated deoxyuridine triphosphate nick end labeling assay
4. Sperm chromatin dispersion assay.

DNA Fragmentation Index and Magnetic Activated Cell Sorting

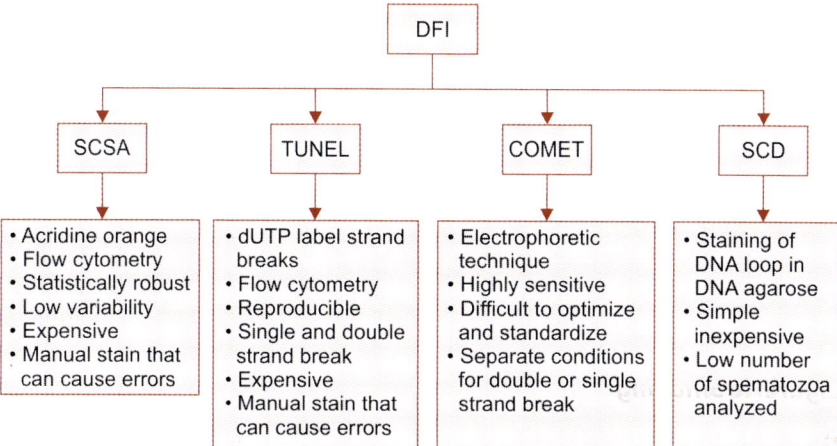

Fig. 1: Techniques for DNA fragmentation index (DFI) determination.
(SCSA: sperm chromatin structure assay, TUNEL: test, terminal deoxynucleotidyl transferase mediated deoxyuridine triphosphate nick end labeling, COMET: single gel electrophoresis, SCD: sperm chromatin dispersion, dUTP: deoxyuridine triphosphate)

■ MAGNETIC ACTIVATED CELL SORTING

Magnetic activated cell sorting is an efficient method that can avoid apoptotic sperm during selection. MACS efficiently reduce sperm DNA fragmentation levels[15] and effectively separates apoptotic from non-apoptotic spermatozoa. This selection leads to an improvement in sperm quality and functionality because MACS positively affects sperm motility and morphology as determined by the sperm deformity index. Several authors reported an improvement in fertilization rates and embryo quality[16] because the best sperms were selected using MACS compared with standard selection methods.

Another benefit of MACS, which may improve ART results, is the efficient removal of the caspases that are present in human spermatozoa, which represent the main pathway of apoptosis.[17] Their removal enhances human sperm motility and cryosurvival rates following cryopreservation. An ideal sperm preparation method should select the best sperm from the ejaculate. Most studies demonstrated that double density gradient centrifugation (DGC) combined with MACS was the more advantageous sperm selection method.[15]

To date, one of the most promising results of MACS was observed in the outcomes of couples with previous assisted reproduction failure. Studies that included IUI in couples with unexplained infertility[18] and ICSI in patients with high sperm DNA fragmentation[15] concluded that the use of MACS would improve the results for couples with repeated assisted reproduction failure (Fig. 2).

Magnetic activated cell sorting separates apoptotic spermatozoa from non-apoptotic spermatozoa. During apoptosis (programmed cell death), phosphatidyl serine residues are translocated from the inner membrane of the

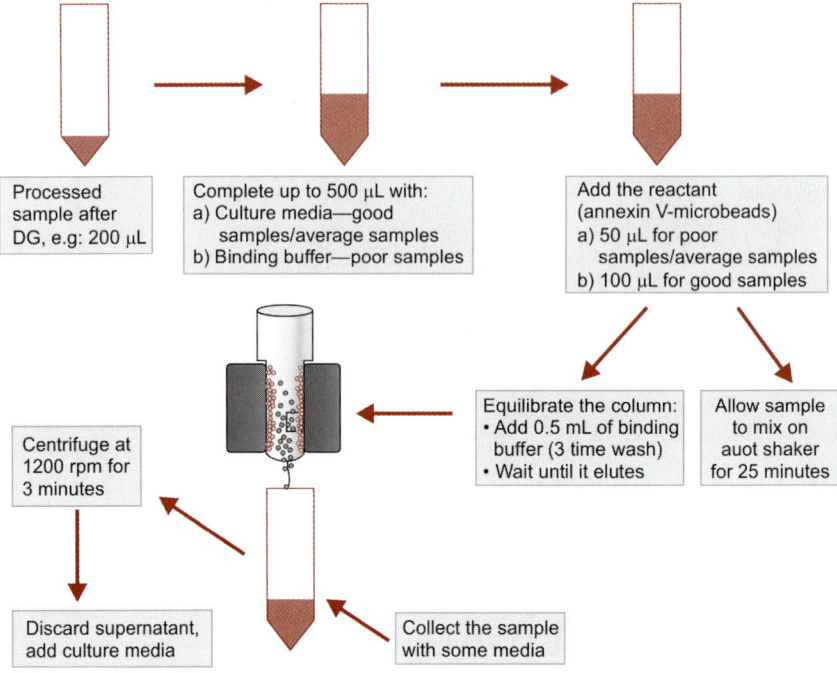

Fig. 2: Technique of magnetic activated cell sorting.

spermatozoa to the outside. Annexin V has a strong affinity for phosphatidyl serine but cannot pass through the intact sperm membrane.

Colloidal superparamagnetic beads (~50 nm in diameter) are conjugated to highly specific antibodies to annexin V and used to separate dead and apoptotic spermatozoa by MACS. Annexin V binding to spermatozoa indicates compromised sperm membrane integrity. A 100 µL sperm sample is mixed with 100 µL of MACS microbeads and incubated at room temperature for 15 minutes. The mixture is loaded on top of the separation column which is placed in the magnetic field [0.5 Tesla (T) between the poles of the magnet and 1.5 T within the iron globes of the column]; 1 Tesla = 10,000 gauss (Fig. 2). The column is rinsed with buffer. All the unlabeled (annexin V-negative) non-apoptotic spermatozoa pass through the column (Fig. 3C). The annexin V-positive (apoptotic) fraction is retained in the column. The column is removed from the magnetic field, and annexin V-positive fraction is eluted using the annexin V-binding buffer (Figs. 3 and 4). The advantages and disadvantages of magnetic activated cell sorting are outlined in Table 1.

DNA Fragmentation Index and Magnetic Activated Cell Sorting

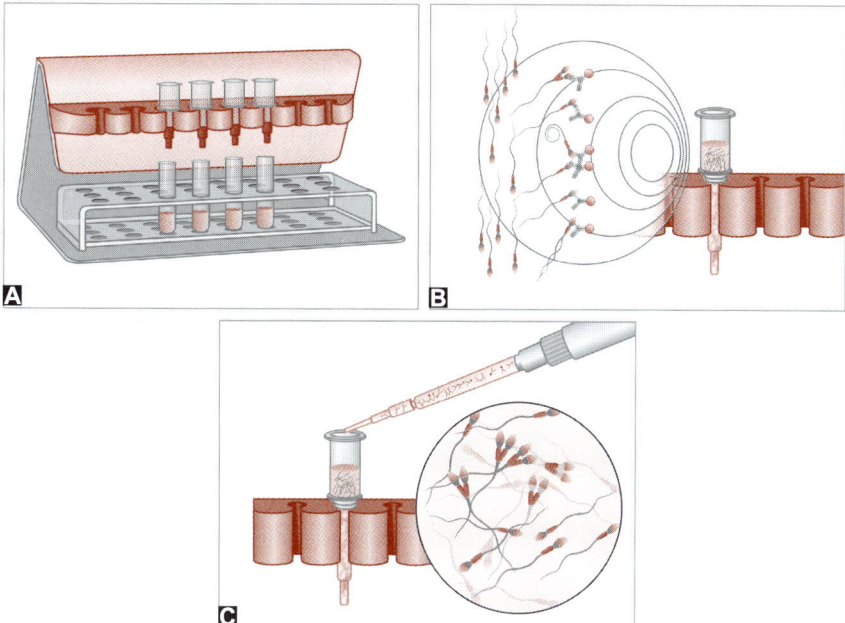

Figs. 3A to C: Magnetic activated cell sorting: (A) The octatet magnetic collection device can be used for loading up to a maximum of 8 samples. The tubes are placed between each open slot surrounded by the magnetic field, (B) The apoptotic and the non-apoptotic cells are labeled with the annexin V antibody beads (magnetic). These attach to the outer surface of the sperm that are apoptotic. Annexin V beads (magnetic) do not bind to the sperm that are non-apoptotic and have intact membranes; (C) Apoptotic sperm with annexin V beads (magnetic) are retained in the column while the non-apoptotic sperm are eluted out and collected in a tube below the collection device.[19]

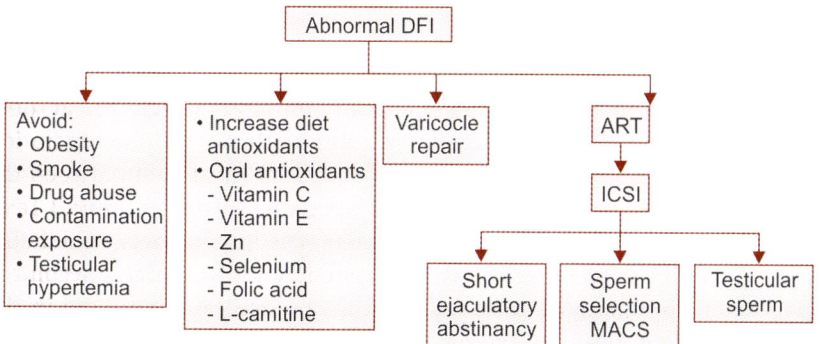

Fig. 4: Summary of management of abnormal DNA fragmentation index (DFI).
(ART: assisted reproductive technology, ICSI: intracytoplasmic sperm injection, MACS: magnetic activated cell sorting)

Table 1: Advantages and disadvantages of magnetic activated sperm sorting (MACS).

Advantages of MACS	Disadvantages of MACS
MACS acts at the molecular level as opposed to routine sperm preparation techniques that rely on sperm density and motility	Viable spermatozoa ought to be separated from all substances in the ejaculate such as apoptotic spermatozoa, leukocytes, and seminal plasma. MACS, which removes apoptotic spermatozoa, needs to be used in conjunction with other techniques such as density gradient centrifugation to remove the other substances
MACS is the only known technique which separates apoptotic spermatozoa from non-apoptotic spermatozoa	
MACS is rapid, convenient and non-invasive	
Bead detachment after MACS is not necessary	
MACS provides optimal purity and recovery with reliable and consistent results	
MACS can used to optimize the cryopreservation-thawing outcome and enhance cryosurvival rates following cryopreservation	

■ CONCLUSION

In conclusion several strategies are proposed to alleviate sperm DNA fragmentation and select the best quality chromatin content for assisted reproductive techniques: intake of oral antioxidants, varicocele repair, avoiding smoke, correcting obesity, use of recurrent ejaculations, use of ICSI technique and also use of testicular sperm. But in cases of elevated sperm DNA fragmentation index after those implementation actions, there is a possibility of using the MACS technique prior to oocyte microinjection to select non-fragmented spermatozoa. MACS is a promising new technique that helps us to get better fertilization rates as well as better embryos and enables and empowers us to offer better success rates to couples with unexplained infertility as well as previous IVF-ICSI failures and recurrent miscarriages.

KEY POINTS

- Sperm DNA fragmentation is an important factor in the etiology of male infertility.
- Elevated DNA sperm fragmentation is associated with infertility, low results in fertility techniques and also with recurrent pregnancy loss.
- Origin of Sperm DNA fragmentation can be due to varicocele, obesity, age, cigarette smoking, alcohol or cancer.
- One of the early markers of sperm apoptosis is the loss of membrane integrity, which leads to externalization of phospholipid phosphatidylserine (a molecule with a high affinity for annexin V).
- Magnetic activated cell sorting efficiently reduces sperm DNA fragmentation levels and effectively separates apoptotic from non-apoptotic spermatozoa.
- Magnetic activated cell sorting is a promising new technique that helps us get better fertilization rates as well as better embryos and enables and empowers us to offer better success rates to couples with unexplained infertility as well as previous IVF-ICSI failures and recurrent miscarriages.

REFERENCES

1. WHO. WHO laboratory manual for the examination and processing of human semen, 5th edn. Geneva: World Health Organization; 2010. pp. 271.
2. Vermes I, Haanen C, Steffens-Nakken H, et al. A novel assay for apoptosis: flow cytometric detection of phosphatidylserine expression of early apoptotic cells using fluorescein labeled Annexin V. J Immunol Methods. 1995;184(1):39-51.
3. Pesce M, De Felici M. Purification of mouse primordial germ cells by MiniMACS magnetic separation system. Dev Biol. 1995;170(2):722-5.
4. Romany L, Garrido N, Fernandez JL, et al. Assisted reproduction results improvements due to magnetic activated cell sorting (MACS) depletion of apoptotic sperm is not mediated by sperm DNA fragmentation decrease. Hum Reprod. 2012;27(suppl 2):ii121-50.
5. Aitken RJ, De Iuliis GN, McLachlan RI. Biological and clinical significance of DNA damage in the male germ line. Int J Androl. 2009;32:46-56.
6. Oleszczuk K, Augustinsson L, Bayat N, et al. Prevalence of high DNA fragmentation index in male partners of unexplained infertile couples. Andrology. 2013;1:357-60.
7. Alkhayal A, San Gabriel M, Zeidan K, et al. Sperm DNA and chromatin integrity in semen samples used for intrauterine insemination. J Assist Reprod Genet. 2013; 30:1519-24.
8. Kennedy C, Ahlering P, Rodriguez H, et al. Sperm chromatin structure correlates with spontaneous abortion and multiple pregnancy rates in assisted reproduction. Reprod Biomed Online. 2011;22:272-6.
9. Bungum M, Humaidan P, Axmon A, et al. Sperm DNA integrity assessment in prediction of assisted reproduction technology outcome. Hum Reprod. 2007;22: 174-9.

10. Bungum M, Bungum L, Giwercman A. Sperm chromatin structure assay (SCSA): a tool in diagnosis and treatment of infertility. Asian J Androl. 2011;13:69-75.
11. Chambers TJ, Richard RA. The impact of obesity on male fertility. Hormones (Athens) 2015;14:563-8.
12. Schmid TE, Eskenazi B, Baumgartner A, et al. The effects of male age on sperm DNA damage in healthy non-smokers. Hum Reprod. 2007;22:180-7.
13. Anifandis G, Bounartzi T, Messini CI, et al. The impact of cigarette smoking and alcohol consumption on sperm parameters and sperm DNA fragmentation (SDF) measured by Halosperm®. Arch of Gynecol Obstet. 2014;290:777-82.
14. Esteves SC. Novel concepts in male factor infertility: clinical and laboratory perspectives. J Assist Reprod Genet. 2016;33:1319-35.
15. Young E, De Caro R, Marconi G, et al. Reproductive outcome using Annexin V columns for non- apoptotic sperm selection. Hum Reprod. 2010;25(suppl 1):i6-9.
16. Romany L, Meseguer M, García-Herrero S, et al. Magnetic activated sorting of non-apoptotic sperm result in improved embryo quality in ovum donation cycles with intracytoplasmic sperm injection. Hum Reprod. 2010;25(suppl 1):i8.
17. Paasch U, Grunewald S, Agarwal A, et al. Activation pattern of caspases in human. Fertil Steril. 2004;81(Suppl 1):802-9.
18. Lee TH, Liu CH, Shih YT, et al. Magnetic- activated cell sorting for sperm preparation reduces spermatozoa with apoptotic markers and improves the acrosome reaction in couples with unexplained infertility. Hum Reprod. 2010; 25(4):839-46.
19. Chan PJ, Jacobson JD, Corselli JU, et al. A simple zeta method for sperm selection based on membrane charge. Fertil Steril. 2006;85(2):481-6.

CHAPTER 11

Antioxidant or Nutraceutical Therapy as Medical Management in Idiopathic Infertility

Charulata Chatterjee, Lakshmi Krishna Leela B

■ INTRODUCTION

Infertility is defined by World Health Organization (WHO) as the inability of a couple to achieve conception or bring a pregnancy to term after 1 year of regular unprotected sexual intercourse. Infertility affects 13–15% of couples worldwide.

The most common causes of infertility are divided into male, female and unexplained factor. Infertility of unknown origin and is classified as unexplained or idiopathic infertility.

The therapeutic strategies can be classified as etiological or empirical and fertility treatments are classified into medical (hormones for ovulation/spermatogenesis, nutraceutical supplements) and surgical (male/female).

Assisted reproductive technology (ART) refers to treatments used to assist couple in achieving a pregnancy. ART covers a wide spectrum of treatments like intrauterine insemination (IUI), in vitro fertilization (IVF), gamete donation and surrogacy, but ART techniques cannot overcome basic deficiency of gametes. Advanced genetic test like preimplantation genetic diagnosis (PGS) may improve success rate but it does not address the core issue, namely why gametes are deficient in quality and mechanisms that affect gametes. This results in introduction of nutraceutical therapy in treating infertility.[1]

■ TYPES OF NUTRACEUTICALS

Nutraceutical can be grouped into three categories:
1. *Nutrients or Antioxidants:* Substance with established nutritional functions such as vitamins, minerals, amino acids and fatty acids.
2. *Herbals:* Herbs or botanical products as concentrates and extracts.
3. *Dietary substance:* Reagents derived from other sources, e.g. steroid hormone, precursor serving specific functions, such as sports nutrition, weight loss, etc.

■ MALE INFERTILITY

Almost half of the all couples trying to conceive are affected by male infertility.[2] While conditions such as varicocele, cryptorchidism, and hypogonadism are definable causes for infertility, no cause may be determined for an abnormal semen analysis in over 25% of cases.[3] Such idiopathic infertility and oligoasthenoteratospermia (OATs) is a condition in which sperm concentration, the proportion of motile sperms, and the proportion of morphological normal sperms are below the WHO reference values.[4]

The exact reason for the decline in semen quality is not clear, but it may be due to environmental, nutritional, oxidative stress (OS), smoking, socioeconomic or other unknown causes.[5] All external factors ultimately increase OS and impair spermatogenesis or oogenesis.

Oxidative Stress

Oxidative stress is defined as a disturbance in the balance between the production of reactive oxygen species (ROS, free radicals) and the ability of the body to counteract or detoxify their harmful effects through neutralization by antioxidants.

Free radicals are atoms or groups of atoms with an odd (unpaired) number of electrons and can be formed when oxygen interacts with certain molecules. Once formed these highly reactive radicals can start a chain reaction, like dominoes. In the reproductive tract, free radicals also play a dual role and can modulate various reproductive functions. The damage happens when they react with important cellular components such as cell DNA, lipid membrane and protein.

Reactive Oxygen Species and Male Infertility

Human spermatozoa exhibit a capacity to generate ROS and initiate peroxidation of the unsaturated fatty acids in the sperm plasma membrane, which plays a key role in the etiology of male infertility. The short half-life and limited diffusion of these molecules is consistent with their physiological role in key biological events such as acrosome reaction and hyperactivation.[6]

Types of ROS

Reactive oxygen species represent a broad category of molecules that indicate the collection of radicals (hydroxyl ion, superoxide, nitric oxide, peroxyl, etc.) and nonradicals (ozone, single oxygen, lipid peroxides, hydrogen peroxide) and oxygen derivatives.[7] Reactive nitrogen species (nitrous oxide, peroxynitrite, nitroxyl ion, etc.) are free nitrogen radicals are considered a subclass of ROS.[8] Nitric oxide (NO) has been shown to have detrimental effects on normal sperm functions inhibiting both motility and sperm competence for zona binding.

Effects of ROS on Sperm Parameters

Positive Effect
Controlled generation of ROS may function as a signaling molecule in many different cell types and also important as mediators of sperm functions. It is also essential for the development of capacitation and hyperactivation.

Negative Effect

Oxidative stress can lead to sperm damage and infertility through several pathways. When spermatogenesis is impaired, the cytoplasmic extrusion mechanisms are defective. Spermatozoa released from the germinal epithelium carrying surplus residual cytoplasm are thought to be immature and functionally defective.[9] In addition ROS can react with DNA, proteins, carbohydrates and lipids to cause sperm dysfunction and cell death.

Lipid Peroxidation, Decreased Sperm Motility, Sperm DNA Damage

Lipids are found in the sperm plasma membrane in form of polyunsaturated fatty acids (PUFA). These fatty acids contain double bonds that make them susceptible to attack by free radicals. The initial attack by the hydroxyl radical leads to a series of chemical reactions referred to as lipid peroxidation.

Lipid peroxidation results in damage of the axonemal structure by loss of intracellular ATP, which has consequences related to sperm motility and loss of membrane integrity. As a result DNA and proteins can become susceptible to damage.[10,11]

If the amount of oxidative DNA damage is considerable, then apoptosis and embryo fragmentation may also occur. DNA damage and ROS production has also been found to correlate with abnormal head morphology and cytoplasmic retention in immature sperm, but not in mature sperm. This may be a result of OS affecting the regulation of spermiogenesis, the final stage of spermatogenesis where immature spermatids develop into mature spermatozoa.

Measurement of ROS and DNA Fragmentation in Semen

Chemiluminescence method, Cytochrome C reduction or nitroblue tetrazolium (NBT) Reduction method, electron spin resonance and spin trapping-electron spin resonance (ESR) spectroscopy-also known as electron paramagnetic resonance (EPR), and aromatic traps are standard measurement system of ROS. Sperm DNA fragmentation can be checked by sperm chromatin structure assay (SCSA), TUNEL assay, sperm chromatin dispersion (Halo) test and Comet assay.

Role of Nutraceuticals in Treating Idiopathic Male Infertility

Nutrition plays an important role in spermatogenesis. There is a definitive role of micronutrients such as zinc, folate and antioxidants for the normal maintenance of spermatogenesis and sperm maturation, DNA synthesis, repair and transcription. However, knowledge about the effect of paternal malnutrition on sperm aneuploidy is scarce.

Nutraceuticals commonly used are:
1. *Nutritional factors:* Arginine, vitamin B_{12}, Folic acid
2. *Motility enhancers:* L-carnitine, acetyl carnitine, Co-enzyme Q10
3. *Antioxidants:* Enzymatic, nonenzymatic (vitamin C, vitamin E, glutathione, lycopene, selenium, zinc).

Nutritional Factors: Vitamin B_{12}, Arginine, Folic acid

Vitamin B_{12} may increase sperm count, enhance sperm motility and reduce sperm DNA damage. The beneficial effects of vitamin B_{12} on semen quality may be due to increased functionality of reproductive organs, decreased homocysteine toxicity, reduced amounts of generated nitric oxide, decreased levels of oxidative damage to sperm, reduced amount of energy produced by spermatozoa, decreased inflammation-induced semen impairment, and control of nuclear factor-κB activation. However, additional research, mainly clinical, is still needed to confirm these positive effects.[12]

Mixed evidence suggests positive as well as no effect of vitamin B_{12} therapy.

Long-term treatment (>3 months) with methylcobalamin at 1,500 μg/day increased sperm motility in patients with idiopathic oligozoospermia or normozoospermia,[13] whereas a study by Chen et al.[14] demonstrated an insignificant difference in seminal vitamin B_{12} concentrations between fertile and infertile men.

Researchers has evaluated clinical efficacy of arginine in a men with decreased sperm motility and found positive results.

Folic acid or vitamin (B_9) that plays a vital role in nucleic acid synthesis and amino acid metabolism, but no robust evidence exists to support the use of folic acid for the treatment of men with idiopathic infertility.[15]

Motility Enhancers: L-carnitine, Acetyl Carnitine, Coenzyme Q10

Carnitine is water-soluble antioxidant involved in sperm metabolism and involved in sperm motility. The main forms used in the treatment of male subfertility are L-carnitine (LC) and L-acetyl carnitine (LAC). There is no conclusive evidence on the use of carnitine to treat idiopathic male infertility.[16]

Coenzyme Q10 is an essential antioxidant, available at high concentrations in sperm mitochondria playing an integral role in energy production. Two different studies suggest its positive effect in improving sperm motility in OAT men.[17,18]

Antioxidants: Enzymatic, Nonenzymatic (Vitamin C, Vitamin E, Glutathione, Lycopene, Selenium, Zinc)

Vitamin-C neutralizes hydroxyl, superoxide, and hydrogen peroxide radicals, thus providing protection against endogenous oxidative damage. Vitamin C was mainly investigated in combination with other vitamins and minerals and is believed to have a synergistic effect in reducing peroxidative damage on spermatozoa.[19]

Vitamin-E is a well-documented antioxidant and has been shown to inhibit free radical-induced damage to sensitive cell membranes. Again use of vitamin-E in treating unexplained male infertility has mixed evidence.[20,21]

Glutathione is essential for the formation of phospholipid hydroperoxide glutathione peroxidase, an enzyme present in spermatids which becomes a structural protein comprising over 50% of the mitochondrial capsule in the mid-piece of mature spermatozoa. Its deficiency can lead to instability of the mid-piece, resulting in defective motility. Therapy with glutathione helps increasing motility.[22]

Lycopene plays a major role in the human redox defense system as it has the highest quenching ability against singlet oxygen, a high-energy form of oxygen. One study reported statistically significant improvements in sperm concentration and motility in OAT men.[23]

Selenium is an essential trace element involved in spermatogenesis. It provides protection for sperm DNA against OS damage in a mechanism that is not very well-established. Selenium has mainly been studied in combination with other vitamins, specifically with vitamin E.[24]

Zinc is a trace mineral essential for normal functioning of the male reproductive system. Zinc deficiency is associated with decreased testosterone levels and sperm count. Zinc supplementation appears warranted in the treatment of male infertility, especially in cases of low sperm count or decreased testosterone levels.[25]

■ IDIOPATHIC FEMALE INFERTILITY

"Female idiopathic infertility" refers to a condition in which clinical examination does not reveal any pathological finding which might explain the infertility of the couple.

Known causes for female infertility includes vaginal, cervical, tubal or uterine factors, ovarian dysfunction and endometriosis, but there may be some unknown reasons which cannot identified for having such female reproductive abnormalities.

Role of Oxidative Stress in Female Reproductive Tract

ROS and the Ovary

Various biomarkers of OS have been demonstrated in normal cycling human ovaries and a delicate balance exists between ROS and antioxidant enzymes in the ovarian tissue. ROS within the follicular fluid plays a role in modulating oocyte maturation, folliculogenesis, ovarian steroidogenesis, and luteolysis. Antioxidants neutralize ROS production and protect the oocycte.

Endometrium

There is a cyclical variation in the expression of superoxide dismutase (SOD) in the endometrium. In the late secretory phase, SOD activity decreases and levels of ROS increases. It is important for endometrial shedding and the onset of menstruation.

Role of ROS in PCOD: Elevated insulin resistance and hyper homocysteinemia has been proposed to be caused by OS in patients with polycystic ovary syndrome (PCOD).[26] Antioxidant supplementation can improve insulin sensitivity.

ROS in Endometriosis: An increased generation of ROS by pelvic macrophages and increased lipid oxidation in patients with endometriosis is observed.[27] Antioxidant levels of superoxide dismutase (SOD) were noted to be significantly lower in peritoneal fluid in patients of endometriosis. Increased ROS levels in the tubal and the peritoneal environment negatively alter fertilization and embryonic development.

Role of long chain fatty acids in endometriosis: The long chain fatty acids improve quality of oocyte membrane and provide energy for cell metabolism. EPA present in fish oil suppresses activation of nuclear factor kappa. Supplementation with fish oil is useful in women with endometriosis and PID.

ROS and Female Infertility

Oxidative stress induces infertility in women through a variety of mechanisms. Excess ROS in the follicle may damage DNA of oocytes, leading to defective fertilization. Even when fertilization is achieved, OS-induced apoptosis may result in embryo fragmentation, implantation failure, abortion, impaired placentation, and congenital abnormalities. Excess ROS may hinder the endometrium, which normally functions to support the embryo and its development. OS may induce luteal regression and insufficient luteal hormonal support for the continuation of a pregnancy.

Elevated levels of ROS that disturb the redox balance within the body may be the root cause of infertility in women who do not have any other obvious cause.

Elevated ROS levels in patients with unexplained infertility imply exhausted antioxidant defense resulting in the inability to scavenge ROS and neutralize their toxic effect.

Antioxidant to Treat Idiopathic Female Infertility

A number of drugs with antioxidative properties have been postulated to have a possible role in the management of idiopathic problems. Several recent randomized controlled trials (RCTs) have revealed an increased rate of successful pregnancies by antioxidant supplementation in IVF-ICSI levels.

Antioxidants—Astaxanthin, Ubiquinone 10, Anthocyanins, L-Carnitine

Astaxanthin: It is a strong antioxidant which is a lipophilic carotenoid produced by an algae which showed beneficial results in women with infertility.

Ubiquinone Q10: It is a highly active antioxidant which acts at the level of mitochondria. Supplementation will help in reducing the ROS levels.

Anthocyanins: They are extracted from pine bark. These have scavenger effects on intracellular free oxygen radicals and help in reducing OS.

L-Carnitine: In women with infertility, supplementation of L-carnitine has shown to be beneficial in some studies. In vitro maturation of human oocyte could be supported by the addition of L-Carnitine.

Role of Plant Extracts

Curcumin from turmeric, pycnogenol and lepidium were shown to be beneficial because of their antioxidant properties.

Micronutrients: Magnesium/Selenium/Zinc

Few patients with a history of unexplained infertility and abnormal red blood cell-magnesium (RBC-Mg) levels were unresponsive to oral magnesium supplementation and shown to be associated with deficient red blood cell glutathione peroxidase (RBC-GSH-Px) activity.[28] Supplementation of selenium and oral magnesium for a period of 2 months was shown to normalize RBC-Mg and RBC-GPx levels. This improved pregnancy rates in this group of women.

N-acetyl-cysteine

For PCOS patients, insulin resistance and hyperglycemia are established as factors that increase oxidative stress. N-acetyl-cysteine (NAC), known to replenish stores of the antioxidant glutathione, on insulin secretion and peripheral insulin resistance in subjects with PCOS. Patients can be treated for 5–6 weeks with a 1.8 g oral NAC per day.[29]

Vitamins: Folic acid/Zinc/β-Carotene/Vitamin C/Vitamin E

Folic Acid

Women receiving folic acid supplementation had a better quality oocytes and a higher degree of mature oocytes compared with women who did not receive folic acid supplementation.[30]

Zinc

Normal adult women with celiac disease can be benefited with zinc supplementation.

β-Carotene

Higher intakes of β-carotene from dietary supplements is associated with a shorter time to pregnancy in overweight/obese women whose body mass index (BMI) was greater than 25, and also in the younger age group (under 35 years old).

Vitamin C/Vitamin E

Vitamin C slows down free radicals and helps in the recycling of glutathione and vitamin E, thus improving fertility.

CONCLUSION

Many environmental and biochemical factors are involved in male and female reproduction. The importance of many of these factors is not yet clearly understood. Still, numerous couples face unexplained subfertility and can only be treated by ART. However, these treatments do not address the cause of subfertility, for which no therapies are available. A better understanding of underlying mechanisms in (sub)fertility and better study results clarifying the effectiveness of nutritional factors are important to improve diagnosis and treatment. Such aspects include patient selection, study duration, sample size and dosage of the treatment.

Food supplementation with nutraceutical or antioxidants can improve the quantity and functional quality of gametes.

Majority of male infertility cases are due to deficient sperm production of unknown origin. External factors which may adversely affect spermatogenesis should be properly addressed. And based on that nutritional strategies should be made which have a beneficial impact on sperm count, motility, and ultimately, fertility.

OS modulates a range of physiological functions and plays a role in pathological processes affecting female reproduction. Hence a planned strategy should be made to improve female infertility.

By applying this strategy, remarkable results have been obtained in terms of increasing the probability of spontaneous conception or can enhance the success rate of IVF.

KEY POINTS

- Free radicals cause oxidative damage to cells and DNA, which can be reduced by antioxidants.
- About 10–15% of infertility is considered idiopathic, which may be caused by oxidative stress.
- Beside lifestyle modifications nutraceuticals help in maturation of sperm, provide nutrition for motility of sperm, help in improvement in sperm count and motility, help in production of sex hormones and prevent sperm damage.
- Intake of antioxIdant nutrients impacts the generation of reactive oxygen species and may play a beneficial role in female fertility.
- Infertility is a significant public health problem and diagnosis and treatment are stressful, invasive, and costly. Identifying modifiable factors to decrease oxidative stress with antioxidant supplementation will enhance fertility.

REFERENCES

1. Comhaire FH, Decleer W. The benefit of nutraceutical food supplementation and antioxidants for the treatment of the infertile couple and in assisted reproduction. Reproductive Sys Sexual Disord. 2012;S1:4.
2. Sharlip ID, Jarow JP, Belker AM, et al. Best practice policies for male infertility. Fertil Steril. 2002;77(5):873-82.
3. Siddiq FM, Sigman M. A new look at the medical management of infertility. Urol Clin North Am. 2002;29(4):949-63.
4. Cooper TG, Noonan E, von Eckardstein S, et al. World Health Organization reference values for human semen characteristics. Hum Reprod Update. 2009;16(3):231-45.
5. Adiga SK, Jayaraman V, Kalthur G, et al. Declining semen quality among South Indian infertile men: a retrospective study. J Hum Reprod Sci. 2008;1:15-8.
6. Selly MU, Lacey MJ, Bartlett MR, Copeland CM, Ardlie NG Content of significant amounts of a cytotoxic end product of lipid peroxidation in human semen. J reprod Fertil 1991;92:291-8
7. Agarwal A, Prabakaran SA. Mechanism, measurement, and prevention of oxidative stress in male reproductive physiology. Ind J Experiment Biol. 2005;43(11):963-74.
8. Darley-Usmar V, Wiseman H, Halliwell B. Nitric oxide and oxygen radicals: a question of balance. FEBS Letters. 1995;369(2-3):131-5.
9. Huszar G, Sbracia M, Vigue L, et al. Sperm plasma membrane remodeling during spermiogenic maturation in men: Relationship among plasma membrane beta 1,4-galactosyltransferase, cytoplasmic creatine phosphokinase and creatine phosphokinase isoform ratios. Biol Reprod. 1997;56:1020-4.
10. Saleh R, Agarwal A, Kandirali E, et al. Leukocytospermia is associated with increased reactive oxygen species production by human spermatozoa. Fertil Steril. 2002;78(6):1215-24.
11. Kodama H, Yamaguchi R, Fukuda J, et al. Increased oxidative deoxyribonucleic acid damage in the spermatozoa of infertile male patients. Fertil Steril. 1997;68(3):519-24.
12. Moriyama H, Nakamura K, Sanda N, et al. Studies on the usefulness of a long-term, high-dose treatment of methylcobalamin in patients with oligozoospermia. Hinyokika Kiyo. 1987;33:151-6.
13. Iwasaki A, Hosaka M, Kinoshita Y, et al. Result of long-term methylcobalamin treatment for male infertility. Jpn J Fertil Steril. 2003;48:119-24.
14. Chen Q, Ng V, Mei J, et al. Comparison of seminal vitamin B12, folate, reactive oxygen species and various sperm parameters between fertile and infertile males. Wei Sheng Yan Jiu. 2001;30:80-2.
15. Murphy LE, Mills JL, Molloy AM, et al. Folate and vitamin B12 in idiopathic male infertility. Asian J Androl. 2011;13(6):856-61.
16. Cavallini G, Ferraretti AP, Gianaroli L, et al. Cinnoxicam and L-carnitine/acetyl-L-carnitine treatment for idiopathic and varicocele-associated oligoasthenospermia. J Androl. 2004;25:761-70.
17. Safarinejad MR. Efficacy of coenzyme Q10 on semen parameters, sperm function and reproductive hormones in infertile men. J Urol. 2009;182:237-48.

18. Safarinejad MR. The effect of coenzyme Q10 supplementation on partner pregnancy rate in infertile men with idiopathic oligoasthenoteratozoospermia: an open-label prospective study. Int Urol Nephrol. 2012;44:689-700.
19. Greco E, Iacobelli M, Rienzi L, et al. Reduction of the incidence of sperm DNA fragmentation by oral antioxidant treatment. J Androl. 2005;26:349-53.
20. Rolf C, Cooper TG, Yeung CH, et al. Antioxidant treatment of patients with asthenozoospermia or moderate oligoasthenozoospermia with high-dose Vitamin C and Vitamin E: a randomized, placebo-controlled, double-blind study. Hum Reprod. 1999;14:1028-33.
21. Suleiman SA, Ali ME, Zaki ZM, et al. Lipid peroxidation and human sperm motility: Protective role of Vitamin E. J Androl. 1996;17:530-7.
22. Lenzi A, Culasso F, Gandini L, et al. Placebocontrolled, double blind, cross-over trial of glutathione therapy in male infertility. Hum Reprod. 1993;8:1657-62.
23. Gupta NP, Kumar R. Lycopene therapy in idiopathic male infertility: a preliminary report. Int Urol Nephrol. 2002;34:369-72.
24. Burton GW, Traber MG. Vitamin E: antioxidant activity, biokinetics, and bioavailability. Annu Rev Nutr. 1990;10:357-82.
25. Tikkiwal M, Ajmera RL, Mathur NK. Effect of zinc administration on seminal zinc and fertility of oligospermic males. Indian J Physiol Pharmacol. 1987;31:30-4.
26. Gupta S, Agarwal A, Krajcir A, et al. Role of oxidative stress in endometriosis. Reprod Biomed. 2006;13(1):126-34.
27. González F, Rote NS, Minium J, et al. Reactive oxygen species-induced oxidative stress in the development of insulin resistance and hyperandrogenism in polycystic ovary syndrome. J Clin Endocrinol Metab. 2006;91(1):336-40.
28. Howard JM, Davies S, Hunnisett A. Red cell magnesium and glutathione peroxidase in infertile women—effects of oral supplementation with magnesium and selenium. Magnes Res. 1999;7(1):49-57.
29. Fulghesu AM, Ciampelli M, Muzi G, et al. N-acetyl cysteine treatment improves insulin sensitivity in women with polycystic ovary syndrome. Fertil Steril. 2002;77(6):1128-35.
30. Szymanski W, Kazdepka-Zieminska A. (2003) Effect of homocysteine concentration in follicular fluid on a degree of oocyte maturity. Ginekol Pol. 2003;74,1392-6.

CHAPTER
12

Environmental Effect on Male Infertility: Preventive Therapeutic Approach

Sreyashi Mitra, Nabendu Murmu, SM Rahman, Parag Nandi

■ INTRODUCTION

Environmental, lifestyle, dietary or occupational factors play an important role behind the increasing trend of number of human health hazards across the world. Among them, most frequently encountered problems are—reproductive disorders, developmental defects, cancer, etc. In the past few decades, a disturbing trend of declining reproductive capacity has been observed around the globe. Infertility affects an estimated 15% of couples globally, amounting to 48.5 million couples. Males are found to be solely responsible for 20–30% of infertility cases and contribute to 50% of cases overall.[1-4] As per recent reports nearly 50% of infertility cases in India is related to the reproductive anomalies or disorders of the male partner. The overall prevalence of primary infertility ranges between 3.9% and 16.8% (WHO, 2004). The estimates of infertility vary widely among Indian states.

The potential link between the detrimental environmental effects on reproduction and the worldwide increase in testicular cancer evoke huge interest in clinicians, scientists and the public.[5,6]

■ MALE INFERTILITY AND ENVIRONMENTAL FACTORS

There has been long debate over whether male reproductive ability is determined by environmental factors, such as those present in the workplace or area of residence. In 1992, Carlsen et al. reported that the previous 50 years saw a marked decrease in sperm count.[7] That same year, Brake and Krause reported that during the period since 1970 in Scotland, sperm counts had decreased by approximately 25% compared with the period prior to 1959, a mean annual rate of 2.1%.[8] Many researchers and clinicians have asserted that societal progress in advanced countries and worsening of the natural environment have likely resulted in decreased male fertility. Long-reported risk factors include working in high temperatures,[9] noise associated with manufacturing,[10] exposure to radiation,[11] electromagnetic waves,[12] and a variety of chemical substances.[13] Numerous studies have compared patients with male infertility (oligospermia or azoospermia) to healthy subjects (normal sperm count). On the contrary, many reports indicate the absence of a correlation between environmental factors and male infertility.[14,15] Thus, there is presently no consistent view on the role of environmental factors and male infertility. One reason for these discrepancies is that the sample sizes have been insufficient to determine statistically significant differences. The total number of patients with male infertility included in these studies has been small, fewer than 100 patients in nearly all cases. Another reason is that nearly all of these studies have been survey studies using questionnaires, with no objective tests like measuring blood concentrations. Consequently, levels of exposure have been very ambiguous, and selecting healthy men as controls has been problematic. Many recent studies have included a control group consisting of healthy men selected based on semen findings. However, nearly all of these have been patients who desired to have children and had been examined for infertility on an outpatient basis. Thus, even if the semen findings were normal, it is highly questionable whether the male partner of an infertile couple can be considered healthy.

Pesticides and Fertilizers

Over six and a half billion people populating the world today, food production has been engineered to a large degree. While fertilizers and pesticides have revolutionized food production in recent times, both have also introduced new chemicals and possible toxins to millions. Chemical fertilizers such as nitrogen and ammonia are being extensively used in agriculture today. Nitric oxide has been found to reduce sperm motility, viability, and other semen parameters; it also has been found in some cases to impair the ability of spermatozoa to penetrate the oocyte.[16] Jurewicz suggested that there are consistent indications that pesticides like dichlorodiphenyltrichloroethane, better known as DDT, affect sperm counts in humans. Also, herbicides such as lindane, methoxychlor, and dioxin-TCDD have all been linked with testicular oxidative stress and decreased sperm counts.[17,18] Food preservatives are yet another method for toxins to enter the bloodstream and cause fertility issues. Carbendazim is a systemic broad-spectrum fungicide commonly used on fruit and leather.[19] It has been found to have detrimental effects on male reproduction including decreased mean testicular weight and reduced seminiferous tubule diameters.[20,21] The vast prevalence of such pesticides, herbicides, and fertilizers utilized by the food industry today is a major fertility concern, one that will be difficult to overcome due to the necessity of large scale production.

Toxins, Chemicals and Endocrine Disruptors

Environmental chemicals and toxins have the potential to negatively affect fertility. Some of these chemicals have estrogenic properties and thus are considered toxic because they affect the normal functioning state of the endocrine system. Such compounds can affect luteinizing hormone (LH) stimulated Leydig cells which influence androgen secretion and thus interfere with the proper endocrine regulation of spermatogenesis. The ideal ratio of testosterone and estrogen can be shifted as a result of such endocrine disrupters; this can lead to errors in feedback and regulation of the hypothalamus-pituitary-gonadal (HPG) axis. In addition the pro-oxidant and antioxidant system of cells can also be thrown out of harmony. Such a disturbance could lead to the generation of free radicals and reactive oxygen species (ROS). These free radicals could destabilize the electrolytic balance within cells. Spermatozoa are especially susceptible to ROS and lipid peroxidation due to the large amount of polyunsaturated fatty acids found in their membranes. Therefore, chemical toxins that generate ROS in spermatozoa are quite significant.

Heavy Metal Toxicity

According to the International Union of Pure and Applied Chemistry (IUPAC), the term "heavy metal" is a "meaningless term", as there is no standardized definition for a heavy metal. Although in general terms, heavy metals are toxic metallic elements with relatively high density and atomic weight [e.g. Lead (Pb) and Cadmium (Cd), Arsenic (As), Chromium (Cr), Zinc (Zn), Mercury (Hg), etc.]. In India, systemic exposure to Pb and Cd varies with age, ethnicity, area, demography and socioeconomic, occupational status of the subject. Sources of Pb contamination include vehicle emission, industrial effluents, smelting, mining, agricultural wastes, etc. It has been observed that chronic exposure to Pb causes severe neurological, metabolic and hematological impairment.[22,23] On the other hand, the effect of Cd exposure on human health has been studied extensively since 1950s, following the occurrence of *Itai Itai* disease in Japan which occurred due to the ingestion of high amount of cadmium-contaminated rice by postmenopausal women. The gradual accumulation of Cd levels in the water, air, and soil has been particularly observed in industrial areas. People working in the industrial plants that make Cd products such as batteries, coating, plastic, etc. are particularly susceptible to Cd toxicity. Both Pb and Cd are considered to be critical reproductive toxicants and exposure to them has been associated with decreased semen quality and fertility rates along with the increased frequencies of male infertility.[24] In the male body, Cd interferes in testicular steroidogenesis and interferes in the process of spermatogenesis.[25,26] Although the specific sequence of biochemical, cellular and physiological events which followed Pb, Cd exposure that ultimately leads to male reproductive dysfunction are still unclear. Growing evidences indicate oxidative stress (OS) as a mediator of sperm dysfunction. Studies suggest that the damage to spermatozoa by ROS play a key role in the etiology of male infertility.[27,28] The spermatozoa have a high content of polyunsaturated fatty acids (PUFA) within the plasma membrane and a low concentration of scavenging enzymes within the cytoplasm and they are susceptible to the peroxidation in the presence of elevated seminal ROS.[29-31]

Smoking

A meta-analysis of 20 observational studies showed that men who smoked cigarettes were more likely to have low sperm counts.[32] In utero exposure to smoking was studied in 1,770 young, healthy, potential military recruits and results showed the possibility of a small effect.[33] Exposure to smoking in utero was associated with mean sperm concentrations which were 20% lower when compared with unexposed men. In another study, there were no significant differences in mean sperm concentrations in men whose mothers either smoked or did not smoke during pregnancy.[34] However, men whose mothers had smoked more than or equal to 10 cigarettes per day while pregnant were at higher risk of having oligospermia (sperm concentration $<20 \times 10^6$/mL).

On the other hand, Benzo(a)pyrene, a polyaromatic hydrocarbon, which is a result of incomplete combustion of organic matter and is also present in cigarette smoke. Benzo[a]pyrene (BaP) is known for causing cancer and is an aryl hydrocarbon receptor ligand that stimulates the expression of the CYP1 family of P450 monooxygenases. The same enzymes also biotransform BaP into several metabolites,[35] one of which is considered the ultimate carcinogen, due to the formation of a stable epoxide.[36] More recently, BaP has been recognized as a reproductive and developmental toxicant.[37,38]

■ PREVENTION AND THERAPY

There is around 40% infertility cases detected across the globe where the cause of the reduced reproductive health is not diagnosed. This condition is called as idiopathic male infertility. However, for infertility issues caused by sperm production problems due to addiction, infectious diseases and other reversible conditions, treatment will help cure male infertility.

Only lifestyle-related problems that cause male infertility can be prevented by taking better care of the body. The prevention of male fertility problems that are caused by lifestyle issues can be managed by living a healthier life. Below are some suggestions:

- *Avoid being overweight*: Excess weight has often been associated with sperm production problems
- *Overcome additions to alcohol, smoking and drugs*: Addictions tend to disrupt the proper functioning of biological processes
- *Maintain an optimum testicular temperature*: Wearing tight clothes can affect the circulation of blood in the genital region and raise the temperature of the testicles. Higher testicular temperature has been associated with infertility by affecting sperm production

- *Eating nutritious food*: A lack of nutrients, zinc and vitamin C in particular, can cause problems in sperm production. Fresh fruits, vegetables and food rich with vitamins and fibers are essential to maintain healthy reproductive status.
- *Exercise to maintain high immunity*: Infections and inflammations may completely stop the production of healthy sperm. Exercising regularly is a means by which one can ensure a healthy immune system.

Therapeutic Approaches

Hormonal Treatment

Gonadotropin-releasing hormone (GnRH): The release of GnRH in the hypothalamus stimulates the release of follicle-stimulating hormone (FSH) and LH from the anterior pituitary. In men, normal levels of FSH and LH are responsible for induction of spermatogenesis and maintaining high levels of testicular T.[39] Pulsatile administration of GnRH is an effective treatment to replace GnRH deficiency in infertile men with hypogonadotropic hypogonadism (HH) due to a lack of secretion from the hypothalamus (e.g. Kallmann's syndrome, idiopathic HH). Men with HH have reduced fertility that is usually restored by re-establishing the high intra-testicular T and the FSH stimulation of sertoli cells.[40] The goal of GnRH therapy is to stimulate the release of gonadotropins from the anterior pituitary and subsequent pathways in the HPG. The most effective dose for pulsatile GnRH is a dose between 5 µg and 20 µg every 1–2 hours delivered by a subcutaneous pump or needle.[41] GnRH is very effective in inducing spermatogenesis as early as 4 months after the start of therapy.[42] Pulsatile GnRH therapy induces spermatogenesis in about 85% of patients,[43] and on average 60% of couples will achieve pregnancy after 9 months of treatment, and can take up to 2 years.[44] Some men who receive GnRH will see an improvement in their sexual characteristics such as increase in the testicular volume, and other features like pubic hair growth. These changes can be used as clinical markers to monitor treatment. Increase in testicular size, normalization of gonadotropin and T levels, maturation of secondary sexual characteristics, normal baseline inhibin B levels, and absence of cryptorchidism are positive predictors of treatment success.[45] GnRH is successfully used in the treatment of men with HH, but currently there is a lack of evidence to support its use in the treatment of idiopathic infertility. About 10% of patients with HH might not require longtime treatment; there is evidence that the hypothalamus will produce and secret GnRH after treatment is withheld for a short period of time.

Gonadotropins: The treatment of male infertility in men with pituitary insufficiency (e.g. pituitary adenoma, systemic diseases such as hemochromatosis and sarcoidosis) is based on the use of gonadotropins, therefore spermatogenesis and T production cannot be induced by pulsatile GnRH. Gonadotropins were previously extracted from urine. With advancement in laboratory technology, human chorionic gonadotropin (rec-hCG), FSH (rec-hFSH) and LH (rec-hLH) or highly purified urinary gonadotropins are used with superior quality, activity and performance. There have been no confirmed differences in the safety, purity, or clinical efficacy among the various available highly purified or recombinant gonadotropin products.[46]

Surgical sperm extraction with hormonal manipulation: The use of medical therapy to optimize surgical sperm extraction is based also on the concept that spermatogenesis is dependent on high levels of intratesticular T and FSH stimulation of the sertoli cells.[47]

Antioxidant: Increased rates of infertility have been found in men with seminal fluid containing high levels of ROS.[48] These ROS are associated with sperm dysfunction, germ cell DNA damage with the possibility of impaired fertility, but the exact mechanism is not completely understood. These associations have led clinicians to treat infertile men with antioxidant supplements. A variety of clinical trials have suggested that the use of antioxidant supplements have a slight benefit in improving sperm function and DNA integrity. However, most of these studies are not randomized controlled trials, and to date there are no convincing trials that have demonstrated a significantly higher unassisted pregnancy rate after treating men with antioxidant therapy.[48] Moreover, the benefit of antioxidants might be limited to certain groups of patients that is not, as yet, clearly defined. The use of individual antioxidants is very common. These trends have led pharmaceutical companies to produce and market specific combinations of antioxidants and numerous studies have looked at the benefit of these combinations. A study that looked at the use of vitamin E and C in combination found no improvement in semen parameters or pregnancy rates[49] and a similar study using vitamin E and C found a meaningful reduction in DNA fragmentations.[50-52]

Role of Natural Compounds

A diverse range of natural compounds derived from plants or animals or produced by microbes are believed to play critical role in fertility prevention and therapeutics. Several laboratories around the world are dedicated to find out the health benefits of these compounds.

Coenzyme Q10

Coenzyme Q10, is an essential compound found naturally in virtually every cell in the human body. CoQ10 acts as a potent antioxidant which scavenges free radicals. Recent studies suggest that coenzyme Q10 may be useful in treating infertility. The deep involvement of coenzyme Q10 in mitochondrial bioenergetics and its antioxidant properties are at the basis of its role in seminal fluid. Following the early studies addressing its presence in sperm cells and seminal plasma, the relative distribution of the quinone between these two compartments was studied in infertile men, with special attention to varicocele. The reduction state of CoQ10 in seminal fluid was also investigated. After the first in vitro experiments CoQ10 was administered to a group of idiopathic asthenozoospermic infertile patients.[53] Seminal analysis showed a significant increase of CoQ10 both in seminal plasma and in sperm cells, together with an improvement in sperm motility. The increased concentration of CoQ10 in seminal plasma and sperm cells, the improvement of semen kinetic features after treatment, and the evidence of a direct correlation between CoQ10 concentrations and sperm motility strongly support a cause/effect relationship.[54]

Resveratrol

Resveratrol is a naturally occurring polyphenol that provides a number of health benefits including improved metabolism, cardioprotection, and cancer prevention. Resveratrol is known for its anti-inflammatory, antioxidant, analgesic, cardioprotective, antiaging and neuroprotective roles.[55] Studies have demonstrated that resveratrol may inhibit cell apoptosis, thereby providing protection from numerous diseases, including atherosclerosis, cerebral ischemia and myocardial ischemic reperfusion injury.[56] Juan et al.[57] reported that resveratrol is able to decrease germ cell apoptosis in mice and rats, and serves a protective role in the male reproductive tract, as well as enhancing blood testosterone levels, testicular sperm count and epididymis sperm motility in rabbits.

■ CONCLUSION

The increase in defective spermatogenesis, cryptorchidism testicular cancer and numerous other male fertility issues over the course of the past few decades is a great cause of concern and has prompted the investigation of environmental and lifestyle factors that may be responsible. The environmental factors can disrupt endocrine functions eventually leading to fertility problems. This is an issue that both developed and developing countries face. Exposure to certain toxins can lead to DNA damage, oxidative stress, and a host of other issues. Whether it occurred during gestation, the prepubertal age, or during adulthood, such exposure can affect fertility. The effects of exposure during each period are not fully understood, but information from animal models reveals that exposure itself and exposure at certain times is a topic worth investigating. While assisted reproductive techniques have advanced in recent years and allows couples to improve their chance of conception by directly injecting sperm into an egg, this only treats the symptom and not the issue itself. By eliminating or reducing certain environmental or lifestyle factors and by adding proper nutrition to daily food intake routine the status of male reproductive health can be improved.

REFERENCES

1. Agarwal A, Mulgund A, Alaa Hamada A, et al. A unique view on male infertility around the globe. Reprod Biol Endocrinol. 2015;13:37.
2. Kumar N, Singh AK. Trends of male factor infertility, an important cause of infertility: a review of literature. J Hum Reprod Sci. 2015;8(4):191-6.
3. Sharma R, Biedenharn KR, Fedor JM, et al. Life style factors in determining male reproductive health. IJEB. 2009;47:615-24.
4. Skakkebaek NE, Jorgensen N, Main KM, et al. Is human fecundity declining? Int J Androl. 2006;29:2-11.
5. Rocco F, Finkelberg E, Olivia I, et al. Azoospermia and spermatogenesis in testicular cancer. Eur Urol Rev. 2010;5:42-5.
6. Hotaling JM, Walsh TJ. Male infertility: a risk factor for testicular cancer. Nat Rev Urol. 2009;6:550-6.
7. Carlsen E, Giwercman A, Keiding N, et al. Evidence for decreasing quality of semen during past 50 years. Br Med J. 1992;305(6854):609-13.
8. Brake A, Krause W. Decreasing quality of semen. Br Med J. 1992;305(6867):1498.
9. Zorgniotti AW, Sealfon AI, Toth A. Further clinical experience with testis hypothermia for infertility due to poor semen. Urology. 1982;19(6):636-40.
10. Carosi L, Calabro F. Fertility in couples working in noisy factories. Folia Medica. 1968;51(4):264-8.
11. Sandeman TF. The effects of x irradiation on male human fertility. Br J Radiol. 1966;39(468):901-7.
12. Lancranjan I, Maicanescu M, Rafaila E, I. et al. Gonadic function in workmen with long term exposure to microwaves. Health Phys. 1975;29(3):381-3.
13. Kenkel S, Rolf C, Nieschlag E. Occupational risks for male fertility: an analysis of patients attending a tertiary referral centre. Int J Androl. 2001;24(6):318-26.
14. Oldereid NB, Rui H, Purvis K. Life styles of men in barren couples and their relationship to sperm quality. Int J Fertil. 1992;37(6):343-9.
15. Effendy I, Krause W. Environmental risk factors in the history of male patients of an infertility clinic. Andrologia. 1987;19:262-5.
16. Wu TP, Huang BM, Tsai HC, et al. Effects of nitric oxide on human spermatozoa activity, fertilization and mouse embryonic development. Arch Androl. 2004;50(3):173-9.
17. Jurewicz J, Hanke W, Radwan M, et al. Environmental factors and semen quality. Int J Med Environment Health. 2009;22(4):305-29.
18. Chitra KC, Sujatha R, Latchoumycandane C, et al. Effect of lindane on antioxidant enzymes in epididymis and epididymal sperm of adult rats. Asian J Androl. 2001;3(3):205-8.
19. Latchoumycandane C, Mathur PP. Induction of oxidative stress in the rat testis after short-term exposure to the organochlorine pesticide methoxychlor. Arch Toxicol. 2002;76(12):692-8.
20. Selmanoglu G, Barlas N, Songur S, et al. Carbendaziminduced haematological, biochemical and histopathological changes to the liver and kidney of male rats. Hum Experiment Toxicol. 2001;20(12):625-30.

21. Carter SD, Hess RA, Laskey JW. The fungicide methyl 2-benzimidazole carbamate causes infertility in male Sprague-Dawley rats. Biol Reprod. 1987;37(3):709-17.
22. Lockitch, G. Perspectives on lead toxicity. Clin Biochem. 1993;26(5):371-81.
23. Yoshida F, Hata A, Tonegawa H. Itai-Itai disease and the countermeasures against cadmium pollution by the Kamioka mine. Environment Econ Policy Stud. 1999;2(3):215-29.
24. Taha EA, Sayed SK, Ghandour NM, et al. Correlation between seminal lead and cadmium and seminal parameters in idiopathic oligoasthenozoospermic males. Cent European J Urol. 2013;66(1):84-9.
25. Smida AD, Valderrama XP, Agostini MC, et al. Cadmium stimulates transcription of the cytochrome p450 side chain cleavage gene in genetically modified stable porcine granulosa cells. Biol Reprod. 2004;70(1):25-31.
26. Akinloye O, Arowojolu AO, Shittu OB, et al. Cadmium toxicity: a possible cause of male infertility in Nigeria. Reprod Biol. 2006;6(1):17-30.
27. Alkan I, Simsek F, Haklar G, et al. Reactive oxygen species production by the spermatozoa of patients with idiopathic infertility: relationship to seminal plasma antioxidants. J Urol. 1992;157:140-3.
28. Hendin BN, Kolettis PN, Sharma RK, et al. Varicocele is associated with elevated spermatozoal reactive oxygen species production and diminished seminal plasma antioxidant capacity. J Urol. 1999;61:1831-4.
29. Fraczek M, Szkutnik D, Sanocka D, et al. Peroxidation components of sperm lipid membranes in male infertility. Ginekologia Polska. 2001;72:73-9.
30. Agarwal A, Saleh RA, Bedaiwy MA. Role of reactive oxygen species in the pathophysiology of human reproduction. FertilSteril. 2003;79:829-43.
31. Dandekar SP, Nadkarni GD, Kulkarni VS, et al. Lipid peroxidation and antioxidant enzymes in male infertility. J Postgrad Med. 2002;48:186-9.
32. Vine MF, Morrison HI, Hulka BS, et al. Cigarette smoking and sperm density: a meta-analysis. Fertil Steril. 1994;61(1):35-43.
33. Jensen TK, Jørgensen N, Punab M, et al. Association of in utero exposure to maternal smoking with reduced semen quality and testis size in adulthood: a cross-sectional study of 1,770 young men from the general population in five European countries. Am J Epidemiol. 2004;159(1):49-58.
34. Jensen MS, Toft G, Bonde JP, et al. Lower sperm counts following prenatal tobacco exposure. Hum Reprod. 2005;20(9):2559-66.
35. Scornaienchi ML, Thornton C, Willett KL, et al. Functional diferences in the cytochrome P450 1 family enzymes from zebrafish (Danio rerio) using heterologously expressed proteins. Arch Biochem Biophys. 2010;502:17-22.
36. Van CJ, Gielen JE, Nebert DW. Benzo[a]pyrene metabolism in mouse liver. Association of both 7,8-epoxidation and covalent binding of a metabolite of the 7,8-diol with the Ah locus. Biochem Pharmacol. 1985;34:1821-6.
37. Nicolas JM. Vitellogenesis in fish and the effects of polycyclic aromatic hydrocarbon contaminants. Aquat Toxicol. 1999;45:77-90.
38. Pait AS, Nelson JO. A survey of indicators for reproductive endocrine disruption in Fundulus heteroclitus (killifish) at selected sites in the Chesapeake Bay. Mar Environ Res. 2009;68:170-7.

39. Conn PM, Crowley WF Jr. Gonadotropin-releasing hormone and its analogues. N Engl J Med. 1991;324:93-103.
40. Zitzmann M, Nieschlag E. Hormone substitution in male hypogonadism. Mol Cell Endocrinol. 2000;161:73-88.
41. Happ J, Ditscheid W, Krause U. Pulsatile gonadotropin-releasing hormone therapy in male patients with Kallmann's syndrome or constitutional delay of puberty. Fertil Steril. 1985;43:599-608.
42. Blumenfeld Z, Makler A, Frisch L, et al. Induction of spermatogenesis and fertility in hypogonadotropic azoospermic men by intravenous pulsatile gonadotropin-releasing hormone (GnRH). Gynecol Endocrinol. 1988;2:151-64.
43. Liu L, Banks SM, Barnes KM, et al. Two-year comparison of testicular responses to pulsatile gonadotropin-releasing hormone and exogenous gonadotropins from the inception of therapy in men with isolated hypogonadotropic hypogonadism. J Clin Endocrinol Metab. 1988;67:1140-5.
44. Blumenfeld Z, Frisch L, Conn PM. Gonadotropin-releasing hormone (GnRH) antibodies formation in hypogonadotropic azoospermic men treated with pulsatile GnRH--diagnosis and possible alternative treatment. Fertil Steril. 1988;50:622-9.
45. Büchter D, Behre HM, Kliesch S, et al. Pulsatile GnRH or human chorionic gonadotropin/human menopausal gonadotropin as effective treatment for men with hypogonadotropic hypogonadism: a review of 42 cases. Eur J Endocrinol. 1998;139:298-303.
46. Pitteloud N, Hayes FJ, Dwyer A, et al. Predictors of outcome of long-term GnRH therapy in men with idiopathic hypogonadotropic hypogonadism. J Clin Endocrinol Metab. 2002;87:4128-36.
47. Raivio T, Falardeau J, Dwyer A, et al. Reversal of idiopathic hypogonadotropic hypogonadism. N Engl J Med. 2007;357:863-73.
48. Practice Committee of American Society for Reproductive Medicine, Birmingham, Alabama. Gonadotropin preparations: past, present, and future perspectives. Fertil Steril. 2008;90:S13-20.
49. Sharma RK, Agarwal A. Role of reactive oxygen species in male infertility. Urology. 1996;48:835-50.
50. Saleh RA, Agarwal A. Oxidative stress and male infertility: from research bench to clinical practice. J Androl. 2002;23:737-52.
51. Rolf C, Cooper TG, Yeung CH, et al. Antioxidant treatment of patients with asthenozoospermia or moderate oligoasthenozoospermia with high-dose vitamin C and vitamin E: a randomized, placebo-controlled, double-blind study. Hum Reprod. 1999;14:1028-33.
52. Greco E, Iacobelli M, Rienzi L, et al. Reduction of the incidence of sperm DNA fragmentation by oral antioxidant treatment. J Androl. 2005;26:349-53.
53. Paradiso Galatioto G, Gravina GL, Angelozzi G, et al. May antioxidant therapy improve sperm parameters of men with persistent oligospermia after retrograde embolization for varicocele? World J Urol. 2008;26:97-102.
54. Angelitti AG, Colacicco L, Arizzi M, et al. Coenzyme Q: potentially useful index of bioenergetic and oxidative status of spermatozoa. Clin Chem. 1995;41:217-9.

55. Babior BM, Curnette JT, McMurrich BJ. The particulate superoxide-forming system in human neutrophils. J Clin Invest. 1976;58:989-96.
56. Langova M, Polivkova Z, Šmerak P, et al. Antimutagenic effect of resveratrol. Czech J Food Sci. 2005;23:202-8.
57. Athar M, Back JH, Tang X, et al. Resveratrol: a review of pre-clinical studies for human cancer prevention. Toxicol Appl Pharmacol. 2007;224(3):274-83.
58. Juan ME, González-Pons E, Munuera T, et al. Trans-Resveratrol, a natural antioxidant from grapes, increases sperm output in healthy rats. J Nutr. 2005;135:757-60.

CHAPTER 13

Role of Micromanipulation in Recent Advancement of Assisted Reproductive Technology Procedures

Arundhati Athalye, Dattatray Naik, Nandkishor Naik, Prochi Madon, Madhavi Panpalia, Meenal Khandeparkar, Firuza Parikh

■ EVOLUTION OF INTRACYTOPLASMIC SPERM INJECTION

Infertility can be a frustrating experience for a couple. Current procreative technologies have made significant progress in the last decade. More than 5 million babies have been born to date with assisted reproductive technology (ART). Since professor Robert Edwards opened the door to infertile couples with in vitro fertilization (IVF) in 1978 with the birth of Louise Brown,[1] many new technologies have evolved as offshoots of IVF.

To understand the evolution of intracytoplasmic sperm injection (ICSI) technique and other micromanipulation techniques, it would be interesting to go back in time.

In 1935, Gregory Pincus inspired by Heape's results of successfully transferring embryos in a rabbit in 1890, was able to culture rabbit oocytes to the metaphase stage of meiosis II.[2] Professor Robert Edwards discovered that human oocytes required 37 hours for polar body extrusion and having timed each stage of human oocyte maturation, he led the way to human IVF. In 1970, Edwards and Steptoe set up a small laboratory in Manchester. Dr Carl Wood of the Monash IVF team in Melbourne reported the first IVF pregnancy in 1973, although it resulted in early miscarriage. In 1976, Steptoe and Edwards published a case of an ectopic pregnancy following transfer of an early blastocyst. After several failed attempts medical history was made on 25th July 1978 with the birth of the world's first "test tube baby" Louise Brown.[1] The reintroduction of ovarian stimulation by Trounson et al. in 1981,[3] was a major breakthrough that increased the chances of pregnancy in IVF.

Although pregnancy rates improved with time, results of IVF for male factor infertility remained very low with failed fertilization occurring commonly as the sperm of these men did not have the ability to perform all the steps needed for fertilization.

In order to characterize the fertilization potential of human sperm, the hamster egg-human sperm penetration assay was developed.[4] Uehara and

Yanagimachi's classic work in 1976 of injection of human sperm into hamster oocytes showed sperm nuclear decondensation (Fig. 1). The technique of sperm microinjection was pioneered by Hiramoto in the Sea Urchin in 1962[5] and by Lin in 1966 in Mouse oocytes.[6]

The practical use of micromanipulation started in the mid 80's with zona drilling (ZD) and partial zona dissection (PZD) when the sperm count, motility, or morphology were low. Pioneering attempts of ZD on a mouse model were carried out using a micromanipulator to produce holes in the zona pellucida (ZP) of unfertilized mouse oocytes, with acid Tyrode's solution.[7] The first attempts at ZD of human oocytes for the alleviation of male infertility resulted in fertilization, but pregnancy did not ensue in the 10 couples in this report.[8]

The first live birth in the world with embryo micromanipulation techniques was from Singapore, where insemination was done under the ZP.[9] This microinsemination sperm transfer (MIST) technique later became popularly known as subzonal injection of sperm (SUZI).[10] The earlier PZD technique did not give good results and was discontinued as it led to polyspermy, while SUZI gave better results and eventually led to the development of ICSI. Thus, by the end of the 1980's several procedures of assisted fertilization had been developed and used where conventional IVF could not succeed. Microsurgical fertilization techniques helped to remove the barrier presented to the sperm by the ZP. Assisted hatching (AH) was pioneered by Cohen around the same time.[11]

In order to achieve fertilization in nature, the sperm has to penetrate the cumulus cells. This is followed by zona binding and penetration, egg-sperm membrane interaction and oocyte activation. Lanzendorf initiated sperm microinjection but the fertilized oocyte only went up to the pronuclear stage. He therefore abandoned the technique.[12]

In 1992, Gianpiero Palermo in Dr André van Steirteghem's laboratory in Brussels created the first baby by sperm microinjection into the oocyte

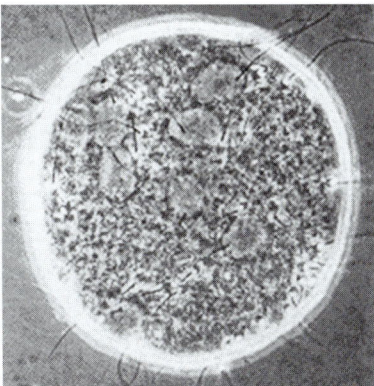

Fig. 1: Sperm nuclear decondensation in zona free hamster oocyte.
Source: Li CY, Jiang LY, Chen WY, et al. CFTR is essential for sperm fertilizing capacity and is correlated with sperm quality in humans. Hum Reprod. 2010;25(2):317-27.

cytoplasm. The team called it ICSI.[13] This discovery got them international acclaim.

In India, the first ICSI baby of South Asia "Luv Singh", was created by our team at Jaslok Hospital, Mumbai, in 1994.[14]

■ TECHNIQUE OF INTRACYTOPLASMIC SPERM INJECTION

Oocytes are mechanically denuded of the granulosa cells and cumulus oophorus cells which are present in the oocyte-cumulus complexes (OCC). Only metaphase II oocytes with one polar body can be utilized for ICSI. The entire process is carried out under 40X magnification on a heated stage of the micromanipulator system. Initially, the oocyte is immobilized using a holding pipette with the polar body either at 12 O'clock or 6 O'clock position. The sperms are immobilized in polyvinylpyrrolidone (PVP). Immobilization of the sperm is done by slicing the sperm tail with the injection pipette which has an internal diameter of 6 µm. The sperm is then gently aspirated tail first into the injection pipette. The injection pipette is then passed through the ZP and the oolemma into the cytoplasm. A tiny portion of the ooplasm is first aspirated into the injection pipette before injecting the sperm into the cytoplasm (Fig. 2). This process causes oocyte activation. The injection pipette is kept far away from the polar body in order not to injure the meiotic spindle. Once the sperm is deposited, the injection pipette is withdrawn. The negative pressure of the holding pipette is released and the injected oocyte is transferred to the fertilization medium.

■ UTILITY OF USING THE SPINDLE VIEW DURING INTRACYTOPLASMIC SPERM INJECTION

It is a tool for looking at the oocyte chromosome spindle prior to ICSI. Spindle view allows the embryologist to localize and identify the meiotic spindle. This

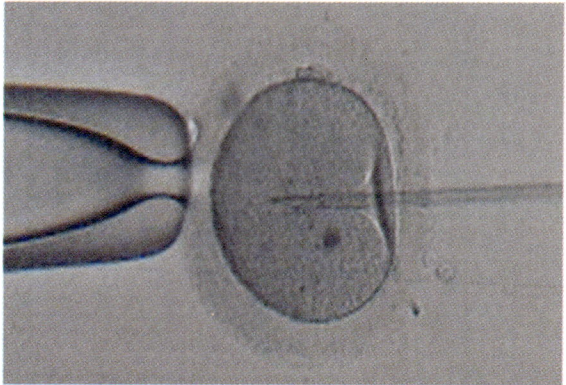

Fig. 2: Intracytoplasmic sperm injection (ICSI)—sperm is microinjected into the cytoplasm of the oocyte in ICSI.

can be used primarily for the purpose of ICSI so that localizing the spindle prior to ICSI allows one to ascertain that the spindle is not damaged during microinjection. There is a significant increase in the fertilization and pregnancy rates in oocytes showing an intact spindle. An abnormal spindle may suggest an abnormal distribution of the microtubules. The capability to look at and measure that can enhance the ability to study oocyte quality.

◼ INDICATIONS FOR INTRACYTOPLASMIC SPERM INJECTION

Although, the current indications for ICSI are not rigid, the initial use of ICSI was restricted by rigid specifications which included:
- Severe oligoasthenoteratospermia
- Presence of acrosomeless sperm
- Presence of completely immotile sperm
- Previous failed fertilization with conventional IVF
- Use of epididymal or testicular sperm
- The use of preimplantation genetic testing (PGT)
- Poor quality and quantity of retrieved oocytes.

As the technique of ICSI evolved, the indications for ICSI increased to include:
- An ejaculation and retrograde ejaculation due to anatomical defects.
- Cancer patients in remission when sperm had been cryopreserved.
- Men with spinal cord injuries.
- Cryopreserved sperm could be used in couples where the man had undergone vasectomy and the couple desired children.
- In conditions of failed vaso-epididymal anastomosis and bilateral obstruction of both ejaculatory ducts in the inguinal canal.
- Thick ZP.

◼ ADVANTAGES OF INTRACYTOPLASMIC SPERM INJECTION

- Intracytoplasmic sperm injection enables:
- Cryopreservation of sperm and embryos
- Use of testicular and epididymal sperm
- Use of ejaculated sperm in cases of oligoasthenospermia (OA)
- Preimplantation genetic testing of embryos
- Use of oocytes in the field of stem cells.

A meta-analysis of sibling oocytes studied in the presence of OA showed that the odds of fertilization after ICSI were 3.9-fold greater than IVF.[15] For this reason many IVF programs have completely switched to using only ICSI in their program. However, caution should be applied while using this as a treatment of choice in all ART cycles as it increases laboratory time, expenses, medical resources, and bypasses the natural selection process.[16]

Men with nonobstructive azoospermia (NOA) have impaired spermatogenesis. Despite severe male factor infertility, most men are reluctant to use donor sperm. With advances in the science of reproduction, testicular sperm retrieval techniques such as testicular sperm aspiration (TESA) and microtesticular sperm extraction (m-TESE), pregnancy can be achieved. The procedures of round spermatid injection (ROSI) and elongated spermatid injection (ELSI) were introduced in 1996 by Fishel et al.[17] Secondary spermatocyte injection (SESI) was developed in 1998 by Sofikitis et al,[18] where round spermatids and secondary spermatocytes were incorporated into the egg using either electrofusion or ICSI.

We have reported successful pregnancies following ICSI for the first time in India using testicular sperm from cryptorchid testis,[19] electroejaculated sperm from a man with paraplegia,[20] and with immotile sperm from a man with the immotile cilia syndrome.[21]

■ REASONS FOR FAILED FERTILIZATION FOLLOWING INTRACYTOPLASMIC SPERM INJECTION

- Less number of oocytes of poor quality
- Immotile or "dead" sperm available for injection
- Acrosomeless sperm
- Abnormal oocyte morphology
- Absence of activation of oocytes
- Absence of decondensation of sperm, or defective deoxyribonucleic acid (DNA) decondensation and aberrant pronuclear development, abnormalities in migration of the pronuclei.
- An abnormal phospholipase C zeta (PLCz) activity within the sperm head or a mutant PLC isoform may cause failed oocyte activation leading to absent Ca^{2+} oscillations and subsequently failed fertilization.[22]
- Defective oocyte cytoplasmic components may also cause failed fertilization.[23] This can be caused by abnormal spindle and interphase microtubules and abnormal chromosome patterns both of maternal and paternal origin.
- Asynchrony between oocyte nuclear and cytoplasmic maturation may prevent decondensation of the sperm nucleus. Although nuclear immaturity is easily measured by the extrusion of the first polar body, early retrieval post human chorionic gonadotropin (hCG) trigger and early denudation following oocyte retrieval can cause cytoplasmic immaturity and therefore failed fertilization.

■ DISADVANTAGE OF USING IMMOTILE SPERM DURING INTRACYTOPLASMIC SPERM INJECTION

Some authors have shown decreased fertility, cleavage, and pregnancy rates with ejaculated immotile sperm.[24] However, for testicular sperm authors have shown that there were no significant differences in fertilization, cleavage, and pregnancy rates when either motile or immotile testicular sperm was used—15.8% pregnancy rate per oocyte retrieval in the immotile testicular sperm group as opposed to 23.5% in the motile testicular sperm group.[25,26]

INTRACYTOPLASMIC MORPHOLOGICALLY SELECTED SPERM INJECTION TECHNOLOGY

Intracytoplasmic sperm injection has been utilized to overcome male infertility since its introduction in 1992. The sperms used for injection into the oocyte are selected by the embryologist based primarily on their motility and gross morphology as seen under the microscope with an optical magnification of 200X or 400X. However, studies have reported the presence of various defects in the spermatozoa, particularly head abnormalities leading to reduced fertilization, implantation rates, pregnancy rates, and increased miscarriage rates.[27] So there developed a need to further improvise the technique such that these defects could be picked up in real time by selecting the most competent gamete to enhance fertilization rates and improved pregnancy outcome. This led to attempts to assess the sperm morphology under high magnification.

In 2001, Bartoov's group developed a new technique known as motile sperm organelle morphology examination (MSOME) which could evaluate the spermatozoa in real time using a much higher magnification (6,600X).[28] It could pick up subtle morphological features, such as abnormal head proportions, presence of vacuoles in the head, and midpiece abnormalities, which could not be picked up under regular optical magnification. This is carried out using an inverted microscope with differential interference contrast (DIC) or Nomarski optics. This technique is now termed as intracytoplasmic morphologically selected sperm injection (IMSI).[29] All the motile sperm are analyzed under a higher magnification (6,600X). The criteria for selecting morphologically competent sperm is smooth, symmetric, oval configuration of the sperm nuclear shape with average length and width, a homogeneous nuclear chromatin mass, with one vacuole not exceeding more than 4% of the nucleus (Fig. 3). However, these vacuoles are ubiquitously present in sperm donors and infertile males and hence their significance is questioned.[30]

The results of IMSI are controversial possibly because of the differences in the design and selection of patients in the different studies. Some studies have shown that IMSI increased pregnancy rates of couples who had previous two or more failed ICSI cycles and of female infertility with no reason for failure. It also resulted in a decrease in the miscarriage rates.[31] However, other studies have not shown any improvement in pregnancy rates in those with repeated ICSI failures in the absence of severe male factor.[32]

Some studies have shown improved clinical pregnancy rates (CPRs), implantation rates, and ongoing pregnancy rates when IMSI is used for oligoasthenoteratozoospermia (OAT). However, there was no difference in the fertilization rate or embryo quality rate of day 3 embryos. This is because

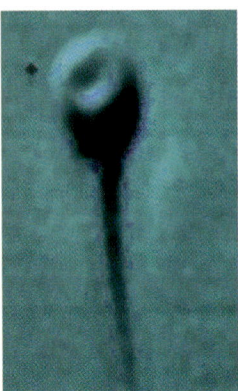

Fig. 3: Sperm visualized at 6,600X magnification for intracytoplasmic morphologically selected sperm injection (IMSI).

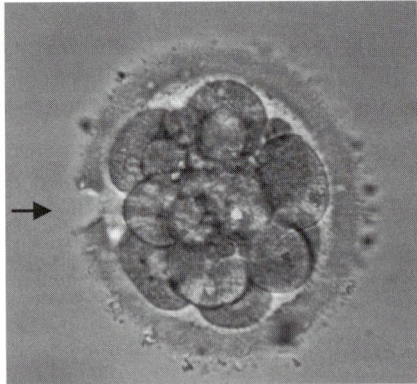

Fig. 4: Laser assisted hatching.

it is the blastocyst formation and quality that is associated with the grade of the sperms. The oocytes injected with sperm with none or one small vacuole have significantly higher rate of blastocyst formation than those with two or more small vacuoles or at least one large vacuole or an abnormal head shape.[31,32] However, some studies have not shown any advantage of IMSI over conventional ICSI in male factor infertility in the first attempt.[33] However, there is a need for more randomized controlled trials.

ASSISTED HATCHING TECHNOLOGY

Assisted hatching (AH) involves the artificial thinning or breaching of the ZP (Fig. 4) and has been proposed as an important technique to improve implantation and pregnancy rates following IVF.[34] The procedure of mechanically opening the ZP was developed in 1990 by Jacques Cohen. This resulted in increased implantation rate.[35] In vivo hatching of the embryo at the blastocyst stage is an essential step resulting in successful implantation. AH is performed prior to embryo transfer on day 3, 5, or 6 after fertilization. Several different methods for AH have been introduced. The various methods include mechanical (PZD with glass microneedles), chemical drilling with acidified Tyrode's solution, and laser.[36] Results have varied and likely reflect variations in the level of expertise in AH. In the limited trials mechanical or laser AH did not show any significant difference in CPRs and live birth rates (LBRs).[34] Laser represents an ideal method for AH as the energy is easily focused on the targeted area producing a controlled and precise opening. The most commonly used laser is the infrared 1.48 μm diode laser. We reported our first pregnancy in India using laser AH in 2000.[37]

Emerging evidence suggests that AH techniques may improve CPRs, particularly in those having poor prognosis including those with prior failed IVF cycles. However, there still remains considerable uncertainty. Meta-analysis of 36 randomized controlled trials supported the association of AH with increased clinical pregnancy and multiple pregnancy rates. However, nonsignificant outcomes were seen in the LBR and miscarriage rates and warrants further investigations. Despite long-term use of AH, there are very few clinical trials assessing the effect of AH on LBR.

Assisted hatching is not recommended routinely for all patients. It may benefit women with age more than 37 years, with elevated follicular phase follicle stimulating hormone (FSH), with previous failed IVF/ICSI cycles, with poor embryo quality and with thick ZP more than 15 μm. Most studies support the hypothesis that AH improves CPRs in these patients. However, there is insufficient evidence that AH improves LBRs in these populations.[34]

Assisted hatching may be associated with specific complications like lethal damage to the embryo, damage to the individual blastomeres, and reduction of the embryo viability, independent of the IVF procedure. A hole in the ZP may deprive the embryo of its protective coat, which shields it from the deleterious factors in the female genital tract. Blastomeres may also get trapped in the smaller holes and may fail to hatch completely. AH appears to be associated with an increased risk of multiple pregnancies, but there is insufficient evidence that it is associated with an increased risk of monozygotic twin pregnancy. AH is not associated with an increased risk of major congenital or chromosomal abnormalities. Further studies including different types of AH and other covariates like maternal age, infertility factors, and embryo quality are needed to evaluate the safety of AH and its potential impact on the offspring's long-term development.

■ CONSEQUENCES OF INTRACYTOPLASMIC SPERM INJECTION

During ICSI, since the acrosome reaction is skipped, altered sperm function may be the major important cause of failed ICSI. Male infertility can be caused by environmental factors, physical factors, or genetic factors. Currently, ICSI is commonly carried out around the world as the method for fertilizing the egg where IVF fails due to nonavailability of normal sperm.

Once ICSI was introduced, there were major concerns about the safety of this technique. The major points were use of artificially chosen spermatozoa for this invasive procedure and use of nonejaculated sperm either from the epididymis or the testis. It was observed that men with NOA may show more chromosomal aberrations, whereas with testicular sperms imprinting may be partially completed at the time of fertilization. This may not hamper fertilization and early embryonic development, but problems may occur in later postnatal life. Latham et al. suggested from their studies on mice that after fertilization, prior to syngamy, parental genomes keep on modifying.[38]

In many studies the safety of the ICSI procedure has been examined.[39,40] None of the studies showed any significant increase in major congenital malformations after use of ICSI compared to natural conception. But these studies found that there was an increased risk in sex chromosomal aneuploidies and other chromosomal aberrations. Bonduelle et al. in their follow-up study of children born using cryopreserved ICSI embryos, showed that the slight increase in chromosomal aberrations (5.8%) may be due to male factor infertility rather than the effect of the ICSI technique.[41]

In men with severe OAT or nonobstructive azoospermia, chromosomal analysis, and Y chromosome microdeletion testing should be performed. In such cases, male children conceived after ICSI will inherit the same Y chromosome deletion as their fathers.[42] In men with congenital bilateral absence of the vas deferens (CBAVD), mutations in the cystic fibrosis transmembrane conductance regulator (CFTR) gene should be looked for.[43] Some facts are:

- Chromosomal aberrations increase in oligospermia
- Risk of sex chromosomal aneuploidies is higher in azoospermia
- Robertsonian and reciprocal translocations are more frequently seen in oligozoospermia.

The ICSI/IVF children have double the risk of having major birth defects such as cardiovascular, urogenital, chromosomal, and musculoskeletal defects as compared to children conceived naturally.[44]

Devroey and Steirteghem described the results of different studies showing an increased risk of imprinting disorders in ICSI children, like Angelman syndrome, a neurogenetic disorder (1/10,000) and childhood cancers of kidney, liver or muscle due to Beckwith–Wiedemann syndrome, a human overgrowth syndrome (1/13,000). Only a few observations in the literature provide data on possible frequencies of these events. Sandin et al. in their study showed that there were significant increased risks in autistic disorders and mental retardation in the children born after ICSI using surgically extracted sperm or frozen embryos.[45] Sutcliffe et al. compared children born through ICSI, IVF, and natural conceptions in a multicentric international study and concluded that ICSI/IVF born children differ only in minor ways with bodily malformations as compared to children born naturally.[46]

Intracytoplasmic sperm injection can cause increased risk of miscarriage as low-quality sperm or sperm with fragmented DNA may be used to fertilize the egg.[47]

Transferring more than one ICSI embryo may lead to twin pregnancy in 30–35% of women and triplets or more in 5–10%. Multiple gestation may cause complications during pregnancy and at the time of delivery such as gestational diabetes, premature delivery, and increase in congenital malformations.[48,49]

■ OTHER OFF-SHOOTS OF INTRACYTOPLASMIC SPERM INJECTION

Preimplantation Genetic Testing

Preimplantation genetic testing was introduced clinically in the early 90s. Handyside et al. in 1990 were the first to describe pregnancies from biopsied human preimplantation embryos that were selected for gender by Y-specific DNA amplification in order to avoid the transmission of sex-linked disease in boys called adrenoleukodystrophy and X-linked mental retardation.[50] The first report on polar body biopsy and successful embryo transfer was by Verlinsky et al. in 1990.[51] Pregnancy after embryo biopsy and coamplification of DNA from X and Y chromosomes was reported by Grifo et al.[52] Munné et al published the first report of aneuploidy testing by fluorescence in situ hybridization (FISH).[53] The first live birth following blastocyst biopsy and preimplantation genetic diagnosis (PGD) analysis was reported in 2002 by de Boer et al.[54] The first clinical experience of preimplantation human leukocyte antigen (HLA) matching was reported by Verlinsky et al. demonstrating the feasibility of this novel approach for stem cell transplantation in siblings with bone marrow failure.[55]

We reported the first PGD live births in India after FISH for a Robertsonian translocation in 2010,[56] reciprocal translocation in 2012,[57] and an inversion in 2016.[58] We also have successfully treated couples with their chromosomal abnormalities and single gene disorders like β-thalassemia, sickle cell anemia, Leigh syndrome, Duchenne muscular dystrophy, neurofibromatosis type 1, heredity inclusion of body myopathy (HIBM), cardiac disorder, and *BRCA1* carrier state.

Our Results with ICSI and PGS-PGD

In our latest series of 112 cycles, pregnancy rates for PGT-A were 41%. Our miscarriage rate was 11%.

■ CONCLUSION

The science of assisted reproduction has moved forward by leaps and bounds. It is however imperative to study its implications so that future generations born through this technology are healthy and have their full potential of life.

KEY POINTS

- Intracytoplasmic sperm injection technology has revolutionized ART.
- It has a learning curve and needs expertise in the laboratory.
- Intracytoplasmic morphologically selected sperm injection technology is helpful to identify morphologically normal sperm for microinjection.
- Assisted hatching, IMSI, and PGT are off-shoots of ICSI and they enhance pregnancy rates in ART.
- Couples need genetic counseling prior to ICSI for severe male factor infertility and other genetic conditions.

REFERENCES

1. Steptoe PC, Edwards RG. Birth after the reimplantation of a human embryo. Lancet. 1978;12(2):366.
2. Heape W. Preliminary note on the transplantation and growth of mammalian ova within a uterine foster-mother. Proc R Soc Lond B Biol Sci. 1890;48:457-8.
3. Trounson AO, Leeton JF, Wood C, et al. Pregnancies in humans by fertilization in vitro and embryo transfer in the controlled ovulatory cycle. Science. 1981;212:681-2.
4. Binor Z, Joseph E, Sokoloski JE, et al. Penetration of the Zona-Free Hamster Egg by Human Sperm. Fertil Steril. 1980;33(3):321-7.
5. Hiramoto Y. Microinjection of the live spermatozoa into sea urchin eggs. Exp Cell Res. 1962;27:416-26.
6. Lin TP. Microinjection of mouse eggs. Science. 1966;151:333-7.
7. Gordon JW, Talansky BE. Assisted fertilization by zona drilling: A mouse model for correction of oligospermia. J Expl Zoo. 1986;239(3):347-54.
8. Gordon JW, Grunfeld L, Garrisi GJ, et al. Fertilization of human oocytes by sperm from infertile males after zona pellucida drilling. Fertil Steril. 1988;50(1):68-73.
9. Ng SC, Bongso TA, Chang SI, et al. Transfer of human sperm into the perivitelline space of human oocytes after zona-drilling or zona-puncture. Fertil Steril. 1989;52(1):73-8.
10. Laws-King, Trounson A, Sathananthan AH, et al. Fertilization of human oocytes by microinjection of a single spermatozoon under the zona pellucida. Fertil Steril. 1987;48:637.
11. Cohen J. Assisted hatching of human embryos. J In Vitro Fertil Embryo Transf. 1991;8:179-90.
12. Lanzendorf SE, Maloney MK, Veeck LL, et al. A preclinical evaluation of pronuclear formation by microinjection of human spermatozoa into human oocytes. Fertil Steril. 1988;49(5):835-42.
13. Palermo G, Joris H, Devroey P, et al. Pregnancies after intracytoplasmic injection of single spermatozoon into an oocyte. Lancet. 1992;340:17-8.
14. Parikh FR, Kodwaney G, Kamat S, et al. Successful human micromanipulation with subzonal sperm insemination and intracytoplasmic sperm injection. J Obstet Gynaecol India. 1994;44(3):458-63.

15. Tournaye H. Management of male infertility by assisted reproductive technologies. Baillieres Best Pract Res Clin Endocrinol Metab. 2000;14(3):423-35.
16. Oehninger S. Strategies for the infertile men. Semin Reprod Med. 2001t;19(3):231-7.
17. Fishel S, Aslam I, Tesarik J. Spermatid conception: A stage too early, or a time too soon? Hum Reprod. 1996;11:1371-5.
18. Sofikitis NY, Yamamoto I, Miyagawa I, et al. Ooplasmic injection of elongating spermatids for the treatment of non-obstructive azoospermia. Hum Reprod. 1998;13:709-14.
19. Parikh FR, Kamat SA, Nadkarni S, et al. Successful pregnancy from testicular sperm obtained from cryptorchid testis having undergone orchiopexy. Ind J Urol. 1997;13:97-8.
20. Parikh FR, Kamat SA, Shah R, et al. Successful pregnancy following Intracytoplasmic sperm injection using electroejaculated spermatozoa from a man with paraplegia. Indian J Urol. 1998.
21. Kamat SA, Kodwaney G, Chitale AR, et al. Pregnancy and birth after intracytoplasmic sperm injection with immotile spermatozoa from a patient with the immotile cilia syndrome: a case Report. Indian J Urol. 1998;69-71.
22. Kashir J, Heindryckx B, Jones C, et al. Oocyte activation, phospholipase C zeta and human infertility. Hum Reprod Update. 2010;16(6):690-703.
23. Eichenlaub-Ritter U, Schmiady H, Kentenich H, et al. Recurrent failure in polar body formation and premature chromosome condensation in oocytes from a human patient: indicators of asynchrony in nuclear and cytoplasmic maturation. Hum Reprod. 1995;10:2343-9.
24. Nijs M, Vanderzwalmen P, Vandamme B, et al. Fertility ability of immotile spermatozoa after intracytoplasmic sperm injection. Hum Reprod. 1996;11:2180-5.
25. Flaherty SP, Payue D, Swann NJ, et al. Aeitiology of failed & abnormal fertilization after Intracytoplasmic Sperm Injection. Hum Reprod. 1995;10:2623-9.
26. Sousa M, Tesarik J. Ultrastructural analysis of fertilization failure after intracytoplasmic sperm injection. Hum Reprod. 1994;9:2374-80.
27. Cassuto NG, Bouret D, Plouchart JM, et al. A new real-time morphology classification for human spermatozoa: a link for fertilization and improved embryo quality. Fertil Steril. 2009:92:1616-25.
28. Bartoov B, Berkovitz A, Eltes F. Selection of spermatozoa with normal nuclei to improve the pregnancy rate with intracytoplasmic sperm injection. N Engl J Med. 2001;345(14):1067-8.
29. Bartoov B, Berkovitz A, Eltes F, et al. Pregnancy rates are higher with intracytoplasmic morphologically selected sperm injection than with conventional intracytoplasmic injection. Fertil Steril. 2003;80:1413-9.
30. Fekonja N, Štrus J, Žnidarič MT, et al. Clinical and structural features of sperm head vacuoles in men included in the in vitro fertilization programme. Biomed Res Int. 2014;2014:927841.
31. Hyung JK, Hye JY, Jung MJ, et al. Comparison between intracytoplasmic sperm injection and intracytoplasmic morphologically selected sperm injection in oligoastheno teratozoospermia patients. Clin Exp Reprod Med. 2014;41(1):9-14.

32. Laïla EK, Charlotte D, Nathalie S, et al. Is intracytoplasmic morphologically selected sperm injection effective in patients with infertility related to teratozoospermia or repeated implantation failure? Fertil Steril. 2013;100(1):62-8.
33. Leandri RD, Gachet A, Pfeffer J, et al. Is intracytoplasmic morphologically selected sperm injection (IMSI) beneficial in the first ART cycle? A multicentric randomized controlled trial. Andrology. 2013;1:692-7.
34. Practice Committee of the American Society for Reproductive Medicine, Practice committee of the Society for Assisted Reproductive Technology. Role of assisted hatching in in vitro fertilization: a guideline. Fertil Steril. 2014;102(2):348-51.
35. Cohen J, Elsner C, Kort H, et al. Impairment of the hatching process following IVF in the human and improvement of implantation by assisted hatching using micromanipulation. Hum Reprod. 1990;5:7-13.
36. Obruca A, Strohmer H, Sakkas D, et al. Use of lasers in assisted fertilization and hatching. Hum Reprod. 1994;9:1723-6.
37. Parikh FR, Nadkarni S, Naik N, et al. Laser assisted embryo hatching—A ray of hope for the infertile. J Obstet Gynaecol India. 2000;50(6):98-9.
38. Latham KE, Rambhatla L. Expression of X-linked genes in androgenetic, gynogenetic, and normal mouse preimplantation embryos. Dev Genet. 1995;17(3):212-22.
39. Van Steirteghem AC, Nagy Z, Joris H, et al. High fertilization and implantation rates after intracytoplasmic sperm injection. Hum Reprod. 1993;8(7):1061-6.
40. Devroey P, Liu J, Nagy Z, et al. Pregnancies after testicular sperm extraction and intracytoplasmic sperm injection in non-obstructive azoospermia. Hum Reprod. 1995;10:1457-60.
41. Bonduelle M, Wilikens A, Buysse A, et al. A follow-up study of children born after intracytoplasmic sperm injection (ICSI) with epididymal and testicular spermatozoa and after replacement of cryopreserved embryos obtained after ICSI. Hum Reprod. 1998;13(1):196-207.
42. Kent-First MG, Kol S, Muallem A, et al. The incidence and possible relevance of Y-linked microdeletions in babies born after intracytoplasmic sperm injection and their infertile fathers. Mol Hum Reprod. 1996;2:943-50.
43. Lu S, Cui Y, Li X, et al. Association of cystic fibrosis transmembrane-conductance regulator gene mutation with negative outcome of intracytoplasmic sperm injection pregnancy in cases of congenital bilateral absence of vas deferens. Fertil Steril. 2014;101(5):1255-60.
44. Hansen M, Kurinczuk JJ, Bower C, et al. The risk of major birth defects after intracytoplasmic sperm injection and in vitro fertilization. N Engl J Med. 2002;346(10):725-30.
45. Sandin S, Nygren KG, Iliadou A, et al. Autism and mental retardation among offspring born after in vitro fertilization. JAMA. 2013;310(1):75-84.
46. Sutcliffe A, Loft A, Wennerholm UB, et al. International collaborative study of ICSI-child and family outcomes–physical development at 5 years. Madrid: 19th Annual Meeting of the EHSRE; 2003. pp. 97-98.

47. Steward RG, Zhang CE, Shah AA, et al. High Peak estradiol predicts higher miscarriage and lower live birth rates in high responders triggered with a GnRH agonist in IVF/ICSI Cycles. J Reprod Med. 2015;60(11-12):463-70.
48. Svobodová M, Brezinová J, Oborná I, et al. Prevention of multiple pregnancy after IVF/ICSI by elective single embryo transfer pilot study. Ceska Gynekol. 2005;70(4):343-7.
49. Zhu L, Zhang Y, Liu Y, et al. Maternal and live-birth outcomes of pregnancies following assisted reproductive technology: a retrospective cohort study. Sci Rep. 2016;6:35141.
50. Handyside AH, Kontogianni EH, Hardy K, et al. Pregnancies from biopsied human preimplantation embryos sexed by Y-specific DNA amplification. Nature. 1990;344(6268):768-70.
51. Verlinsky Y, Ginsberg N, Lifchez A, et al. Analysis of the first polar body: preconception genetic diagnosis. Hum Reprod. 1990;5:826-9.
52. Grifo JA, Tang YX, Cohen J, et al. Pregnancy after embryo biopsy and coamplification of DNA from X and Y chromosomes. JAMA. 1992;268:727-9.
53. Munné S, Dailey T, Sultan KM, et al. The use of first polar bodies for preimplantation diagnosis of aneuploidy. Hum Reprod. 1995;10(4):1014-20.
54. de Boer KA, McArthur S, Murray C, et al. First live birth following blastocyst biopsy and PGD analysis. Reprod Biomed online. 2002;4:35.
55. Verlinsky Y, Rechitsky S, Schoolcraft W, et al. Preimplantation diagnosis for Fanconi anemia combined with HLA matching. JAMA. 2001;285(24):3130-3.
56. Madon PF, Athalye AS, Naik NJ, et al. PGD for a Robertsonian translocation by FISH: first successful pregnancy from India. J Prenat Dig Ther. 2010;1(1):20-2.
57. Madon PF, Naik NJ, Athalye AS, et al. PGD by FISH in India: first live birth after PGD for a reciprocal translocation. Reprod Biomed Online. 2012;24(2):15-51.
58. Sanap RR, Athalye AS, Madon PF, et al. First successful pregnancy by pre-implantation genetic diagnosis by FISH for an inversion together with a cryptic translocation in India. J Fetal Med. 2016;3:25-30.

CHAPTER 14

Intracytoplasmic Morphologically Selected Sperm Injection

Sudesh A Kamat, Hrishikesh Pai

■ INTRODUCTION

In conventional in vitro fertilization (IVF), the zona pellucida functions as biological barrier against abnormal sperm, so that in most cases only "normal" sperm is able to fertilize an oocyte. Since intracytoplasmic sperm injection (ICSI) bypasses the natural sperm selection process, there is an increased risk of genetic abnormalities being transmitted to the offspring. Hence, several sperm selection methods have been developed to select the most normal spermatozoa, prominent among which is the intracytoplasmic morphologically selected sperm injection (IMSI) technique.

Intracytoplasmic sperm injection is normally performed at a 200–400X magnification which enables the observation of major sperm morphological defects, such as head abnormalities (round, tapering, etc.), midpiece defects (bent neck, thick mid piece), tail defects (short stubby, double) whereas minor morphological defects, such as vacuoles in the sperm head, which seem to be related to the ICSI outcome are not identified (Figs. 1A and B).

The IMSI technique, developed by Bartoov et al.[1,2] is the new modified version of ICSI, wherein the sperms are magnified to about 6,600 times and subjected to the Motile Sperm Organelle Morphology Examination (MSOME criteria) in order to select the most morphologically normal sperm prior to performing the ICSI procedure. *IMSI is performed with an inverted light microscope equipped with high-power Nomarski optics enhanced by digital imaging to achieve a magnification of 6,600X.* Using IMSI, the spermatozoon can be evaluated for fine integrity of its nucleus and the injection of a normal spermatozoon with a vacuole-free head can be assured (Figs. 2A and B).

■ IMSI EQUIPMENT

The apparatus used for sperm evaluation comprises of:
- Inverted microscope (micromanipulator)
- Nomarski differential interference contrast (DIC) system

Intracytoplasmic Morphologically Selected Sperm Injection

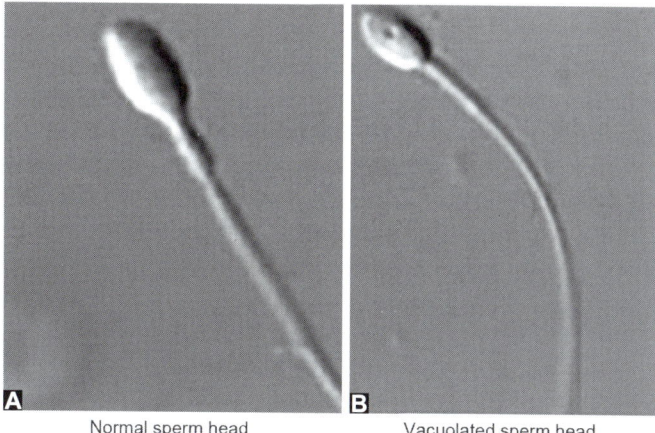

Figs. 1A and B: Difference between head of a normal sperm and vacuolated sperm.

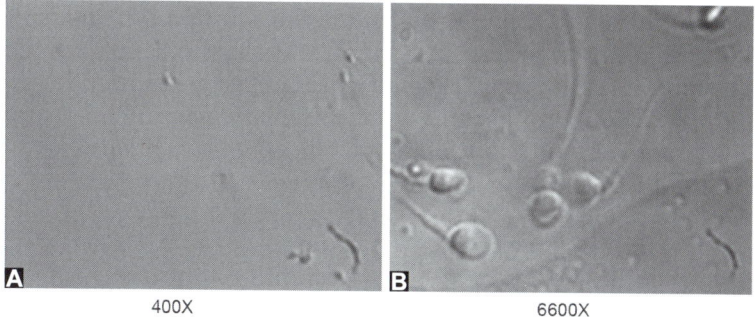

Figs. 2A and B: Regular (ICSI) versus ultra-high magnification (IMSI) sperm selection.

- Images are captured by a three-charge-coupled device (CCD) video camera
- Monitor screen.

Once assembled, the equipment is capable of high magnification over 6,600X, required to achieve a detailed visualization of the sperm subcellular organelles.

In 2007, OCTAX, Microscience GmbH showed the first oil-free IMSI system called *Cytoscreen*. This system was able to significantly improve image quality and at the same time target the practical needs of the embryologist, offering a system which could work without DIC and oil immersion.

CALCULATION OF MAGNIFICATION

Calculation of the "total reached magnification" may vary depending upon the system components, but usually it is as follows:

Microscope magnification (100X objective magnification × 1.5X magnification selector)
- Video coupler magnification (1X)
- Video magnification (CCD × monitor diagonal dimension) (44.45X)

$$\text{Total magnification} = 100 \times 1.5 \times 1 \times 44.45 = 6{,}600X$$

■ MSOME CRITERIA FOR IMSI

The MSOME criteria are based on a morphological analysis of isolated motile spermatozoa in real-time at high magnification (up to 6,600X). MSOME is able to identify not only conventional morphological sperm alterations with a definition close to that of SEM, but also more specifically sperm head vacuoles, considered by Bartoov et al.[1,2] as nuclear defects. The MSOME method has been combined with the ICSI technique, giving rise to IMSI.

MSOME criteria are applied exclusively to the motile spermatozoa fraction. Moreover, sperm cells with severe malformations that are already evident at low magnification are excluded because they are not routinely used for microinjection. Each sperm cell is evaluated according to the morphological status of six subcellular organelles comprising the acrosome, post-acrosomal lamina, neck, mitochondria, tail and nucleus. Nuclear normality appeared to be the most important parameter to influence fertilization and pregnancy rates whereas other morphological characteristics of spermatozoa (acrosome, post-acrosomal lamina, neck, mitochondria and tail) examined did not seem to influence the final ICSI outcome.

As per the MSOME criteria, a spermatozoa is classified as morphologically normal when the sperm head exhibits a normal nucleus shape (smooth, symmetric and oval nucleus) and chromatin content (homogeneity of the chromatin mass containing no extrusion or invagination of nuclear chromatin). The criterion for normality of chromatin content is the absence of vacuoles occupying more than 4% of the sperm nuclear area. The average length and width limits are estimated to be 4.75 ± 0.28 and 3.28 ± 0.20 μm.

■ IMSI DISH PREPARATION

In order to achieve the best optical quality, at high magnification, a glass bottom Petri dish (Willco-dish; Willco wells BV, Amsterdam, The Netherlands) is used for IMSI and is prepared as follows:
1. In the center, three 5 μL observation droplets of polyvinyl pyrrolidone medium (7% PVP) are made.
2. Surrounding the PVP drops are 7 μL drops of HEPES buffered medium to host the oocytes that are to be injected with the selected sperm.
3. The droplets are overlaid with sterile liquid paraffin oil.

The sperm cell suspension obtained after semen preparation is used for *real-time* high magnification MSOME that is performed on the observation droplets by means of a Narishige micromanipulator, with attached inverted microscope (Nikon Eclipse, TE2000S, Tokyo, Japan). The images are captured by a high definition USB2.0 camera 3 MPx and visualized on a monitor screen with diagonal dimension of 42 cm.

■ MODIFIED IMSI TECHNIQUE

Morphology analysis mainly involves three elements such as the absence of sperm head vacuoles; sperm head size and head shape. Selection of sperm according to these standards will take between 30 minutes to 120 minutes. In order to minimize the time taken to perform the IMSI procedure, the Bloom IVF center, Mumbai has modified the IMSI procedure. Two embryologists work together for analyzing the sperms to minimize the chances of human error. 20–30 morphologically normal motile sperm are selected and immobilized at 200X magnification. Sperms with obvious defects like pin head, amorphous head, large mid-piece, double tail/head are not evaluated. To minimize the oocyte exposure outside the incubator, the IMSI dish contains only the spermatozoa and not the oocytes. The selected sperms are placed in a row one below the other in the microscopic field. They are then magnified real time (6,000X), and then an image is clicked. With the help of the computer program, the measurement of the image of the sperm head is performed. The selected spermatozoa are subjected to the MSOME criteria, the length and breadth of the sperm head is measured. Sperm which fulfill the MSOME criteria are magnified further to 6,600X and evaluated for presence of vacuoles. The spermatozoa are graded into four groups according to the presence and size of the vacuoles: (1) grade I, no vacuole; (2) grade II, a maximum of two small vacuoles (<4% head surface); (3) grade III, at least one large vacuole; and (4) grade IV, a large vacuole and abnormal head shapes or other abnormalities.[3] The morphologically normal sperm, free of vacuoles are separated out, the oocytes are loaded into the IMSI dish, and ICSI is performed at 200X.

INDICATIONS FOR IMSI

Following are the conditions that can be successfully treated using the IMSI sperm selection technique:
- Severe male factor infertility cases such as teratozoospermia, severe oligoasthenoteratozoospermia.
- Aging male.
- Patients with high degree of sperm DNA fragmentation rate.
- Couples with previous conventional ICSI failures.
- Repeated poor quality embryo development rate after ICSI cycle.
- Unexplained infertility who failed in previous IVF attempts.
- Surgically retrieved sperm from testis especially micro-TESE.
- Recurring abortion in the first trimester with MSOME showing nuclear defects.

SPERM MORPHOLOGY AND VACUOLES

Sperm morphology has been recognized to have an impact on fertilization in IVF treatments. Presence of nuclear vacuoles is associated with decreased fertility potential.[4] Several studies have shown that high magnification selection of morphologically normal motile spermatozoa, free of head vacuoles, is positively associated with increased pregnancy rates in couples with previous and repeated implantation failures[5,6] suggesting that vacuolization reflects some underlying chromosomal DNA defects. Several studies have reported lower miscarriage rate in the IMSI group,[7-9] others have reported that the IMSI procedure improved laboratory and clinical outcomes without compromising the aneuploidy rate when compared to the classical ICSI procedure.[10,11]

Garolla et al. demonstrated that sperm with vacuoles were related to the integrity of sperm DNA fragmentation, and abnormal chromosomes.[12] Recently, Hammoud et al. noted that the presence of large or multiple vacuoles was associated with a higher amount of DNA fragmentation in sperm than that which lacked vacuoles.[13] A recent study has demonstrated that morphologically normal spermatozoa, with an absence of vacuolization, selected using IMSI, is free of DNA damage, thereby establishing a direct relationship between a good morphological pattern on the sperm and a good DNA quality. Furthermore, results showed spermatozoa presenting a normal morphology and no traces of vacuolization to be fully free of DNA damage. However, traces of vacuolization and more severe morphological alterations were accompanied by significant increases in the proportion of sperm containing a damaged DNA molecule.[14]

In a major study 1,891 IVF-ICSI cycles were compared with 577 IVF-IMSI cycles. In first IVF cycles, either technique was equally effective in producing pregnancies and life births so first cycles saw no difference. However, in second cycles after the first ICSI cycle failed, using IMSI to identify normal sperm showed a better pregnancy rate (56% vs 38% PRs) and delivery rates (28% vs 18%) in the IMSI group.[15]

In another study, fertilization rate, embryo development, implantation, pregnancy and abortion rates were compared. With IMSI, there were more blastocysts per cycle than in the ICSI group at day 5 and fewer cycles with arrested embryos, suggesting that better embryo quality was achieved with use of high power morphological selection.[16] There was a trend toward higher implantation and pregnancy rates, although the results were not statistically significant.

In a retrospective study conducted at Bloom IVF Center, Mumbai, it was observed that in cases of recurrent implantation failures, there was a significantly higher implantation and pregnancy rate in the IMSI group as compared to the ICSI group.[17]

■ CONCLUSION

Among the different malformations identified by MSOME, those affecting sperm nuclear structure, such as large vacuoles, have been demonstrated to be correlated to male reproductive impairment. Current literature agrees on the presence of higher decondensed DNA levels corresponding to vacuolated regions. Although, IMSI is not an effective frontline treatment for all patients, it does allow *real-time* selection of the best available morphologically normal motile spermatozoa before oocyte injection. Only extensive use and availability of large amount of data will help us understand the feasibility, effectiveness and safety of the IMSI technique.

REFERENCES

1. Bartoov B, Berkovitz A, Eltes F. Selection of spermatozoa with normal nuclei to improve the pregnancy rate with intracytoplasmic sperm injection. N Engl J Med. 2001;345:1067-8.
2. Bartoov B, Berkovitz A, Eltes F, et al. Real-time fine morphology of motile human sperm cells is associated with IVF-ICSI outcome. J Androl. 2002;23:1-8.
3. Vanderzwalmen P, Hiemer A, Rubner P, et al. Blastocyst development after sperm selection at high magnification is associated with size and number of nuclear vacuoles. Reprod Biomed Online. 2008;17:617-27.
4. Bartoov B, Berkovitz A, Eltes F, et al. Pregnancy rates are higher with intracytoplasmic morphologically selected sperm injection than with conventional intracytoplasmic injection. Fertil Steril. 2003;80:1413-9.
5. Berkovitz A, Eltes F, Lederman H, et al. How to improve IVF-ICSI outcome by sperm selection. Reprod Biomed Online. 2006;12:634-8.
6. Hazout A, Dumont-Hassan M, Junca AM, et al. High-magnification ICSI overcomes paternal effect resistant to conventional ICSI. Reprod Biomed Online. 2006; 12:19-25.
7. Souza Setti A, Ferreira RC, Paes de Almeida Ferreira Braga D, et al. Intracytoplasmic sperm injection outcome versus intracytoplasmic morphologically selected sperm injection outcome: a meta-analysis. Reprod Biomed Online. 2010;21:450-5.
8. Balaban B, Yakin K, Alatas C, et al. Clinical outcome od intracytoplasmatic injection of spermatozoa morphologically selected under hogh magnification: a prospective randomized study. Reprod Biomed Online. 2011;22:472-6.
9. Antinori M, Licata E, Dani G, et al. Intracytoplasmic morphologically selected sperm injection: a prospective randomized trial. Reprod Biomed Online. 2008;16:835-41.
10. Figueira Rde C, Braga DP, Setti AS, et al. Morphological nuclear integrity of sperm cells is associated with preimplantation genetic aneuploidy screening cycle outcomes. Fertil Steril. 2011;95:990-3.
11. Luna D, Hilario R, Dueñas-Chacón J, et al. The IMSI procedure improves laboratory and clinical outcomes without compromising the aneuploidy rate when compared to the classical ICSI procedure. Clin Med Insights Reprod Health. 2015;9:29-37.
12. Garolla A, Fortini D, Menegazzo M, et al. High-power microscopy for selecting spermatozoa for ICSI by physiological status. Reprod Biomed Online. 2008;17:6106.
13. Hammoud HC, Albert MF, Vialard F, et al. Can IMSI be efficient in situation of ICSI failure and teratospermy, with special study of macrocephaly? Fertil Steril. 2008;90:192.
14. Gosálvez J, Migueles B, López-Fernández C, et al. Single sperm selection and DNA fragmentation analysis: The case of MSOME/IMSI. Natural Science Vol.5 No.7A(2013)

15. Klement AH, Koren-Morag N, Itsykson P, et al. Intracytoplasmic morphologically selected sperm injection versus intracytoplasmic sperm injection: a step toward a clinical algorithm. Fertil Steril. 2013;99(5):1290-3.
16. Knez K, Zorn B, Tomazevic T, et al. The IMSI procedure improves poor embryo development in the same infertile couples with poor semen quality: a comparative prospective randomized study. Reprod Biol Endocrinol. 2011;9:123.
17. Dalal R, Pai H, Palshetkar N, et al. Intracytoplasmic morphologically selected sperm injection vs intracytoplasmic sperm injection: a retrospective analysis. Int J Infertil Fetal Med. 2011;2(3):1-9.

CHAPTER
15

Male Sexual Dysfunction

Milind R Shah, Kunal A Doshi

■ INTRODUCTION

Assessing sexual function of couple is a real task and one needs to spend several hours in sexual history and has to gain confidence of couple to elicit any dysfunction. Especially when it comes to males, they are always shy and consider it inferior to tell about their sexual problems. Its clinician's acumen to elicit these problems tactfully to decide on further management. Else, many of them land up in either donor sperm program or intracytoplasmic sperm injection (ICSI) with various sperm retrieval techniques. But, it is quite often a rewarding experience if clinician is able to detect male sexual dysfunction and manages it well to get pregnancy in that couple. It is not only pregnancy but it also saves marriages getting broken due to misconceptions and inability to detect and treat these male dysfunction issues. While research suggests that sexual dysfunction is common (43% of women and 31% of men report some degree of difficulty), it is a topic that many couple are hesitant to discuss. Fortunately, most cases of sexual dysfunction are treatable, so it is important on couple's part to share their concerns with each other and doctor.[1]

A sexual problem, or sexual dysfunction, refers to a problem during any phase of the sexual response cycle that prevents the man or couple from experiencing satisfaction from the activity. The sexual response cycle has four phases—(1) excitement; (2) plateau; (3) orgasm; and (4) resolution.

Sexual disorders in men are categorized according to their occurrence in the cycle of sexual response into disorders of desire, arousal (erectile dysfunction), or orgasm (premature or delayed ejaculation, or anorgasmia), albeit with considerable potential for overlap and concurrence between these disorder groups.

A wealth of information is presented on erectile dysfunction, its development through time, and its correlates. The field is still in need of more epidemiological studies on the men's sexual dysfunction.[2]

■ CAUSES OF MALE SEXUAL DYSFUNCTION

Sexual activity involves coordination between various systems of the body. Hormones and neurological pathways must be in sync for sexual desire to be present. Blood vessels, nerves, and penile integrity must all be present for an adequate erection and its maintenance during the sexual relation. Muscles and nerves coordinate ejaculation achieved, when the physiological passageway for sperm that is from the testicles to the urethra is present. Orgasm is a complex phenomenon that is not completely understood but it involves the coordination of muscles and nerves. When sexual dysfunction is present, the physician must evaluate all the possible problems in this chain of events (Fig. 1).[3]

Sexual dysfunction in men can be a result of a physical or psychological problem:

- *Physical causes*: Many physical and medical conditions can cause problems with sexual function. These conditions include diabetes, heart and vascular disease, neurological disorders, hormonal imbalances, chronic diseases such as kidney or liver failure, and alcoholism and drug abuse. In addition, the side effects of certain medications, including some antidepressant drugs, can affect sexual desire and function.
- *Psychological causes*: These include work-related stress and anxiety, lack of time, concern about sexual performance, marital or relationship problems, depression, feelings of guilt, and the effects of a past sexual trauma.[4]

It is very important to take detailed history and good physical examination to clinch the diagnosis. Multidisciplinary approach with the help of dedicated andrologists, urologists, or psychologists can help for this exercise.

In India, in approximately 1% of infertile couples with male factor, there are factors other than seminal abnormalities. Commonly seen problems in males leading to infertility are:

- No consummation of marriage
- Ejaculatory disturbances
- Erectile dysfunction.

Extensive research results from the last 15 years and the introduction of selective phosphodiesterase type-5 (PDE5) inhibitors have led to changes

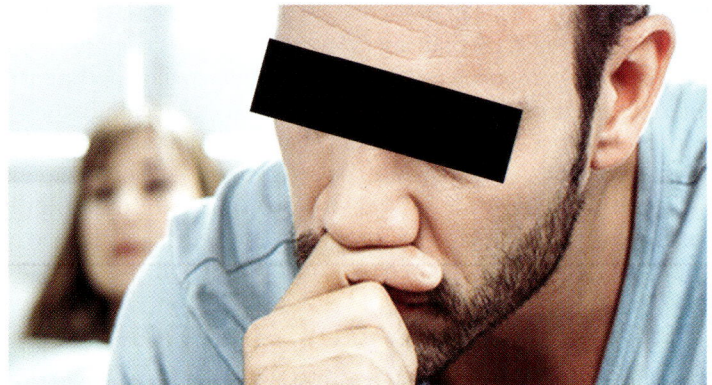

Fig. 1: Male sexual dysfunction.

in the diagnostics and treatment of male sexual dysfunction. Invasive investigation is now almost obsolete. Medication is introduced early. Success is measured in terms of function, which in turn is measured using questionnaire instruments such as the International Index of Erectile Function (IIEF), its short version (IIEF-5), or the Cologne Erectile Dysfunction Questionnaire (Kölner Erfassungsbogen der Erektilen Dysfunktion, KEED).[5] The spectrum of sexual dysfunction is wide ranging, and inadequately captured by the International Classification of Diseases (ICD)-10 and Diagnostic and Statistical Manual, Fourth Edition (DSM-IV) classifications. In addition to functional sexual disorders, which may or may not be associated with organic pathology, disorders of sexual development, gender identity, sexual preference (paraphilia) and sexual behavior can occur in men.

No Consummation of Marriage

The main factor associated with an unconsummated marriage is the intense social pressure to accomplish hasty sexual activity with an unfamiliar woman and in the presence of relatives waiting nearby for evidence of the bride's virginity and confirmation of sexual act. This initial problem will then be further compounded with resultant erectile failure caused by anxiety about sexual performance. These are very common in India due to lack of sexual knowledge in adolescents or sometimes few myths, which are commonly spread by peers of those boys. We have seen occasionally couples with total ignorance of penetration act and feel that just rubbing on thighs is sexual act. Extreme end of this could be when it lands up in crime of even killing female partner to avoid revealing this problem in society.

Inability to consummate marriage is caused by:
- Premature ejaculation (PE) in 23%
- Erectile dysfunction in 61%
- Combination in 16%.

Tests for diagnosing for erectile dysfunction are:
- *Combined injection and stimulation test or pharmacotesting*: It consists of intracavernous injection and visual rating of the subsequent erection. It is simple, minimally invasive, and performed without monitoring equipment.
- *Blood flow studies*: Inefficient penile blood flow and inefficient corporal veno-occlusion is implicated in up to 30%. Duplex ultrasound, which measures penile blood flow, provides an objective minimally invasive evaluation of arterial pattern in a suboptimal or equivocal erectile response.
- *Neurological assessment*: Sacral reflex arc of erection consists of somatosensory afferents via the dorsal and pudendal nerves and autonomic efferent via the pelvic and cavernous nerves.

Erectile dysfunction evaluation is based on clinical judgment and not all these tests may be necessary for evaluation. Most cases respond to medications and good counseling.

Ejaculatory Disturbances

Due to underlying conditions so simple such as undiagnosed diabetes, or problem with erection such as that might be caused by a significant smoking history, severe hypercholesterolemia or to the further extent of hypogonadism.

Ejaculatory disorders include:
- Premature ejaculation
- Retrograde ejaculation
- Anejaculation
- Deficient or retarded ejaculation.

Premature Ejaculation

Premature ejaculation is the most common form of sexual dysfunction in men. It is defined as the persistent or repeated occurrence of ejaculation before, during, or shortly after penetration, over which the individual has little or no control and not accompanied by a feeling of orgasmic satisfaction. Around 20–25% of surveyed adult men in modern industrialized nations report PE associated with distress. In seeking to present valid prevalence data, one encounters two problems: On the one hand, the normal interval between penetration and ejaculation is to a large extent a subjective judgment, and subject to wide individual and cultural variation; and on the other hand, this is an area in which it is particularly clear that biological dysfunction is not synonymous with a clinically relevant disorder (Fig. 2).

No strict time parameters have been defined, but an intravaginal ejaculatory latency time (IELT), that is, penetration to ejaculation of less than 2 minutes is generally accepted as defining PE.[6] Use of this broad definition has contributed to the large range in prevalence, from 5–30%. New definitions for PE are being considered for the DSM-V and ICD-11. PE can be divided into—primary PE, which begins when the patient becomes sexually active, and secondary PE, which is acquired later in life. Additional subclasses include global and situational PE. Global PE is present in all circumstances, whereas situational

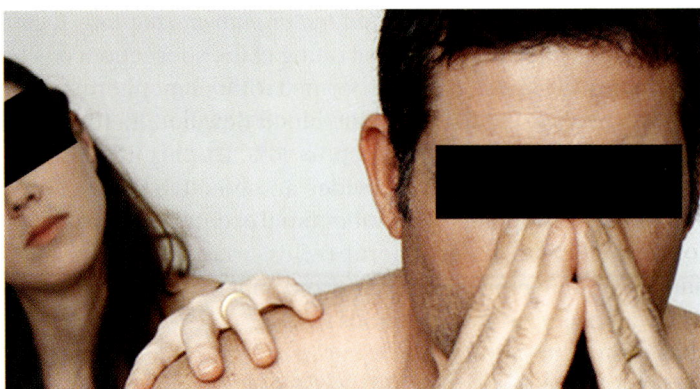

Fig. 2: Premature ejaculation.

PE occurs only with certain partners and situations. This itself emphasizes its psychological component.

Deficiency in ejaculation appears to be caused by sympathetic motor pudendal or suprasacral lesion. With proper assessment and identification, a specific diagnosis of PE can be made and accurate treatment designed. Commonly used medications are fluoxetine, paroxetine and clomipramine, either singly or in combination.

Retrograde Ejaculation

It can be described as an escape of seminal fluid from the posterior urethra into the bladder. The etiology may be anatomic, neurogenic, pharmacologic or idiopathic. It is suspected in any case of persistent low ejaculate volume (<1.5 mL), absent ejaculate or rarely in cases of azoospermia. Typical history of male getting orgasm without obvious semen seen coming out of urethra clinch the diagnosis.

But, investigations which will aid in the diagnosis are:
- Demonstration of sperm in the post masturbation urine
- Analysis of the ejaculate
- Ultrasonographic (abdominal and transrectal) examination of the genital organs.

Principles of management of retrograde ejaculation:
- Conversion of retrograde to antegrade ejaculation by drug therapy
- Harvesting those sperm from post ejaculatory urine or using it for assisted reproductive technology (ART)
- Surgical treatment.

Medical therapy includes agents like ephedrine, pseudoephedrine, imipramine and phenylpropanolamine. When pharmacologic attempts fail, the spermatozoa should be recovered from post ejaculation urine. The successful recovery of viable spermatozoa from the urine is dependent upon careful regulation of pH and osmolarity of the urine at the time of ejaculation.

Anejaculation

Inability of a man to have an ejaculation is not very uncommon in infertility practice, which could be due to variety of causes like as a result of spinal cord injury, retroperitoneal lymph node dissection, or other retroperitoneal surgeries, diabetes mellitus, transverse myelitis or multiple sclerosis.

Treatment generally is by vibratory stimulation and electroejaculation. Many of so-called participants of donor sperm program could achieve pregnancy with their own sperms with the use of vibrators.

Retarded Ejaculation

It is a persistent difficulty or inability to ejaculate despite the presence of adequate sexual desire, erection and stimulation.

Erectile Dysfunction (Fig. 3)

Virtually, every male can regain sexual function, if he chooses. The silent suffering experienced by over 50% of males can come to an end with a wide spectrum of treatment forms from well-known means like Viagra to not so commonly used implants.

The prevalence of erectile dysfunction has been well researched. The Massachusetts Male Aging Study (MMAS) (Feldman, et al. 1994) found minimal erectile dysfunction in 17% of the 40–70 years old respondents, moderate erectile dysfunction in 25%, and complete erectile failure in 10%. Braun and colleagues (2000) found erectile dysfunction in 19.2% of their 4,489 respondents over 30 years, although the authors demonstrated that not all participants with erectile dysfunction reported distress.

Sexual dysfunction can also be due to drugs like antihypertensives, antipsychotics, and antidepressants, but reaching root cause is the skill of treating infertility specialist or andrologist. Erectile dysfunction is generally regarded in the literature primarily as a vascular disorder, acting as a first sign of generalized atherosclerosis. The view of this disorder has changed from an almost entirely psychogenic to an organically dominated, multifactorial etiology. A large proportion of studies on male sexual dysfunction is directed at the effects of pharmacological treatment on desire, erection and ejaculation, and remains purely at the level of the functional disorder. The discovery of highly effective oral medications by the pharmaceutical industry has quite literally created a "potent" new market. It is true that the predominantly somatically focused literature alludes in general terms to the role played by psychological and relational factors, and consensus statements emphasize the importance of a full sexual history taking into account the relationship. In clinical practice, however, the norm is to focus in a shorthand way on "functional repair," marginalizing or completely neglecting psychosocial relationship aspects. There may be underlying cause like a condition called Peyronie's disease (scar tissue in the penis) also can cause erectile dysfunction.[7]

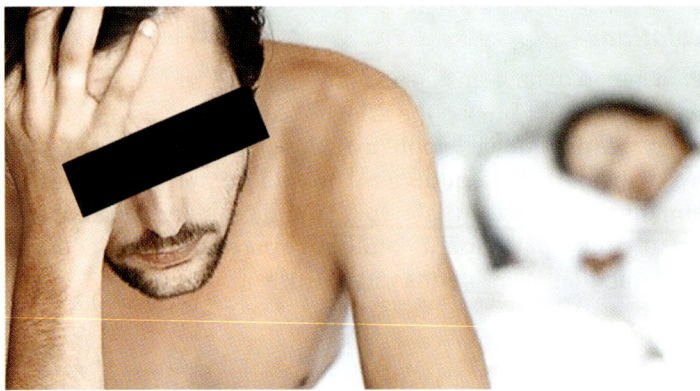

Fig. 3: Erectile dysfunction.

Though underlying cause is not known exactly, it could be because of possible causes of plaque or scar formation in the penile shaft like vitamin E deficiency, beta-blocking drugs, elevation in serotonin levels, genetic causes and trauma to the penis. Obesity is one of the commonly found but not well-addressed causes of erectile dysfunction.[8]

Erectile dysfunction can broadly be classified as organic, psychogenic or mixed.

Two most common risk factors for organic erectile dysfunction are aging and diabetes.

There is a growing recognition that erectile dysfunction is an important marker of vascular disease. A recent study by Sun et al. showed that erectile dysfunction was a significant marker for diabetes particularly in younger patients. Men 45 years old or younger with erectile dysfunction were more than twice as likely to have diabetes as men without erectile dysfunction.

Thus, markers of erectile dysfunction may represent an early warning for the development of diabetes which is particularly important considering many patients remain undiagnosed for many years.

Oral PDE-5 inhibitors have emerged as the preferred first-line treatment of erectile dysfunction worldwide due to their efficacy, ease of use, and patient safety. Erectile function can now be evaluated by the response to these agents at home or intracavernous injection of vasoactive agents in the office, and improved diagnostic tests can differentiate among types of impotence. Patient satisfaction with penile prostheses is high, as the latest generation of devices is more sophisticated and durable than ever. Current treatments continue to evolve and new therapies such as stem cells and gene therapies may represent the next generation of more physiologic and disease-specific solutions to various types of erectile dysfunction.

Desire Disorders

Lastly, we cannot complete this article unless we address desire disorders increasingly present as a problem among men seeking medical help for sexual difficulties. Erectile dysfunction is often presented as the primary complaint, but it is not uncommon for this to mask other problems such as exhaustion (with or without substance abuse), relationship difficulties, and, more rarely, disorders of sexual preference. Inhibited desire, or loss of libido, refers to a decrease in desire for, or interest in sexual activity. Reduced libido can result from physical or psychological factors. It has been associated with low levels of the hormone testosterone. It also may be caused by psychological problems, such as anxiety and depression; medical illnesses, such as diabetes and high blood pressure; certain medications, including some antidepressants and anti-androgens, 5-alpha-reductase inhibitors, opioid analgesics; and relationship difficulties. Organic causes like testosterone deficiency, hyperprolactinemia, and medication-related side effects are important, but at times overemphasized in the somatic medical literature.

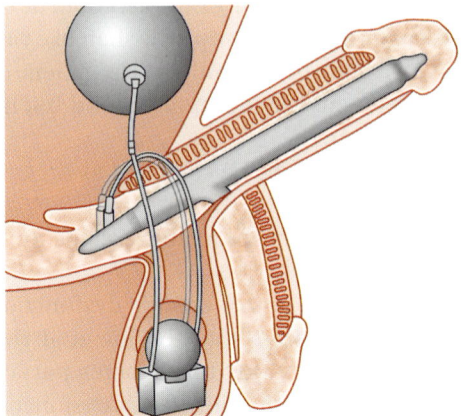

Fig. 4: Penile implants.

CONCLUSION

Male sexual dysfunction can be treated by:
- *Medical treatment*: This involves treatment of any physical problem that may be contributing to a man's sexual dysfunction.
- *Medications*: Medications such as sildenafil may help improve erectile function in men by increasing blood flow to the penis. However, its injudicious use may not give results as expected.[9] Promescent is a drug used to treat PE. The topical spray is applied to the penis and contains lidocaine, reducing sensitivity and allowing for more ejaculation control.
- *Hormones*: Men with low levels of testosterone may benefit from testosterone replacement therapy.
- *Psychological therapy*: Therapy with a trained counselor can help a person address feelings of anxiety, fear, or guilt that may have an impact on sexual function.
- *Mechanical aids*: Aids such as vacuum devices and penile implants (Fig. 4) may help men with erectile dysfunction.
- *Education and communication*: Education about sex and sexual behaviors and responses may help a man overcome his anxieties about sexual performance. Open dialogue with partner about needs and concerns also helps to overcome many barriers to a healthy sex life.

REFERENCES

1. Web MD. Medical Reference Reviewed by Joseph Goldberg on September 21, 2016.
2. Lewis RW, Fugl-Meyer KS, Corona G, et al. Definitions/Epidemiology/Risk Factors for Sexual Dysfunction. J Sex Med. 2010;7(4 Pt 2):1598-607.
3. Shifren JL. (2017). Patient information: Sexual problems in men (Beyond the Basics). [online] UptoDate website. Available from https://www.uptodate.com/

contents/sexual-problems-in-women-beyond-the-basics. [Accessed February 2018].
4. Zorn KC. (2016). Sexual Problems in Men. [online] Available from https://www.medicinenet.com/sexual_sex_problems_in_men/article.htm. [Accessed February 2018].
5. IIEF (International Index of Erectile Function), its short version (IIEF-5), or the Cologne Erectile Dysfunction Questionnaire (Kölner Erfassungsbogen der Erektilen Dysfunktion, KEED)
6. Victor A. Diaz VA, Close JD. Male sexual dysfunction. Prim Care. 2010;37:473-89.
7. MedicineNet. Erectile dysfunction (ED) causes and treatment (Davis CP). [online] Available from https://www.medicinenet.com/impotence_pictures_slideshow_erectile_dysfunction/article.htm#what_drugs_treat_erectile_dysfunction. [Accessed March, 2018].
8. Esposito K, Giugliano F, Di Palo C, et al. Effect of lifestyle changes on erectile dysfunction in obese men: A randomized controlled trial. JAMA. 2004;291:2978-84.
9. Hatzichristou D, Moysidis K, Apostolidis A, et al. Sildenafil failures may be due to inadequate patient instructions and follow-up: A study on 100 nonresponders. Eur Urol. 2005;47:518-22.

CHAPTER

16

Semen Banking

Soumojit Paul, Zeba Ali Jahangir, Rohit Gutgutia

■ INTRODUCTION

Semen banking is a process of freezing sperm at very low temperatures and storing it for future use in assisted conception. The process was first used in the 1950s to freeze and store bull semen in an effort to improve dairy cow breeding.[1,2] In 1963, Schermann et al. were first to apply the technology to human-assisted conception.[3] In their breakthrough study, artificial insemination utilizing human sperm, frozen in dry ice with glycerol (10%), resulted in three successful pregnancies with viable embryo development. One of Schermann's discoveries was that storing human sperm at liquid nitrogen (LN_2) temperature (–196°C) was superior to storage at –75°C. In addition, no loss of motility was observed when the sperm were stored in LN_2 for 1 year; however, there was a decline in motility after storage at –75°C (Schermann, 1963). Prior to 1964, all pregnancies were produced from short-term storage of sperm; however, Perloff et al. (1964) reported pregnancies from insemination with frozen-thawed sperm stored for 1–5.5 months. It was not until 1964, however, when the first live birth was reported using thawed ejaculated sperm, preserved in glycerol-freezing media, and embedded in LN_2.[4]

Currently, sperm banking is used to preserve fertility in a variety of men, including those with cancer. In fact, it has garnered a lot of attention in recent years largely because cancer cure rates have dramatically improved along with reproductive medicine technology. As a result a new field called "oncofertility" has been created to focus on fertility preservation and quality of life issues for cancer survivors. Additionally as male reproductive health has deteriorated during the past century, the indication for sperm banking have become more broadly implemented.

■ THEORY OF CRYOPRESERVATION

Cryopreserved cells are stored in LN_2 at –196°C. At this temperature, no physiological processes take place, meaning that cells can be stored almost indefinitely. However, the freezing processes themselves can cause stress, compromising survival. The main risk is mechanical damage from ice crystal formation, and the larger the cell the more likely it is that ice crystals form in the cytoplasm. Dehydration of the cells can help to prevent damage during the cryopreservation process. In order to achieve this, two complementary factors need to be considered—these are the chemical properties of cryoprotectants and the physical properties involved in the rate of cooling. Injury to the cell can also be caused by osmotic stress and "cold shock" injury. Cold shock injury may result in membrane permeability and cytoskeletal structural changes.

Cryoprotectants

Cryoprotectants are important for the prevention of ice crystal formation and can be separated into cryoprotectants that penetrate through the cell membranes and those that do not penetrate, or "permeable" cryoprotectants are completely miscible with water and because they can pass through the cell membrane they have the effect of displacing water from the cell. They also help to stabilize the cell membranes and protect the cytoskeleton. At high concentrations, many of the commonly used penetrating cryoprotectants, such as DMSO (dimethyl sulfoxide), are cytotoxic. Nonpenetrating cryoprotectants tend to be high-molecular weight sugars such as sucrose and trehalose. As they are unable to pass through the cell membrane, they act by increasing the osmolarity of the medium outside the cell and aid dehydration in that way. They are also important during thawing when they prevent damage, which would otherwise be caused by excessive swelling, due to water re-entering the cells faster than permeating cryoprotectants can diffuse out.

■ SEMEN BANKING: REASON AND BENEFITS

Cancer patients of reproductive age are most commonly referred for sperm banking, comprise about 44% of all referrals worldwide.[5] However, other male patients may benefit from this service including adolescents, prepubertal cancer patients, men with severe oligozoospermia or other rheumatic, neurodegenerative or hematologic diseases, those with occupational risks and limitations, and biological males undergoing sex change surgery.

In general, users of sperm banking are divided into two categories—(1) donors group and (2) autoconservation group.

Sperm Donors Group

Sperm donors are recruited to become surrogate fathers for couples suffering from refractory male infertility problems, planning to prevent transmission of certain genetic or infectious diseases in the husband, or for single or lesbian women planning to mother a baby. These donors donate their semen to be preserved in sperm banks for future use in assisted reproductive techniques.

In order to ensure that donor semen is free from bacterial and viral infections, the samples are routinely quarantined for at least 180 days, as it may take this length of time for an infected donor to become seropositive. At the end of this time, the sperm donor is rescreened before the samples are released for use.[6]

Autoconservation Group

Patients who belong to the autoconservation group often preserve their sperm or testicular tissue for the purposes of fertility preservation or fertility treatment. This group can be divided into two major subgroups based on the purpose of sperm cryopreservation—(1) fertility preservation and (2) fertility treatment.

Fertility Preservation Group

Adult oncology patients: In 2011, the American Cancer Society reported that the 5-year relative survival rate for all cancers was 68% (based on data gathered between 1999 and 2006). This is a significant improvement, above 50% which was in the 1970s,[7] and is due to the wide use of reliable screening procedures for earlier detection and successful application of aggressive cancer therapy. As such, more cancer patients are younger when first diagnosed and are more often cured, culminating into a larger number of cancer survivors than ever before.[8] Thus, the landscape of patient priorities surrounding cancer management is changing as there is a greater concern for the treatment's effect on fertility.

The most common cancers that affect males of reproductive age include testicular cancer, Hodgkin's disease, acute leukemia, non-Hodgkin's lymphoma, and soft tissue tumors, such as sarcomas.[7] Cancer affects the body in many negative ways, systemically and locally, and it particularly impairs spermatogenesis.[9,10] Meanwhile, cancer therapies are also quite toxic to reproductive health, hindering normal testicular function, and decreasing sperm quality.[8] As such, high incidence of poor semen quality is observed among referred men, with asthenospermia being the most common finding (64.2–86.3%).[11,12] Other common semen abnormalities among cancer patients who are referred to sperm banking include oligozoospermia (49.8–53%),[13-15] severe oligozoospermia (<1 million sperm/mL) (22.6%),[15] azoospermia (9.7–21%)[13-15] and abnormal sperm morphology (22.8%).[12] Alternatively, a recent study showed that teratozoospermia is the most common abnormality (93.2%) among pretreatment cancer patients.[11] Interestingly, most of these semen abnormalities resolve after cancer therapy. Moreover, the chromosomal aneuploidy rate in germ cells (as detected by fluorescent in situ hybridization) is increased in men with testicular cancer and Hodgkin's disease before they start therapy.[16]

Testicular cancers have local and systemic influences on spermatogenesis, perhaps because they are associated with the production of the local paracrine factors, such as β-human chorionic gonadotropins (enhances estrogen production and suppresses gonadotropin levels)[17] and cytokines,[18] and the cancer itself disrupts the blood testis barrier, resulting in abnormal immune sensitization against sperm.[19] Systemic effects of malignant disease include fever (Hodgkin's disease, non-Hodgkin disease, and leukemia), malignancy-related malnutrition, abnormal immune response (lymphoma), altered hormonal milieu (testicular cancer and central nervous system tumors), and a generalized stress and inflammatory response leading to the production of cytokines, such as interleukins and tumor necrosis factors all of which can have consequences on testicular and sperm function.[10,20] These substances damage sperm before treatment and may result in chromosomal aneuploidy in the germ cells.[16]

In addition to cancer itself, modern oncologic treatments are also highly toxic to the body and the testes. Gonadotropic therapies are particularly harmful to the early stages of spermatogenesis, specifically to proliferating and differentiating spermatogonia and could cause permanent damage.[21] In general, effects of oncologic treatment on fertility are quite unpredictable. A common side effect of toxic treatment is temporary or permanent azoospermia and severe oligozoospermia.[22] Although spermatogenesis can resume after treatment, practitioners do not know how much time that may take or when it does happen, if and when it does happen. For instance, in men with testicular cancer, it takes at least 2 years after cessation of (etoposide + bleomycin) therapy for spermatogenesis to recover. Ultimately, recovery occurs in 80% of patients within 8 years of treatment,[23,24] while normal parameters may recover, the ability to fertilize an oocyte may still be affected as has been observed with the use of vincristine.[25] Due to the uncertain nature of cancer treatment, it is prudent to bank sperm before the start of treatment to insure against potentially permanent loss of fertility. It has been widely accepted that the pretreatment sperm cryopreservation is the most effective method for preserving fertility in young cancer patients.

Chemotherapy, which is generally considered a highly toxic treatment, specifically affects spermatogenesis. Chemotherapy regimen consisting of either a single or multiple therapeutic medications have various effect on testicular function based upon the toxicity profile of each agent, cumulative dose, coexistent radiotherapy, and treatment duration. Alkylating agents, such as nitrogen mustard, cyclophosphamide, ifosfamide, busulfan, procarbazine, and chlorambucil, are notorious for having the most harmful effects on the body organs including the testes. The more toxic regimen used in therapy for Hodgkin's disease, which consists of nitrogen mustard, vincristine (Oncovin), procarbazine, and prednisone (MOPP) should be less commonly used and reserved for mostly for advanced stages of diseases. Six cycles or more of MOPP that contain two alkylating agents, mustard and procarbazine, result in a high incidence of prolonged azoospermia in 83–97% of patients post-therapy.[26,27] Fortunately, the use of adriamycin, bleomycin, vinblastine, and dacarbazine (ABVD) is less toxic and causes significantly less damage to reproductive organs.[28] In testicular cancer, 53% and 44% of men receiving a regimen consisting of bleomycin, etoposide, and cisplatin (BEP)—the most commonly used regimen, develop oligozoospermia and azoospermia, respectively, after 2–4 cycles.[29]

Radiotherapy is similarly harmful to spermatogenesis. While damage to the testicles depends on the dose and method of exposure, the risk is high when treatment is targeted directly at the testicles.[30] Radiotherapy occasionally causes persistent sperm DNA fragmentation and reduced semen volume and damages cells in all areas of male reproductive organ. Moreover, radiotherapy can obstruct the ejaculatory ducts and access to mature sperm.

The amount by which spermatogenesis is affected depends on the dosage. 4 Gy appears to be the threshold for permanent azoospermia, and anything less presumably only causes temporary variations in semen parameters.[30] Radiation-induced transient alterations in spermatogenesis may disappear within 2 years. For Leydig cells, the toxic dosage is 20 Gy or more for prepubertal boys and more than 30 Gy in adult males, which will render men testosterone deficient.[28] The detrimental effects of chemotherapy and radiotherapy are increased when the two are used in combination.[31] During combined therapy, the body is exposed to a variety of toxins that affect the male gonads differently depending on whether the treatment is localized or general.

Pediatric and adolescent cancer patients: Sperm banking is also a viable option for many adolescent cancer patients whose fertile years are still ahead of them at time of diagnosis. Cure rates for pediatric cancers have dramatically improved over recent years and are currently approaching 80%. With the increasing number of cancer survivors living today, long-term quality-of-life concerns are becoming an important part of pretreatment discussions.[32] As a result, adolescent and pediatric cancer patients are increasingly being provided with opportunities for sperm cryopreservation. Adolescents, who have already achieved sexual maturity (at least Tanner stage 2, and testicular volume of 5 mL) are interviewed regarding their ability to masturbate.[33] If masturbation is not feasible, other methods are offered, such as penile vibratory stimulation and electroejaculation under general anesthesia.[33] Semen quality is also influenced by cancer in the same way as in adults and probably through the same mechanism.

When azoospermia is encountered, oncotesticular sperm extraction (TESE) is a reasonable choice. In prepubertal males, fertility preservation is a challenging situation as there are no haploid sperm or even spermatids in testicular tissues. In these cases, testicular tissue freezing opens the door for preserving fertility after iatrogenic sterilization, hopefully through stem cell isolation and transplantation or through in vitro maturation and induced spermatogenesis.

Impaired fertility resulting from other disease-related factors: Patients with other diseases can also benefit from sperm banking before serious treatment or before the disease becomes so debilitating that it disrupts spermatogenesis. For example, men with lupus, rheumatoid arthritis, ulcerative colitis, multiple sclerosis, or hematologic diseases that are treated with bone marrow transplants may also consider sperm banking early in the disease process.[34] Many experts suggest that healthcare providers offer sperm cryopreservation to patients with nonmalignant diseases and urological pathologies, such as bilateral varicocele, testis torsion, or necrosis, particularly when they are about to undergo surgery.[35] A systemic disease that damages the entire body is likely to affect testicular function. Men who are awaiting surgery, such as urogenital procedures or vasectomy should preserve their sperm as a precautionary measure.

Occupational risks: Some healthy men may wish to consider using sperm banking for fertility preservation to counteract certain occupational risks. Gupta et al. recommended that men who work with toxic chemicals, ionization radiation, or biological hazards "consider banking sperm as these exposures may jeopardize their reproductive potential".[36] Radiation, a known carcinogen, may damage the germ cells and cause birth defects in offspring. Working with glycol ethers also poses a threat to male fertility and is associated with low-motile sperm count.[37] To avoid such outcomes, men in high-risk occupations should bank sperm before these negative effects accumulate.

Sex change and gender reassignment: Biological males, who are undergoing gender reassignment through hormonal or surgical therapy may also benefit from sperm banking. Estrogen has been shown to have detrimental effects on spermatogenesis and overall semen parameters,[38] and sex change surgery includes orchiectomy and penectomy, which renders the male sterile, as they are no longer able to ejaculate. After male-to-female sex change surgery, two-thirds of patients identify as lesbians and some may want to have biological children with their partner—either via the biological female partner or a surrogate. For this reason, it would be beneficial to counsel such patients on fertility preservation before irreversible biological changes are made with surgery.

Prior to undergoing surgical procedures for treating or induced infertility: Certain surgeries performed to cure infertility, such as bilateral varicocele ligation and surgical relief of seminal duct obstruction, may be complicated postoperatively by reduced testicular blood supply or inadvertent vasal transaction, particularly when the surgery is performed on both sides of the testes. Fertility preservation may also be an option for men planning to do a surgical contraception via bilateral vasectomy, as they may change their mind regarding having children in future.

Fertility Treatment Group

This group includes the following indications (Table 1):
- *Severe oligozoospermia*: Severe, very severe, and extreme oligozoospermia are defined by a very low-sperm count of less than 5 million/mL, less than 1 million/mL, and less than 10,000 sperm/mL, respectively. Technically, cryobanking is conducted in these patients to preserve existing spermatozoa

Table 1: Indications for sperm cryopreservation.

Fertility preservation:

Patient condition	Reasons for sperm banking	Sperm collection method
Adult cancer	Cancer and related therapies damage the gonads and impair spermatogenesis	Frequent ejaculation
Adolescent cancer	Same as above	Frequent ejaculation (when they are sexually mature), penile vibratory stimulation, electroejaculation
Cancer in prepubescent males	Cancer treatment negatively affects spermatogenesis; testicular tissue extraction is a promising experimental procedure	Testicular tissue freezing
Preoperative surgical procedure to treat or induce infertility	Bilateral varicocele ligation; prior to vasectomy	Frequent ejaculation
Nonmalignant disease	Systemic stress may impair spermatogenesis; gonadotoxic therapies affects semen quality	Frequent ejaculation
Occupational risks	Exposure to harmful chemicals may decrease fertility or cause chromosomal damage in the germ cells; facing hazardous situations that may result in an accident that causes infertility	Frequent ejaculation
Posthumous sperm cryopreservation	Performed at the time of brain death—based upon the patient's will or family request	Electroejaculation; surgical removal of testis and epididymis
Sex change/gender reassignment	Hormone therapy damages spermatogenesis; gender reassignment surgery sterilizes the male	Frequent ejaculation; removal of testicular tissue

Fertility treatment:

Patient condition	Reasons for sperm banking	Sperm collection method
Severe oligozoospermia (<5 million/mL)	Progressive decline in sperm production and high chance of azoospermia	Frequent ejaculation

Contd...

Contd...

Obstructive and nonobstructive azoospermia	Absence of sperm in ejaculate; benefit from sperm extraction technique for ART	Surgical retrieval techniques from testis or epididymis
Spinal cord injuries	Anejaculation and poor semen quality with difficulty in transportation	Assisted ejaculation and sperm retrieval from testis and epididymis
Donor semen insemination	Donor sperm use as therapeutic measure in a couple with sterile men; men with genetic or infectious diseases such as HIV; for insemination of single or lesbian women	Frequent ejaculation
Absence of male factor during conduction of ART cycle	Frequently traveling husband; husband staying abroad	Frequent ejaculation

(ART: assisted reproductive technology; HIV: human immunodeficiency virus)

to ensure adequate sperm supply for multiple assisted reproductive technology (ART) cycles and to eliminate the possibility of not finding fresh sperm in the ejaculate on the day it is needed for ART. Moreover, recent reports have suggested that a significant proportion of men with severe oligozoospermia will ultimately become azoospermic and experience a loss of testicular germ cells, which further supports the use of sperm banking in this population.[39,40]

- *Azoospermia*: Azoospermia is the condition of not having sperm in the ejaculate. There are two kinds of azoospermia—obstructive and nonobstructive. Obstructive azoospermia (OA) is usually caused by post-testicular congenital or acquired obstructive lesions. In such conditions, spermatogenesis is often normal. For this reason, viable sperm can still be obtained through various extraction methods from the testes or epididymides, and testicular sperm retrieval is successful in almost 100% of cases. Nonobstructive azoospermia (NOA), on the other hand, usually implies the presence of a sperm production defect, and its cause is often more difficult to identify and treat. For men with NOA, TESE and microsurgical TESE are the preferred methods for obtaining sperm.

Men with temporary azoospermia (perhaps due to systemic disease or acute testicular insults) may wish to cryopreserve their semen as soon as possible to ensure against further loss of fertility.[41] If the transient azoospermia is due to a disease, it is recommended that semen be banked before the start of any potentially gonadotoxic treatment. Furthermore, men who experience periodic azoospermia and are undergoing ART procedures

with their partners may wish to bank sperm before the procedure, so that the sample is available on the day it is needed, thereby minimizing the chance of any delays or fertilization failure.
- *Absence of male partner during assisted reproductive technology cycles*: This indication applies for men, who are absent from home for long periods because of military service or frequent travel overseas.
- *Ejaculatory dysfunction and spinal cord injured men*: More than 90% of men with spinal cord injury are infertile and have poor semen quality due to combination of adverse factors, such as anejaculation, retrograde ejaculation, semen stagnation, frequent genital infections, and increased levels of seminal oxidative stress.

■ SPERM CRYOPRESERVATION PROTOCOL

Commercially bought sperm cryopreservation media consists of a basic culture medium with glycerin (15%) as the main cryoprotectant and a small amount of sucrose (<2%). This is slowly added to the sperm sample at a ratio of 0.7 mL of cryopreservation media to 1.0 mL of sperm sample. After mixing, it is loaded into labeled straws, sperm straws, which are then heat sealed at both ends. The straws are suspended in nitrogen vapor for 30 minutes before plunging into LN_2.

■ SPERM THAWING

Sperm is thawed rapidly by removing it from LN_2 and allowing it to warm to room temperature. If the sample is to be used for intrauterine insemination or in vitro fertilization (IVF), it should first be prepared. This may be done by slow dilution with medium followed by centrifugation and further washing, or by layering onto a density gradient. The method used for post-thaw preparation will depend on whether there was any prefreeze preparation and also the overall quality of the sample.

■ SAFETY ISSUES INVOLVED WITH CRYOPRESERVATION

Transmission of Pathogens

It is known that viruses and bacteria can survive in LN_2; therefore, there is a risk that pathogens could be transmitted from one patient to another during storage. This risk can be minimized by screening patients for viruses such as HIV, hepatitis B, and hepatitis C prior to treatment, and only storing screened patients in the same tank. As the patient could be infective but not seropositive, this only reduces risk, rather than avoiding it altogether. As semen has higher risks of infection, it should be stored in separate tanks to oocytes and embryos. The type of containers used for storage of the gametes or embryos will also affect the risks of infection; "open" systems, where the gametes come into direct contact with the LN_2, provide more of an opportunity for cross-contamination than "closed" systems. Sterile cryovials can be used with tightly placed caps but risk involved in LN_2 seeping in and the vial getting contaminated or exploding while thawing cannot be avoided. Sperm straws are safer and allow for sterile filling of the straws, which are then heat sealed at both ends. Finally, storage in vapor phase of the LN_2 avoids the risk of transmission and has proved safe for sperm. However, the increased temperature fluctuations in vapor phase make it less attractive.

Traceability and Witnessing

It is essential that sperm straws are correctly identified during the cryopreservation process and accurately labeled for future use. Robust witnessing protocols should be in place at each stage during all laboratory procedures, from the initial retrieval of semen sample to the final placement in the storage tanks. The samples themselves should be easily identifiable and at the minimum should be labeled with the patient's full name, date of freeze, and a unique identifier (identification number or patient ID). Documentation of the samples in storage should be properly maintained such that samples can be easily located and that those reaching legal storage limits can be easily identified.

Operator Safety

Hazards to the laboratory staff should be taken into account when handling samples stored in LN_2, with suitable training and provision of appropriate safety equipment being essential. The main risks can be summarized as follows:

- Injury from samples exploding due to LN_2 in the container rapidly expanding when removed from storage
- Freeze burns due to bodily contact with LN_2 or chilled surfaces
- Suffocation due to handling of LN_2 in poorly ventilated areas.

■ CONCLUSION

Cryopreservation has become an integral part of the modern ART laboratory, increasing the efficiency of the service provided, helping to reduce the multiple pregnancy rate, and giving hope to cancer sufferers whose chance of parenthood may otherwise be destroyed. Although enormous strides have been made in technologies of assisted reproduction, cryopreservation protocols, cancer research, and in the new field of oncofertility, there are still many unknowns to be determined. Primarily, there is still much to be learnt about what causes semen quality to decrease in patients with cancer and the mechanism of how cancer affects spermatogenesis both locally and systemically.[42] Experimental procedures, such as testicular tissue extraction and freezing for prepubertal cancer patients, require more formidable translation from animal research to real clinical human practice.[32] The safety of children born from cryopreserved gametes and embryos is of paramount importance. There are few studies comparing the obstetric and neonatal outcomes of children born from the different methods of cryopreservation, but again the results that are available are reassuring.[43] It is the responsibility of the embryologist to provide the highest possible standard of practice in order to ensure the best possible outcomes from the cryopreservation procedures.

■ REFERENCES

1. Bratton RW, Foote RH, Cruthers JC. Preliminary fertility results with frozen bovine spermatozoa. J Diary Sci. 1955;38:40-6.
2. Polge C, Smith AU, Parkes AS. Revival of spermatozoa after vitrification and dehydration at low temperature. Nature. 1949;164:666.
3. Bunge RG, Keettel WC, Sherman JK. Clinical use of frozen semen: report of four cases. Fertil Steril. 1954;5(6):520-9.
4. Sherman JK. Cryopreservation of Human Semen. In: Keel BA, Webster BW (Eds). CRC Handbook of the laboratory diagnosis and treatment of Infertility. Boston: CRC Press; 1990. pp. 229.
5. Tomlinson M. Therapeutic sperm cryopreservation. In: Björndahl L, Giwercman A, Tournaye L (Eds). Clinical Andrology EAU/ESAU Course Guidelines. London: Informa Health Care; 2010. pp. 124-33.
6. Association of Biomedical Andrologists, Association of Clinical Embryologists, British Andrology Society, et al. UK guidelines for the medical and laboratory screening of sperm egg and embryo donors. Hum Reprod 2008;11(4):201-10.
7. American Cancer Society. (2011). Cancer facts and Figures, US, 2011. [online] Available from www.cancer.org/acs/groups/content/@epidemiologysurveilance/ documents/document/acspc029771.pdf. [Accessed March, 2018].
8. SteliarovaFoucher E, Stiller C, Kaatsch P, et al. Geographical patterns and time trends of cancer incidence and survival among children and adolescents in Europe since the 1970s (the ACCIS project): an epidemiological study. Lancet. 2004;364:2097-105.
9. Ragheb AM, Jones S, Sabanegh, et al. Implications of cancer on male fertility. Arch Med Sci. 2009;5(1A):S63-9.
10. Agarwal A, Allamaneni SS. Disruption of spermatogenesis by the cancer disease process. J Nat Can InstMonogr. 2005;34:9-12.
11. Amirjannati N, Sadeghi M, Hosseini Jadda SH, et al. Evaluation of semen quality in patients with malignancies referred for sperm banking before cancer treatment. Andrologia. 011;43(5):31720.
12. Crha I, Ventruba P, Petrenko M, et al. Cryopreservation of sperm before neoplasm therapy—7 years' experience. Ceska Gynekol. 2002;67(6):3248.
13. Lass A, Akagbosu F, Abusheikha N, et al. A programme of semen cryopreservation for patients with malignant disease in a tertiary infertility centre: lessons from 8 years' experience. Hum Reprod. 1998;13:3256-61.
14. van Casteren NJ, Boellaard WP, Romijn JC, et al. Gonadal dysfunction in male cancer patients before cytotoxic treatment. Int J Androl. 2010;33(1):739.

15. Crha I, Ventruba P, Zakova J, et al. Survival and infertility treatment in male cancer patients after sperm banking. Fertil Steril. 2009;91(6):23448.
16. Tempest HG, Ko E, Chan P, et al. Sperm aneuploidy frequencies analysed before and after chemotherapy in testicular cancer and Hodgkin's lymphoma patients. Hum Reprod. 2008;23:2518.
17. Morrish DW, Venner PM, Siy O, et al. Mechanisms of endocrine dysfunction in patients with testicular cancer. J Natl Cancer Inst. 1990;82:412-8.
18. Ho GT, Gardner H, DeWolf WC, et al. Influence of testicular carcinoma on ipsilateral spermatogenesis. J Urol. 1992;148:8215.
19. Foster RS, Rubin LR, McNulty A, et al. Detection of antispermantibodies in patients with primary testicular cancer. Int J Androl. 1991;14:17985.
20. Perdichizzi A, Nicoletti F, La Vignera S, et al. Effects of tumour necrosis factoralpha on human sperm motility and apoptosis. J Clin Immunol. 2007;27:15262.
21. Bucci LR, Meistrich ML. Effects of busulfan on murine spermatogenesis: cytotoxicity, sterility, sperm abnormalities, and dominant lethal mutations. Mutat Res. 1987;176:25968.
22. Ragheb AM, Sabanegh ES. Male fertility implications of anticancer treatment and strategies to mitigate gonadotoxicity. Anticancer Agents Med Chem. 2010;10:92102.
23. Howell SJ, Shalet SM. Spermatogenesis after cancer treatment: damage and recovery. J Natl Cancer Inst Monogr. 2005;34:127.
24. Petersen PM, Skakkebaek NE, Giwercman A. Gonadal function in men with testicular cancer: biological and clinical aspects. APMIS. 1998;106(1):2434.
25. Dobrzyńska MM, Czajka U, Slowikowska MG. Reproductive effects after exposure of male mice to vincristine and to a combination of Xrays and vincristine. Reprod Fertil Dev. 2005;17(8):75967.
26. Viviani S, Santoro A, Ragni G, et al. Gonadal toxicity after combination chemotherapy for Hodgkin's disease. Comparative results of MOPP vs ABVD. Eur J Cancer Clin Oncol. 1985;21(5):6015.
27. Ortin TT, Shostak CA, Donaldson SS. Gonadal status and reproductive function following treatment for Hodgkin's disease in childhood: the Stanford experience. Int J Radiat Oncol Biol Phys. 1990;19(4):87380.
28. Shalet SM, Tsatsoulis A, Whitehead E, et al. Vulnerability of the human Leydig cell to radiation damage is dependent upon age. J Endocrinol. 1989;120:1615.
29. O'Flaherty C, Hales BF, Chan P, et al. Impact of chemotherapeutics and advanced testicular cancer or Hodgkin lymphoma on sperm deoxyribonucleic acid integrity. Fertil Steril. 2010;94(4):13749.
30. Wallace WH. Oncofertility and preservation of reproductive capacity in children and young adults. Cancer. 2011;117(10 Suppl):230110.
31. Colpi GM, Contalbi GF, Nerva F, et al. Testicular function following chemo-radiotherapy. Eur. J Obstet Gynecol Reprod Biol. 2004;113(Suppl 1):S26.
32. Ginsberg JP, Carlson CA, Lin K, et al. An experimental protocol for fertility preservation in prepubertal boys recently diagnosed with cancer: a report of acceptability and safety. Hum Reprod. 2010;25(1):3741.

33. Hagenäs I, Jørgensen N, Rechnitzer C, et al. Clinical and biochemical correlates of successful semen collection for cryopreservation from 1218 year old patients: a single center study of 86 adolescents. Hum Reprod. 2010;25(8):20318.
34. Ranganathan P, Mahran AM, Hallak J, et al. Sperm cryopreservation for men with non-malignant, systemic diseases: a descriptive study. J Androl. 2002;23:715.
35. Anger JT, Gilbert BR, Goldstein M. Cryopreservation of sperm: indications, methods and results. J Urol. 2003;170(4 Pt 1):107984.
36. Gupta S, Agarwal A, Sharma R, et al. Recovery, preparation, storage and utilization of spermatozoa for fertility preservation in cancer patients and sub-fertile men. J Reprod Stem Cell Biotech. 2011;1:15068.
37. Cherry N, Moore H, McNamee R, et al. Occupation and male infertility: glycol ethers and other exposures. Occup Environ Med. 2008;65(10):70814.
38. Mishra DP, Shaha C. Estrogeninduced spermatogenic cell apoptosis occurs via the mitochondrial pathway: role of superoxide and nitric oxide. J Biol Chem. 2005;18:280(7):618196.
39. Bak CW, Song SH, Yoon TK, et al. Natural course of idiopathic oligozoospermia: comparison of mild, moderate and severe forms. Int J Urol. 2010;17(11):93743.
40. Song SH, Bak CW, Lim JJ, et al. Natural course of severe oligozoospermia in infertile male: influence on future fertility potential. J Androl. 2010;31(6):5369.
41. Walters EM, Benson JD, Woods EJ, et al. The history of sperm cryopreservation. In: Pacey AA, Tomlinson MJ (Eds). Sperm Banking: Theory and Practice. Cambridge: Cambridge University Press; 2009. pp. 110.
42. Woodruff TK. The oncofertility consortium—addressing fertility in young people with cancer. Nat Rev Clin Oncol. 2010;7:46675.
43. Wikland M, Hardarson T, Hillensjö T, et al. Obstetric outcomes after transfer of vitrified blastocysts. Hum Reprod. 2010;25(7):1699-707.

CHAPTER
17

Basic Requirement to set up an IVF Laboratory

Virendra Shah, Anjali Joshi

■ INTRODUCTION

The aim of a well-designed in vitro fertilization (IVF) laboratory set up is to provide an environment that provides both good-working condition and air-quality management, resulting in excellent IVF outcome. This chapter focuses on the critical aspects of building a laboratory in a private practice setting as part of an assisted reproductive technology (ART) clinic. Knowledge of these factors is essential for ART professionals, planning a new facility, or redesigning an existing one.[1]

The general organization of an IVF laboratory includes laboratory design, staffing, quality management, laboratory safety, and the specific aspects of the procedures performed in IVF laboratory (identification of patients and traceability of their reproductive cells, consumables, handling of biological material, oocyte retrieval, sperm preparation, insemination of oocytes, scoring for fertilization, embryo culture and transfer, and cryopreservation). The bench marking parameters such as record keeping, data analysis, and an emergency plan for IVF laboratories play a significant role.

■ LABORATORY DESIGN

The IVF laboratory must have adequate functionalities to minimize any damaging effects upon the gametes and embryos, and ensure good laboratory practice. The laboratory should be adjacent to the operating room where clinical procedures are performed.[2]

While setting up the IVF laboratory, the most recent developments in facilities, equipment, and procedures should be considered. Attention should be given to operator comfort to provide a safe working environment that minimizes the risk of distraction, fatigue, and thereby making a mistake. The main considerations should include bench height, adjustable chairs, adequate work space per person, microscope eye height, efficient use of space and surfaces, sufficient environmental lighting and air-conditioning with controlled humidity and temperature.[3]

- Laboratory design should ensure optimal workflow over minimal distances while handling reproductive cells during all treatment phases.
- Laboratory access should be restricted to authorized personnel.
- A system for clean access of personnel and materials to the laboratory is highly recommended.
- Rooms for changing clothes should be separate from the laboratory.
- Hand-washing facilities should be placed outside the laboratory.
- Separate office space for administrative work should be available outside the laboratory.
- A separate laboratory with a safety fume hood should be provided for analyses using fixatives and other toxic reagents.
- The area for cleaning and sterilization of materials, if present, should be separate from the laboratory (Fig. 1).

■ MATERIALS USED IN LABORATORY CONSTRUCTION

Painting, flooring, and furniture should be appropriate for clean room standards, minimizing volatile organic compounds (VOCs) release and embryo toxicity. All the interior paintings should be done with water-based paints formulated for low VOCs like formaldehyde, acetaldehyde, toluene, benzene, and styrene.[4] Sealing of the joints and surfaces must be done with the silicone materials free of VOCs. The walls and ceilings of the ART laboratories should be solid with minimum penetrations, with sealed lighting, and airtight utility connections. Doors should also have seals and sweeps with locking system.

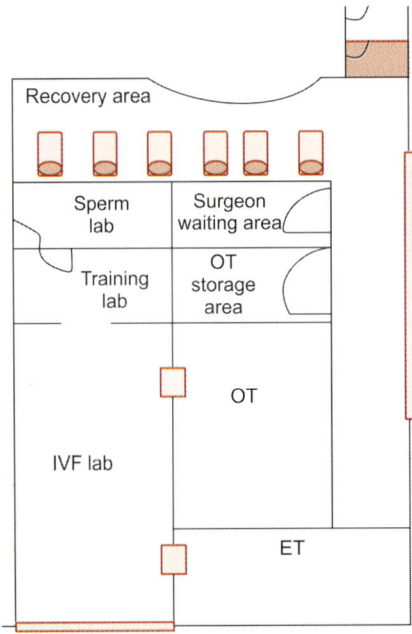

Fig. 1: Basic layout plan of in vitro fertilization (IVF) laboratory.

Ducts and gas connections should be laid out with a view to perform all the routine and emergency work with minimum disruption in the ART laboratory.[5] The choice of flooring is standard for operating rooms and clean rooms, seamless sheet vinyl flooring should be used and the ends where the pieces of flooring meet should be sealed. Flooring should be flashed onto the base of cabinets in the laboratory to prevent the contamination by microbes.

■ BASIC COMPONENTS OF ART LABORATORY

The basic components of IVF set up include the following:
- *Andrology laboratory*: Semen analysis and processing
- *Embryology laboratory*: Oocyte retrieval, fertilization, embryo culture, and transfer
- Micromanipulation; intracytoplasmic sperm injection (ICSI), assisted hatching, preimplantation genetic diagnosis (PGD), and preimplantation genetic screening (PGS)
- *Cryopreservation unit*: Sperms, embryos, blastocysts, oocytes, ovarian, and testicular tissue.

Andrology Laboratory

Description and Function

The andrology laboratory will include benches and storage units for examination of specimens. The space will be enclosed for specialty laboratory functions.

Location and Relationships

- The andrology laboratory has a close working relationship with the IVF/ICSI laboratories.
- The collection room should be located in close proximity.

Considerations

Fittings and equipment to be located in this laboratory will include:
- Laboratory benches and storage units
- Laminar flow IVF workstation cabinets
- Benchtop microscopes
- Automatic sperm analyzing units
- Carbon dioxide (CO_2) incubators
- Electrical pipettes
- Variable pipettes
- Mackler cell
- Fyrite analyzer (CO_2 and O_2 gas analyzer)
- Laboratory refrigerator
- Hand basin and staff change area at entry.

Laboratory equipment will require emergency power, temperature monitoring, and alarms. The construction of the laboratory should ensure aseptic and optimal handling of reproductive tissue during all stages of the process. Air conditioning for the laboratory will include high-efficiency particulate air (HEPA) filters, controlled humidity (20%), and controlled temperature (22–24ºC). Access to the laboratory should be limited.[6]

Embryology—IVF/ICSI Laboratory

Description and Function

Refer to functional areas for a description and functions of the IVF/ICSI laboratory. The space will be enclosed for specialty laboratory function.[7]

Location and Relationships

The IVF/ICSI laboratory should be located with a direct relationship to the operating room for oocyte collection and reimplantation. A pass through hatch from the laboratory to each operating room is recommended. Staff change and hand wash areas should be located at the laboratory entry.

Considerations

- Fittings and equipment to be located in this laboratory will include:
  - Laboratory benches and storage units
  - Laminar flow IVF workstation cabinets
  - Benchtop microscopes, inverted microscope, and stereo microscope
  - CO_2 incubators
  - Micromanipulator
  - Electrical pipettes
  - Variable pipettes
  - CO_2 and O_2 gas analyzer
  - Laboratory refrigerator.
- Hand basin and staff change area must be before the entrance.
- Laboratory equipment will require emergency power, temperature monitoring, and alarms.
- The construction of the laboratory should ensure aseptic and optimal handling of reproductive tissue during all stages of the process. Air conditioning for the laboratory will include HEPA filters.
- Controlled humidity (20%) and controlled temperature (22–24ºC)
- Access to the laboratory should be limited.

Cryopreservation Unit

Description and Function

Storage room for liquid nitrogen (LN_2) tanks containing frozen gametes. Nitrogen tanks should be stored in an enclosed space in case of nitrogen leakage.

Location and Relationships

The cryopreservation storage area should be located in close proximity to the laboratory areas, in an area with controlled access.

Considerations

A monitoring system is required for low levels of LN_2 in the storage tanks and for high levels of nitrogen in the air.

Strict cryopreservation protocols are required and will include:

- Infection control (minimizing the risk of cross contamination of frozen gametes, zygotes, and embryos)
- Labeling, packaging, and documentation of tissue frozen provide controlled access to the room.

Cryopreservation can be performed for gametes, embryos, and tissues. Facilities should be available to cryopreserve and store biological material. Different cryopreservation approaches, including slow freezing and vitrification, can be used according to the type of biological material. For sperm, slow freezing is still the method of choice, but rapid cooling is a possible alternative. For oocytes, vitrification has been reported to be highly successful and is recommended. For cleavage-stage embryos and blastocysts, high success rates have been reported when using vitrification. For tissues, the method of choice is slow freezing, but vitrification of ovarian tissue is an option. In order to minimize any risk of transmission of infection via LN_2—contamination of the external surface of cryo-devices should be avoided when loading them with samples. Safety issues have been raised regarding direct contact of the biological material with the LN_2; however, at this point, closed devices cannot be favored over open devices. Laboratories should make decisions based upon their results, risk analysis, and regulations in place. Specimens from seropositive patients should be stored in high-security closed devices. Dedicated vapor phase tanks are recommended. At cryopreservation, documentation on biological material should include:

- Labeling of devices
- Cryopreservation method
- Date and time of cryopreservation
- Operator
- Embryo quality and stage of development
- Number of oocytes or embryos per device
- Number of devices stored per patient
- Location of stored samples (tank and canister).

Cryo-devices must be clearly and permanently labeled with reference to patient details, treatment number and/or a unique identification code. A periodic inventory of the contents of the cryobank is recommended, including cross-referencing contents with storage records.

Thawing method: At thawing, documentation on biological material should include:
- Date and time of thawing
- Operator
- Post-thawing sample quality.

A double check of patient identity is recommended in the following steps—transfer of samples into labeled cryo-dish, loading of the labeled device, deposition in the cryobank, and removal from the cryobank. During storage and handling of cryopreserved material, care should be taken to maintain adequate and safe conditions. Temperatures should never rise above −130°C.

■ LABORATORY EQUIPMENT

- The laboratory equipment used should be adequate for laboratory work and easy to clean and disinfect.
- Critical items of equipment, including incubators and frozen embryo storage facilities, should be appropriately alarmed and monitored.
- All embryo laboratories should have an automatic emergency generator backup in the event of power failure.
- A minimum number of two incubators are recommended. Gas cylinders should be placed outside or in a separate room with an automatic backup system.
- Incubators should be frequently cleaned and sterilized. Nitrogen tanks should be cleaned and sanitized at least every year (Figs. 2 and 3).

- CO_2 (5–7%) required for:
  1. Maintain pH of bicarbonate buffered media
  2. Incorporate into protein and nucleic acids by the embryos.
- In vivo, oocytes and embryos are exposed to a maximum of ~5–8% O_2 in the reproductive system.
- Atmospheric O_2 may lead to supraphysiological ROS levels, potentially causing oxidative stress (damage to cell organelles, lipids, membranes, DNA, gene expression), and ultimately poor embryo development.
- Reduced O_2 concentration results in enhanced development in vitro.
- Management,—in a separated gas room, alarm system, regulators, responsible personnel, spare line and cylinders, clean the room and cylinders, color of cylinders, time and date of change

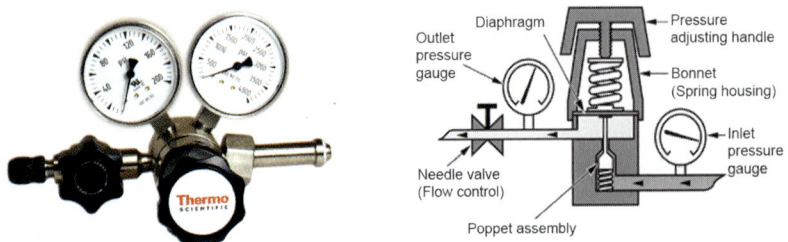

Fig. 2: Gas cylinders.
(ROS: reactive oxygen species; DNA: deoxyribonucleic acid)

- Embryos spend the majority of their time within incubator
- Function—Provides a stable and appropriate culture environment required for optimizing embryo development and clinical outcomes.
- Selection—Type of gas sensors, temperature regulation methods and size of the incubator are different variables and important for selecting the working incubator.
- Management—Air quality, temperature, humidity, gas monitoring and recovery, sterilization

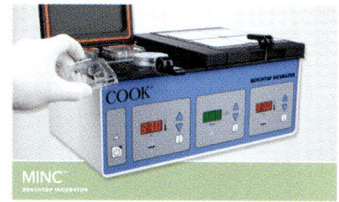

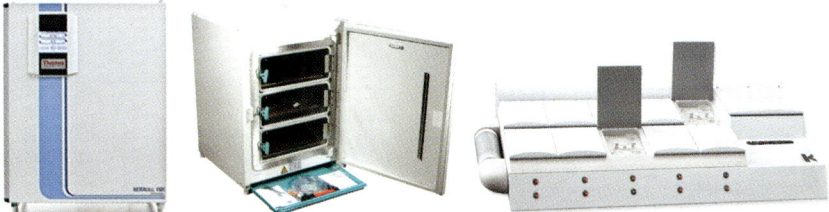

Fig. 3: Incubators.

Essential Equipment

CO_2 Incubator (Fig. 4)

The CO_2 incubators allow to closely, reliably, and repeatedly mimicking the environmental conditions that sperm, oocytes, blastocysts and developing embryos encounter in vivo.[7]

Benchtop Incubator

This kind of bench top incubators is ideal for existing laminar flow hood environment in IVF laboratories.

37°C Incubator

These simple incubators can warm up hydroxyethyl piperazineethanesulfonic acid (HEPES)-buffered media in IVF and can be used to warm up the disposables. A minimum of two CO_2 incubators are essential in any program. One is exclusively for media equilibration and another one for fertilization/embryo culture.

Triple Gas Incubator

Research has shown that incubators with an atmosphere comprising CO_2, O_2, and N_2 provide a more natural environment than a plain CO_2 incubator, giving better embryo quality and higher success rate. It could be a good investment, if going for blastocyst culture.

Vertical Laminar Flow Hoods (Fig. 5)

This HEPA-filtered working environment provides clean air for gamete/embryo handling. This could be an integrated laminar flow hood with two stereo zoom

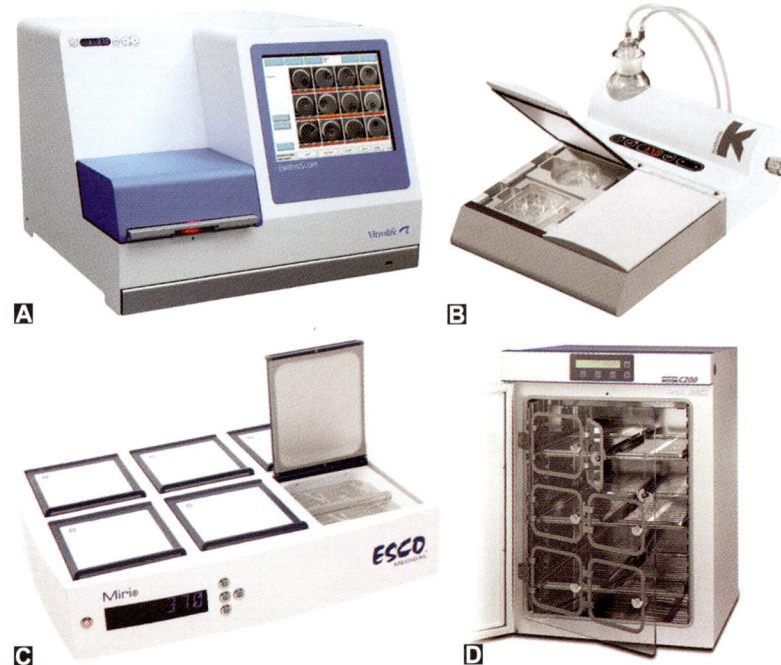

Figs. 4A to D: Various types of incubator: (A) Time lapse incubator; (B) Mini-incubator; (C) Benchtop; (D) Middle-size

- Function:
  1. Clean work station for gametes and embryos manipulation
  2. Media preparation.
- Management:
  Air quality, temperature, decontamination, UV, humidity and gases if close chamber

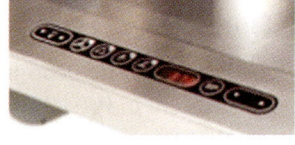

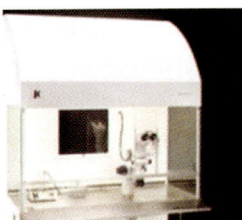 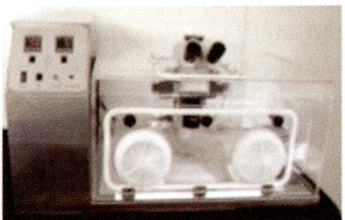 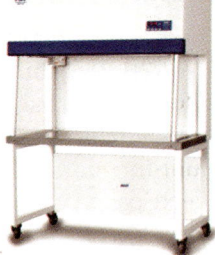

Fig. 5: Laminar flow.
(UV: ultraviolet)

microscopes, a bench top triple gas incubator and an imaging device/monitor with recording facility.[8]

Stereo Zoom Microscopes
Stereo microscopes produce three-dimensional, laterally correct, and upright images. Their major benefits include large object fields and large working

distances. Stereo microscopes, also called dissecting microscopes, are really two compound microscopes, which focus on the same point from slightly different angles. This allows the specimen to be viewed in three dimensions. As opposed to compound microscopes, the image is upright and laterally correct (not upside down and backwards). Stereo microscopes are relatively low power compared with compound microscopes, usually below 100×. They can have a single fixed magnification, several discrete magnifications, or a zoom magnification system. Working distance is much longer than with a typical compound microscope as well allowing work to be done on the specimen while it is being observed through the microscope (hence the name "dissecting microscope"). Many stereo microscopes are modular in design allowing a variety of stands, eyepieces, objectives, and lighting techniques to be implemented depending on the intended use.

Stereo zoom microscope is used in IVF laboratory for egg harvesting during ovum pick up, for insemination, embryo changes from media to media, embryo loading to embryo transfer (ET) catheter, vitrification device, etc.

Stereo zoom microscope is usually integrated into the heated laminar flow table. For a busy IVF laboratory 2–3 stereo zoom microscopes are essential. One can be dedicated exclusively for vitrification of oocytes/embryos with the base where dishes are kept having no-heating plate.

ICSI Workstation

The ICSI for male factor infertility is widely practiced in most of the IVF clinics. To perform ICSI, one need an inverted microscope fitted with a micromanipulator.

Inverted microscopes are available from Nikon, Olympus, Leica, Carl Zeiss, etc. The micromanipulators those are available in the market are Narishige, Eppendorf, research instruments (RI), cell robotics, etc.

IVF Workstation

These are specifically designed for aseptic handling of oocytes and embryos to minimize microbial contamination. Built-in liquid-based heating system, built-in stereomicroscope fitting, transmitted light source, heated plate by electrical heating, or water circulation heating (Fig. 6). The IVF chambers provide a triple gas incubator kind of environment.

Centrifuges

Centrifuge machine with swing-out rotor is ideal from the sperm preparation in IVF.

Liquid Nitrogen Cans

Enough number of liquid nitrogen Dewars are essential for storage of sperm and embryos. One with wide mouth is ideal.

- Separated unit or included in the laminar flow
- Function—are used for maintaining the temperature at 37°C
- Management—routinely and sent for recalibration to ensure that the temperature level is accurate, calibration if not accurate

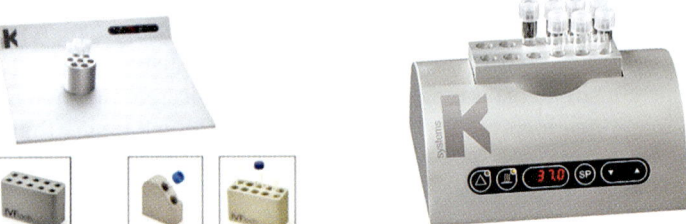

Fig. 6: Heating surface.

■ LABORATORY STAFFING

Personnel are one of the most important parts of an IVF laboratory. The number of laboratory staff should reflect the number of cycles performed per year. As an approximate guide, clinics that perform up to 150 retrievals and/or cryopreservation cycles per year should have always a minimum of two qualified clinical embryologists. This initial number will increase depending not only on the number of treatments, but also on the complexity of the procedures, techniques, and tasks undertaken within the laboratory. Other duties such as administration, training, education, quality management, and communication also need consideration.

As per Indian Council of Medical Research (ICMR) guidelines, the practice of ART requires a well-orchestrated teamwork between the gynecologist, the andrologist, and the clinical embryologist supported by a counselor and a program coordinator/director.

Appropriate human resources should provide an adequate climate to perform all laboratory tasks in a timely manner, to ensure patient safety and quality care. Sufficient qualified personnel should be available to provide back-up for the laboratory staff.

■ "BURNING IN" OF THE FINISHED IVF FACILITY

New IVF set up has high levels of VOCs from the chemicals released by new constructions and furnishings.[9] The ambient levels of many of these materials can be reduced by "burning in" the new construction by raising the temperature of new area by 10–20°C and increasing the ventilation rate, the temperature can be increased higher than this also. The combination of increased temperature and higher air exchange rate results in the removal of volatile compounds. The burn-in period can be from 10 days to 28 days, the laboratory should be closed during this procedure.

After the burn-in is complete the ventilation and air quality in the laboratory should be verified by series of tests using basic airflow measurements and tracer gas studies. The particulate levels should be determined to verify that the HEPA system is functional.

The same burn-in principle is applicable to the newly purchased incubators. Removal of volatile organics is essential for the critical microenvironment of the incubator. It is recommended to purchase incubators months in advance of their intended initial use, and to operate them at elevated temperature in a clean and protected location.

■ LABORATORY AIR QUALITY (FIGS. 7 AND 8)

In designing the laboratory, ensure that the volume of the air entering the facility is sufficient to place the laboratory under a slight positive pressure relative to outside. This will reduce the migration of the materials that can penetrate the laboratory. To optimize environmental conditions, laboratory air should be subjected to HEPA and VOC control. Positive pressure is recommended to minimize air contamination (Fig. 9). Procedures involving gamete or embryo manipulation should be performed in a controlled environment.[10]

■ MAINTENANCE PLANNING: MAINTAINING STABILITY IN THE LABORATORY

A daily, weekly, and yearly maintenance schedule should be made for each equipment and procedure in the system. A checklist for records should be reviewed on weekly, monthly, and annual basis.[11]

* Personal hygiene and changing of scrub, wearing headgears, mask, and proper foot wear should be strictly maintained.

* Importance of air quality in IVF
    - High levels of VOC in unfiltered IVF lab air
    - Efficient particle and VOC removal by air filtration
    - Embryo development inversely correlated with VOC
    - Better outcome (PR, IR, miscarriage) in IVF cycles performed laboratories with air particle and VOC filtration
* Types of filters
    1. HEPA (High efficiency particulate air) filters
    2. ULPA (ultra-low penetration air) filters
    3. VOC (volatile organic compound) filters

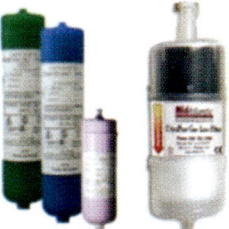

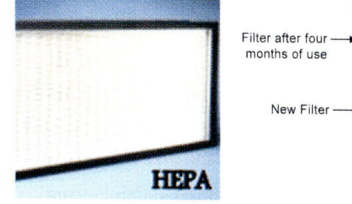
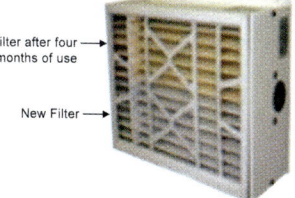
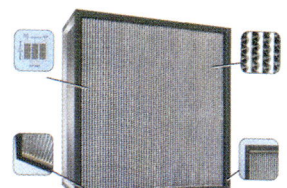

Fig. 7: Air quality equipment.
(IVF: in vitro fertilization; IR: implantation rate, PR: pregnancy rate)

- Function—Clean air pollutants, dust particles, mould spores, dander, pollen, dust mites, cleaning chemicals, volatile organic compounds (VOCs), chemically active compounds (CACs), aldehydes, carcinogenic materials, carbon monoxide, viruses and bacteria
- Mostly portable
- Air filters + UV lamp
- Management—Daily check, change filters and UV lamp, increase velocity according to the level of pollution

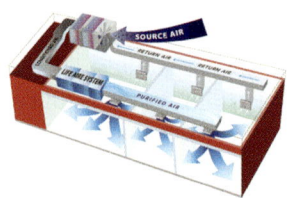

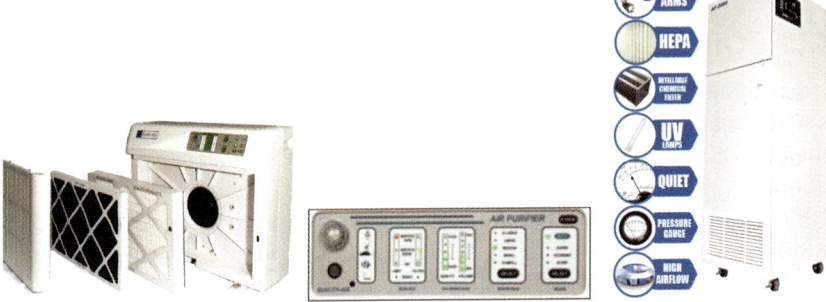

Fig. 8: Air purification system.
(UV: ultraviolet)

- The laboratory should be pressurized to prevent air from adjacent rooms entering the laboratory
- Function
  - Reduce microbial flora to minimum
  - Reduce VOC
  - Exclude contamination coming from surrounding areas with the provision of fresh air intake to replace CO_2 gas released in the IVF lab
  - Protect not only the embryos but also the embryologist
- 4-stage filtration
- Management—Change filters, maintenance, choice the time and frequency of switch on

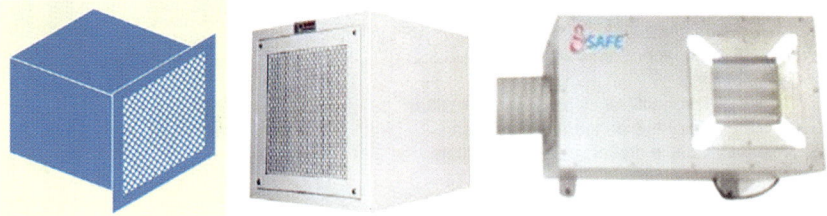

Fig. 9: Positive pressure system.
(VOC: volatile organic compound; IVF: in vitro fertilization; HEPA: high-efficiency particulate air)

- Toxic floor or furniture cleaners should not be used. No detergents or alcohols should be used while handling the oocyte and embryos.
- Strict cleanliness of the laminar flow hoods, work benches, and all equipment with solution of sterile water and 7× laboratory detergents

should be used. A 70% ethanol can be used at the end of the day when all the embryology work is finished and no further opening of incubators or handling of gametes is left.
- CO_2 levels and temperature of the incubators should be monitored daily (Fig. 10A).
- Daily monitoring of temperature of water bath, stage warmers, heating blocks, and other heated surfaces should be monitored routinely (Fig. 10B).
- Measurement of pH of the culture media equilibrated inside the incubator should be done twice week to confirm the correct percentage of CO_2 chambers. The ideal pH should be within the range of 7.2–7.4 (Fig. 10C).
- Carbon filters should be replaced every 10 months before complete exhaustion of these filters.
- Off-gassing of all plasticware utilized in the IVF laboratory should be done by removing them from their packing. This allows volatile gases to escape from polystyrene-based plastics.

PROTECTIVE MEASURES IN THE IVF SET UP

All body fluids (blood, follicular fluid, semen, etc.) should be treated as potentially contaminated. Protective measures for laboratory staff to ensure aseptic conditions for tissue, gametes, and embryos include:
- Strict adherence to staff hygiene regulations and aseptic techniques.
- Use of protective laboratory clothing, preferably with low-particle shedding.
- Use of nontoxic, nonpowdered gloves, head gears, and masks, where appropriate.

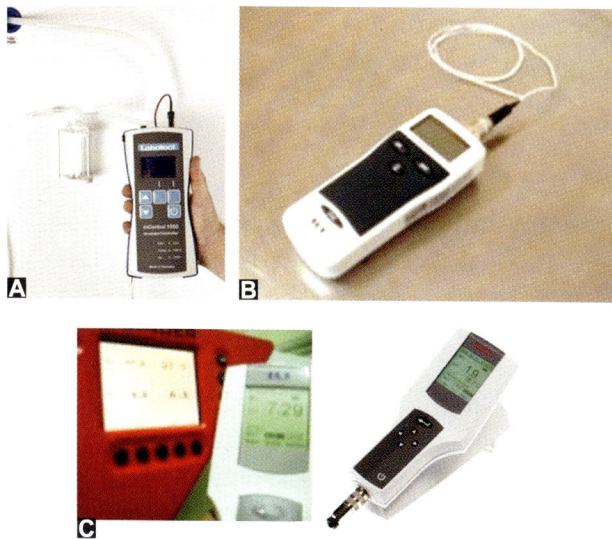

Figs. 10A to C: Quality control (QC) and monitoring equipment: (A) CO_2, O_2 temperature analyzer for incubators; (B) Thermometer; (C) pH meter

- Use of appropriate vertical laminar flow benches for handling biological material.
- Use of mechanical pipetting devices.
- Disposal of single-use consumables immediately into proper waste containers. Potentially infectious materials must be disposed of in a manner that protects laboratory workers and other staff from exposure. Viral-positive waste is segregated into a separate bin, labeled, and disposed of according to biosafety policies.
- Needles, glassware, and other sharps should be handled with extreme caution and discarded into sharps containers.
- Disinfectants with proven compatibility and efficacy for an IVF laboratory should be used.
- Food, gum, drinks, and tobacco are strictly forbidden.
- Use of cosmetics should be minimized and perfumes should be avoided.
- Staff should be appropriately attired to diminish possible sources of contamination.

Emergency Plan

As a part of the general emergency plan of clinic, all IVF laboratories should develop and implement an emergency plan with specific procedures in case of an exceptional failure of infrastructure and facilities, either of natural or human origin.

Emergency planning aims to describe the actions to be taken for (in order of importance):
- Safety of personnel and patients
- Protection of all fresh and cryopreserved human material
- Limitation of damage to equipment and medical records.

The following factors should be considered:

Communication Measures in Emergency Situation
- Contacts (responsible persons, technical services, and contact numbers) should be clear for all personnel.

Facilities
- *Electricity*: Loss of electrical power should be compensated by generators or uninterrupted power supply (UPS) systems.
- LN_2: In case of failure of automatic supply lines, tanks should be filled manually. A fully filled reserve LN_2 tank should be available.

Equipment

- In case of power failure, critical equipment should be prioritized.
- A second item of critical equipment should be available, if the first item fails. All reserve equipment should be fully validated and ready for use.
- *Freezer (–20°C) and refrigerator*: Back-up cooled freezers and refrigerators should be available.
- *Cryopreservation vessels*: It may be necessary to move tanks to another location.
- *Medical records*: Records to identify the ownership of human tissue should be kept on a secure web server.
- Regular revision of the emergency plan is necessary.
- Third-party arrangements should be in place with another IVF laboratory for emergency transfer of gametes and embryos (fresh and cryopreserved).

POLICIES AND PROCEDURES

All laboratory procedures must include provision for unique patient identification while retaining patient confidentiality.[12] Laboratory results should be reported according to a written procedure. They should be validated, dated, and included unique patient identity. Any interpretation of results should be accurate, comprehensive, and clinically relevant. There is a record of all reagents, calibration, and quality control material. There is a written, signed, and dated protocol for every procedure, written transmission of results and regular maintenance of equipment. All the procedures should be gathered in a manual kept in the laboratory and available for consultation. A log book should be maintained in the form of quality system requirement for regular evaluation of the results (Fig. 11)

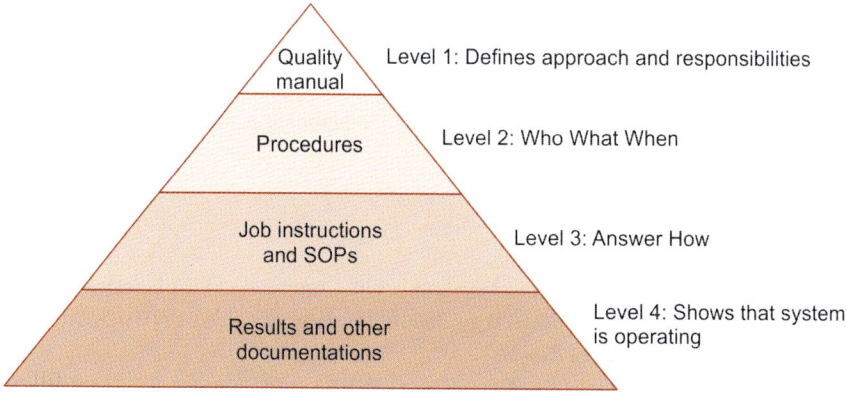

Fig. 11: Quality system requirement.
(SOP: standard operating procedure)

CONCLUSION

Creating a new ART clinic, whether as a standalone building, a new construction in an existing building, or even a renovation of an existing clinic, requires a team effort to learn a myriad of new facts about design, construction methods, building materials, ergonomics, wiring, lighting, patient movement pathways, local building regulations, etc. The more the time spent in the planning stage evaluating the many permutations, the greater the chance of creating a clinic that fully meets your current requirements while remaining adaptable for future growth. Proper planning is pivotal to success. The main goal of the IVF set up should be to provide a safe and secure environment while maintaining optimal parameters for embryonic development.

KEY POINTS

- The IVF laboratory design should be done based on the expected patient flow and future expansion plans. The budget might vary depending on the quality of equipment that you wish to purchase and patient load expected.
- The site of laboratory is very important as the outcome of IVF depends on laboratory quality along with other major contributing factors. A pollution-free area is ideal. Make sure that the IVF laboratory area is away from patient traffic locations in the hospital. If the IVF center is in down town areas keep the IVF laboratory region to the 3rd or upper floors. The ground floor invites more air pollution.
- Air quality in the IVF laboratory/OT area is of utmost importance. Pollution status of the air in the vicinity of the IVF clinic also should be taken into consideration. Based on these, more air handling units with HEPA/activated carbon filters should be installed with adequate positive pressure.
- Control and monitoring of equipment installation/validation/calibration should be performed on the routine basis at regular intervals. Proper installation of IVF equipment, proper after-sales service, and proper calibration and continuous updates on the new equipment, etc. are to be taken care.
- Laboratory equipment will require emergency power, temperature monitoring, and alarms. The construction of the laboratory should ensure aseptic and optimal handling of reproductive tissue during all stages of the process. Air conditioning for the laboratory will include HEPA filters, controlled humidity (20%), and controlled temperature (22–24ºC). Access to the laboratory should be limited.

REFERENCES

1. Magli MC, Van den Abbeel E, Lundin K, et al. Committee of the Special Interest Group on Embryology. Revised guidelines for good practice in IVF laboratories. Hum Reprod. 2008;23:1253-62.
2. Giannaroli L, Plachot M, vanKooij R, et al. ESHRE guidelines for good practice in IVF Laboratories. Hum Reprod. 2000;15:2241-6.
3. Boone WR, Higdon HI, Skeleton WD. How to design and implement an assisted reproductive technology (ART) clean room. J Clin Embryol. 2007;10(4):5-15.

4. Hall J, Gilligan A, Schimmel T, et al. The origin, effects and control of air pollution in laboratories used for human embryo culture. Hum Reprod. 1998;13(Suppl 4):146-55.
5. Morbeck DE. Basics of laboratory set-up in the office. In: Collins RL, Seifer DB, (Eds). Office-based Infertility Practice. New York: Springer; 2002. p. 63.
6. Cooke S, Tyler JPP, Driscoll G. Objective assessments of temperature maintenance using in vitro culture techniques. J Assist Reprod Genet. 2002;19;368-75.
7. Barnes FL. Equipment and general technical aspects of micromanipulation of gametes embryos. In: Gardner DK, Weissman A, Howles CM, Shoham Z (Eds). Textbook of Assisted Reproductive Techniques. London: Taylor and Francis; 2004. pp. 163-70.
8. Meintjes M, Chantilis SJ, Douglas JD, et al. A controlled randomized trial evaluating the effect of lowered incubator oxygen tension on live births in a predominantly blastocyst transfer program. Hum Rerod. 2009;24:300-7.
9. Seifert B. Regulating indoor air, presented at the 5th international conference on indoor air quality and climate. Toronto: Canada; 1990;5:35-49.
10. Riggin R, Winberry W, Murphy N. Compendium of Methods for the Determination of Toxic Organic compounds in ambient air. Washington DC: U.S. Environmental Protection Agency; 1984/1988. US EPA 600/4-84-041.
11. Cohen J, Gilligan A, Willadsen S. Culture and quality control of embryos. Hum Reprod. 1998;13 (Suppl 3):137-44.
12. Hughes PM, Morbeck DE, Hudson S, et al. Peroxides in mineral oil used for in vitro fertilization; defining limits of standard quality control assays. J Assist Reprod Genet. 2010;27:87-92.

CHAPTER

18

Recent Advancement in the Maintenance of Laboratory Quality Control

Julia Szeptycki, Alex C Varghese

■ INTRODUCTION

The earliest attempts in research and in vitro culture of mammalian embryos were mainly performed with the use of laboratory animals (mice and rabbits).[1,2] Decades long expansion of technologies now allows us to isolate, culture, analyze and store human embryos providing successful outcomes for even the most challenging patient situations.

The extreme sensitivities of gametes and early embryos to physical and environmental factors highlight the potential compromise of the in vitro fertilization (IVF) laboratory in absence of strict controls. As such, attention to the general components of a quality control (QC) and quality assurance program are necessary for a repeatable process and as such total quality management (TQM) program must be stressed.

■ IN THE BEGINNING

Historically, quality management was to the discretion of a laboratory director and often developed based on individual quality improvement activities and statistical techniques. As reproductive technologies grew worldwide, disparities amongst laboratories practices warranted attention by clinicians and policy makers.

The advent of Clinical Lab Improvement Amendments of 1988 (CLIA'88) established quality standards for all laboratories ensuring the accuracy, reliability, and timeliness of patient test results performed regardless of where the test was performed. Structural, regulatory bodies, and multidisciplinary organizations operate to impose the regulatory standards of CLIA'88 regionally, nationally, and globally.

Governance of IVF laboratories based on established CLIA'88 regulations is hierarchical in both regulatory and nonregulatory aspects. In the US, the USA Food and Drug Administration and Centers for Disease Control are mandated to provide specific outcomes.

Collective organizations [Society for Assisted Reproductive Technologies, (SART); European Society of Human Reproduction and Embryology, (ESHRE)] Act to advocate established regulations through monitoring and guidelines related laboratory performance compliance.

Membership organizations including the American Society for Reproductive Medicine (ASRM) and the Canadian Fertility and Andrology Society (CFAS) provide information, education, and advocacy of minimum standards and guidelines.

For Canadians specifically, the Assisted Human Reproduction (AHR) Act helps to ensure the safe and ethical use of assisted reproductive technologies. Unlike the US and Europe, Canadian IVF laboratories, operating under the guidelines provided by the CFAS, are free to acquire accreditation status. A potentially cost-prohibitive undertaking those achieving accreditation status often use it as a marketing strategy in the increasingly competitive industry.

The complexity of regulatory and nonregulatory arms necessitates a comprehensive framework for engagement of essential quality management initiatives and their associated factors.

What is total quality management and quality management culture?

The TQM is a global view of QC, quality assurance, and quality initiatives. The oversimplified goal of TQM is to provide an optimal product with process efficiency. This is accomplished by identifying and eliminating problems in work processes and systems.

Implementation involves satisfying customers, system/process, people, and improvement tools. These are further identified as the five pillars of TQM—product (service), process, organization, leadership, and commitment.[3]

Such an undertaking requires an organizational culture change involving a major staff learning and training program followed by pilot quality initiatives in a number of major areas including human, financial, technological, and natural resources.

Diverging from the traditional top-down approach, knowledge sharing is recognized as a key element in enhancing a company's capacity to be more responsive.[4] As such more personal involvement is required by top management to establish effective communication circles with personnel.[5]

■ IMPACT OF TQM ON YOUR DAY TO DAY WORK IN THE ASSISTED REPRODUCTIVE TECHNOLOGY LABORATORIES: EMBRYOLOGY, ANDROLOGY, AND CRYOBIOLOGY LABORATORIES

Several papers examine the complementary of TQM practices on management strategy and its impact on work life, quality, and performance.

The results of TQM implementation are contradictory and inconclusive with the majority of UK and US companies revealing "zero competitive gain" from TQM or mixed findings in relation to the TQM's success.[6]

The main positive impact of TQM concerns job content, job control, global participation, and social relations.[7] At the same time, negative changes are reported for workload and the lack of clarity of duties.[7] These discrepancies may be attributed to a gap about intentions for TQM and the reality of implementation in the various subunits of the organization.

The TQM programs are also charged with failing to create a deep and sustained change in organizations. Communication circles, thought to increase the innovativeness and participation of personnel, reveal only acute, unsustainable effects in altering employees' attitudes, and organizational culture. The importance of organizational culture and attitudes of workforce cannot be understated as being conducive to TQM success.[8,9]

It should be understood that a quality management culture is not a goal, but an ongoing process that requires constant adaptability in human and/or financial resources. A shortage of either of these resources and/or opposition to adopting innovations is barrier to successful TQM implementation, even if their expected values are positive for the organization.[10]

Quality management activities requiring full traceability and documentation are labor intensive. Lacking international standards, and of noteworthy mention, it is an important QC issue to have sufficient number of personnel to perform routine laboratory work without subjecting either personnel or patients to undue stress or risk. The number of personnel should be fixed for routine work, with additional personnel for more complex procedures.[11]

An organization's top management, therefore, plays an important role in promoting quality cultures at all organizational levels. Successful TQM implementation will only persist in a climate of senior leadership capacity to institute an organizational-wide commitment to behavioral changes, cross-functional mechanisms, leadership skills, and dialog needed to not only learn but enable further change.[12]

How to collect and manage the data?

There is general consensus of the value in data reporting of national and clinic-specific outcomes. Performance can be monitored using a QC system in simple tabulated form. For reproductive technologies, at a laboratory level these may include—(1) fertilization rates, (2) cleavage or blastulation rates, and (3) embryo utilization rate. Efficacies as a function of primary endpoint may include rate of—(1) positive β-hCG (human chorionic gonadotropin), (2) gestational sac development, (3) ongoing viable pregnancy (presence of a fetal heartbeat), and (4) live birth.

Data may be further analyzed per treatment—(1) initiation, (2) retrieval, or (3) embryo transfer conventionally as a function of age range demographic.

In smaller data collections, direct cycle-to-cycle comparisons may pose little benefit as cell cycle-specific factors including diagnosis, treatment, stimulation, number of cycles prior to achieving pregnancy, and accurate pregnancy outcome data are numerous and may dilute the observed trend.

Other endpoints including rates of ovarian hyperstimulation syndrome, miscarriage, multiple pregnancy, and ectopic pregnancy may lose value as patient-specific treatment and circumstances may vary.

Industry-wide, arduous and inefficient manual data collection is trending toward internet-based practice management software (e.g. eIVF, Baby Sentry), which integrates all aspects of practice management including treatment and inventory supply chain. Annual reports generated are based on the information collected are pertinent to interpreting trends in the individual practice over time.

These data collections, or registries, extend to regional (BORN, Ontario, Canada), national (CARTR Plus, Canada; SART, USA), and more sophisticated levels (EIM, Europe). On a global level, the International Committee for Monitoring Assisted Reproductive Technology (ICMART) World Reports provide the most comprehensive statistical census and review of assisted reproductive technology (ART) utilization, effectiveness, safety and quality.[7] While this type of data is most desirable, it is expensive to collect and to control for accuracy. But they warn the data presented is reliant on the quality and completeness of data submitted.[7]

■ INTERNAL AND EXTERNAL QUALITY CONTROL FOR IVF, ANDROLOGY, PREIMPLANTATION GENETIC DIAGNOSIS AND CRYOBIOLOGY LABORATORIES

Quality control includes establishing a standard for each aspect of a procedure that will result in a reliably reproducible result. In the case of diagnostic testing, the result may be a predictor of fertility or screening result. In other instances, successful rejuvenation of a cryopreserved sample or in the ART procedure, pregnancy is a measured outcome.

Internal QC provides for full traceability and documentation including standardization of operating procedures with formal training programs for staff within a program.

Ongoing training, tools, and periodic assessments (QA) assure that laboratory- or technician-specific variations are within acceptable tolerance limits, corrected if needed, and that errors are not introduced over time. New tools (QI) including remote monitoring of environment (pH, temperature, and humidity) and technological advancement aim to increase productivities or efficiencies.

In the laboratory, equipment is set at optimal performance, monitored, and recorded at regular intervals. Consumables (e.g. culture media and contact materials) are recorded as traceable by lot number and on a per patient basis. In principle, despite commercial availability of many products, periodic evaluation of all materials and their treatment before introduction into a laboratory is suggested.

Participation in an external quality assurance (EQA) program (e.g. College of American Pathologists) provides for international laboratories to assess accuracies in their methods, individual performance and reporting.[13] This allows a laboratory to evaluate the same samples and procedures as other laboratories and to compare their performance against that of others. The benefit is to help achieve continuous quality improvements and higher standards of care for patients.

■ STANDARDIZED TRAINING PROGRAMS

Assisted reproductive technology is widely practiced worldwide and there is a need for its continuous monitoring to improve the comprehensiveness and quality of ART data and services. Appropriately, there is need for appropriate training and continuing education for technicians of this highly skilled discipline.

Historically, training was performed in laboratory with no specific educational requirements. Under CLIA'88, andrology laboratories, but not embryology laboratories, are required to comply with CLIA'88. Due to the multifaceted role of the technician, it is common practice that all personnel achieve the same training and educational standards.

In general, the minimum educational requirement is a 4-year bachelor degree with advanced degree required for supervisory, managerial, and director level roles. International and online distance learning programs exist such as the Masters in Clinical Embryology (UK, USA, and Australia) although all are not accredited.

In Canada, there are currently no minimum educational requirements to work in ART and more specifically, no formal programs that provide specific learning in the laboratory aspects of ART. Postsecondary institutions are soon to offer advanced degree programs in the discipline and it is anticipated that a specific degree requirement will become the standard in the future.

While the educational requirements vary by country, established guidelines are designed to assist practices by setting criteria that meet or exceed the legislative requirements of each country. Countries lacking legislation may follow the standards established by ESHRE and ASRM.

Several organizations offer Continuing Education courses or certificates specializing in this discipline. The American Board of Bioanalysis (ABB), CFAS, and ESHRE are recognized certifying agencies for directors offering high complexity (HCLD), embryology (ELD), and/or (ALD) Laboratory Directors. Working to standardize the theoretical knowledge and clinical skills of technicians may increase confidence in reliability and outcomes.

■ MONITORING KEY PERFORMANCE INDICATOR

A key performance indicator (KPI) is a measured value evaluating performance outcomes.[14] Strategic goals and performance activities are aligned with a common goal of producing reliably improved outcomes. They must be specific, measurable, attainable, relevant, and time-bound (SMART) and will be short-lived unless they are (SMARTER) evaluated and re-evaluated.

In ART therapeutic procedures, monitoring pregnancy rates as a KPI ensures that pregnancy rates are kept at a maximum level. Pregnancy rates are often viewed at regular time internal, but this form of audit has major limitations, namely—(1) the chance of pregnancy can be influenced by the underlying pathology of the patients; (2) a drop in pregnancy rates means that a problem was encountered at the time of treatment, usually a few weeks before, and (3) the actual problem is not revealed.

Since the embryology laboratory is the epicenter of the IVF unit, the dependence of pregnancy outcome to a greater extend on the laboratory performance highlights the need for ensuring the quality of these services. It is, therefore, essential to lay down certain benchmarks to assess ART laboratory functions.

Any process, whether in a biomedical or nonbiomedical field, can be subjected to inherent deviations from the optimum or from established limits. These deviations may lead to defective end-products or, in the medical field, defective patient care. Monitoring, which is a process able to identify deviations, and then being able to act should such deviation exceed certain limits, plays an important role in avoiding adverse consequences and maintaining optimal performance.[15,16]

If IVF clinician thinks there are fewer pregnancies in recent times, many embryologists might recall that the first thing they use to do is blaming the laboratory. The laboratory may well be the cause of dip in pregnancy rate, but it may well also be other factors external to the laboratory. The best way to respond is with your KPI data. If you make the habit of supplying the clinicians with your basic KPI data regularly, it stops them from even asking the question! More practically though, you should use your KPI data each month to check that the basic embryology is consistent, e.g. the fertilization rate is the same, the number of embryos transferred is constant, etc. This is done each month as a first-line warning of possible problems. Though calculating the implantation rate needs a bit more time.

The very recent Vienna proceedings report presents 19 indicators, including 12 KPIs, 5 performance indicators (PIs), and 2 reference indicators (RIs). This is from an international workshop supported by the ESHRE and Alpha Scientists in Reproduction (Alpha), designed to establish consensus on definitions and recommended values for the ART laboratory.[17] The expert committee is of the opinion that each laboratory should develop its own set of KPIs founded on laboratory organization and processes, and develop a systematic, transparent, and consistent approach to data collection and analysis and calculation of KPIs.

■ DEFINING THE SUCCESS RATES OF CLINIC IN TQM AND THE ROLE OF STATISTICS

The collection of data on the performance of the clinic as a whole, but also of the individuals should be analyzed regularly. Some clinics perform a negative analysis of performance of each month. This will help in discerning any adverse outcomes from any new drugs, procedures, or individuals. Data should be audited, assessed, and structured to discern the input quality, the process quality, and the output quality as appropriate. Moreover, data on the functioning of equipment and culture systems, e.g. temperature, air quality, volatile organic compounds, and level of microbial contamination, must be collected and regularly audited.

Patients considering IVF will want to find the clinic in their area with the highest success rates. Many will search the internet to find the clinic with the "best" statistics even though in India this is not the usual scenario. Traditionally, the success of IVF has been reported on the basis of the outcome of a treatment initiated with the intention of replacing one or more fresh embryos by selecting the best embryo(s) for transfer within the uterus.

Cumulative live birth rate (CLBR) has been suggested as a suitable way of reporting success of an IVF program, which incorporates fresh as well as thawed frozen embryo transfer.[18]

It is important to take account of the total number of cycles for every age group and every medical profile, regardless of their complexity. Some clinics happens to just select easy cases in order to increase its success rate or project the statistics in the web page from a good prognosis IVF batch. Additionally, it is important to present not only positive pregnancy tests but also live births in the statistics.

The parameters that should be considered in the appraisal of statistical success rates are:

- The number of IVF cycles performed—the larger the sample size the more representative and reliable the result will be.
- The rate of pregnancies per age group, as this more accurately classifies an interested party in relation to the overall mean
- Annual updating of statistics
- The rate of positive pregnancy tests does not equal the actual birth rate, since some women with positive pregnancy tests have a miscarriage.
- The rate of multiple pregnancies is important as it reflects the numbers of embryos implanted and the policy of units relating to the prevention of obstetric complications.
- Special categories of IVF must provide the birth rates and health details of newborns, e.g. for preimplant diagnostics.

Honesty is rewarded, and when the success rates are reliably high, their value is significantly increased.

■ NONCONFORMITY IN ART

In quality management, a nonconformity (also known as a defect) is a deviation from a specification, a standard, or an expectation. A nonconformance means that something went wrong—a problem has occurred and needs to be addressed. Nonconformances are addressed with corrective actions.

You may find a nonconformance in a service, a product, a process, from a supplier, or in the system itself. It happens when something does not meet the specifications or requirements in some way. Those requirements might be defined by the customer, a regulatory body, or in the internal procedures of the organization.

A nonconformance could be identified through customer complaints, internal audits, external audits, incoming material inspection or simply during normal testing, and inspection activities. ISO 9001:2008 requires that you document your nonconformance procedure and keep records of nonconformance issues you identify and the actions taken.

You will need to workout a process (documented or not) for how your organization will deal with nonconforming output—how to decide on what immediate actions will be taken to correct the problem and who is responsible for the decision. These immediate actions can be seen as "damage control" and need to stop further nonconformance.

- Assess the effects of the problem—how much, how bad (thawed one embryo instead of two, sperm mixups)
- Contain the effects, e.g. quarantine defective items
- Notify affected customers, if necessary
- How reworked items should be checked (if it is different from normal inspection)
- How and where a nonconformance should be recorded (as incident report)
- What steps should be taken to identify any defective product released to a customer (process mapping)
- What, if any, concessions/discounts will be given to the customer
- How a decision will be made on whether further corrective action is necessary.

The ASRM guidelines on the disclosure of medical errors involving human gametes and embryos states that clinics have an ethical obligation to disclose errors out of respect for patient autonomy and in fairness to patients. Errors that affect the number or quality of gametes or embryos should be disclosed unless they clearly have a minimal effect on patient interests.[19]

It is obligatory to disclose immediately errors in which the wrong sperm is used for insemination, or gametes or embryos are mistakenly switched resulting in embryo transfer, conception, or the birth of a child with a different genetic parentage than intended. Clinics should promote a culture of truth telling and should establish written policies and procedures regarding disclosure of errors to patients. Fertility programs should have in place rigorous procedures to prevent the loss of gametes and embryos and to ensure proper identification of all gametes, embryos, and patients.

Honest-full report of all adverse incidents is part of a proper total quality management system. A "no-blame" and truth-telling culture should prevail it the IVF environment, so that when a mistake is made it is not hidden but brought forward for preventive or corrective actions.

PREPARATION, IMPLEMENTATION, AND REVIEW OF STANDARD OPERATING PROCEDURES

A standard operating procedure (SOP) is a document, which contains detailed written instructions describing the stepwise process and technique of performing a test/procedure in the laboratory. Standard operating procedures represent the sequence of steps that have been standardized to execute a task, and are used every time a given task is performed to ensure that it is executed in the same way every time and by every staff member.

The main reasons why fertility centers need SOPs as integral elements of the QC system are—(1) IVF involves repetitive high-complex critically important tasks; (2) variation must be controlled; (3) more than one person often perform the same task; (4) safety risks are present; and (5) QC must be ensured.[20] SOPs are dynamic and should be constantly reviewed/updated based on new knowledge and variation/errors detected after implementation.

The SOP should be strictly adhered to and no deviation should be permitted. The SOP should specify the persons authorized to perform each test, their qualification, and training. It also provides safety instruction, troubleshooting, waste disposal, etc. The SOP should be available to the staff in the working area itself and should be reviewed periodically by competent personnel. There are well-documented formats in which SOPs can be prepared. An SOP should also be prepared for staff training, equipment care, operation and calibration, cleaning, sterilization and disinfecting procedures, handling and disposal of waste, internal audit, participation in QC program, etc.

MONITORING THE LABORATORY EQUIPMENT AND AIR QUALITY: TEMPERATURE, GASES, PH, PARTICLE COUNT, VOLATILE ORGANIC COMPOUNDS, MICROBIAL COUNT, ETC.

The implanting blastocyst derived in vivo from the human oocyte and sperm traverses the Fallopian tube and uterine endometrium during its preimplantation development. A perfect homeostasis is provided by the in vivo microenvironment during the course of blastocyst development. However, the scenario is of stark difference when the in vitro-derived embryo develops in the confinement of a culture droplet in a petri dish. Several physical parameters need to be controlled meticulously to obtain a healthy embryo in vitro. Physical parameters pertaining to preimplantation embryo development in vitro does not limit to the integrity and complexity of culture media or the type of the incubators.

The major parameters to be controlled are—temperature, pH, osmolarity, humidity, air quality, etc. Even though several electronic gadgets are currently available to measure each of the parameters, devices used for checking physical parameters need proper QC. The Table 1 shows a list of available gadgets for routine quality checks.

Table 1: List of commercially available quality control (QC) devices.

pH meter	Orion Star™ A111 pH Benchtop Meter (Thermo Fisher USA)	LAQUA PH1200 Bench top meter (Horiba Scientific, Japan)	pH Meter-3 (Real time pH measurement) (ORIGIO, Denmark)	PetriSense®—Single sensor for monitoring of pH or CO_2 (Planer PLC, UK)	pH Online™ (MTG, Germany)	IVF-Safe sens continuous pH monitoring system (Safe Sens, USA)
Temperature	RI-IVF Thermometer (ORIGIO, Denmark)	K-System thermometer (ORIGIO, Denmark)	Solid temperature sensor (ORIGIO, Denmark)	GMH 3230 electronic thermometer (MTG, Germany)		
VOC	RI-VOC meter (ppm measurement ORIGIO, Denmark)	Sparmed VOC meter (ppb measurement; Denmark)	GrayWolf VOC meter (ppb measurement; USA)	VOC meter (ppm measurement; S-tech associates, India)		
CO_2/O_2	G-100 (Geotech, UK)	In Control 1050 (Labotect, Germany)				
Microbial air sampling	MAS-100® Microbial Air Monitoring Systems and ICR/ICRplus Settle Plates (Merck Millipore)					

(pH: potential of hydrogen; VOC: volatile organic compound; IVF: in vitro fertilization)

Table 2: Equipment requiring maintenance at 37°C.					
IVF laboratory	Incubators	IVF workstation bench	Stereo zoom heat plates	ICSI workstation stage	Test tube warmer
Oocyte retrieval suite	Test tube warmer	Heated trolley top	—	—	—
Andrology laboratory	Test tube warmer	Incubator	—	—	—

(IVF: in vitro fertilization; ICSI: intracytoplasmic sperm injection)

Maintaining the oocytes and embryos at a constant temperature is of vital importance for the successful outcome and health of implanting blastocysts. Table 2 shows the devices/equipment, which need to be maintained at a physiological temperature. Many laboratory accredited agencies require a secondary validation of temperature and will not allow you to rely solely on a digital reading from the instrument itself. There exist several different temperature measuring devices on the market today, from electronic thermometers with thermocouples to data loggers, temp-tracers, and continuous temperature monitoring probes that can be connected to an IT network and the internet of clinic for instant access and easy monitoring and adjustment.

Thermochrons are button-sized and stainless steel devices that can be placed directly into your testing environment without the need for external probes. The Thermochron devices are calibrated by Thermodata using a system accredited to ISO/IEC 17025 and traceable to National Institute of Standards and Technology (NIST) standards. The monitoring device was adapted for use in incubator environments to continually read temperature and humidity in small areas. The continual monitoring allows the user to validate the external display readings; assess incubator usage during the daytime so as to distribute usage more evenly over time; gauge recovery times of different types of incubators (Figs. 1 and 2); challenge incubators with alterations in temperature to examine whether the Thermochron ibuttons detected any anomalies (Fig. 3). Moreover thermocoins are useful to monitor the temperature in actual working condition such as culture media (Fig. 4).

Continuous temperature and humidity monitoring is critical for proper medical laboratory operation from a quality perspective. The information collected will facilitate strict QC of routine IVF instrumentation; and in particular, benchtop incubators provides the clinical user with a means for challenging the response time of incubators to fluctuations in environment and can help to maintain a constant and regulated state of control for temperature sensitive areas.

Recently, preliminary data have suggested that even slight rises in extracellular pH (pHe) during brief manipulations outside the laboratory

Recent Advancement in the Maintenance of Laboratory Quality Control

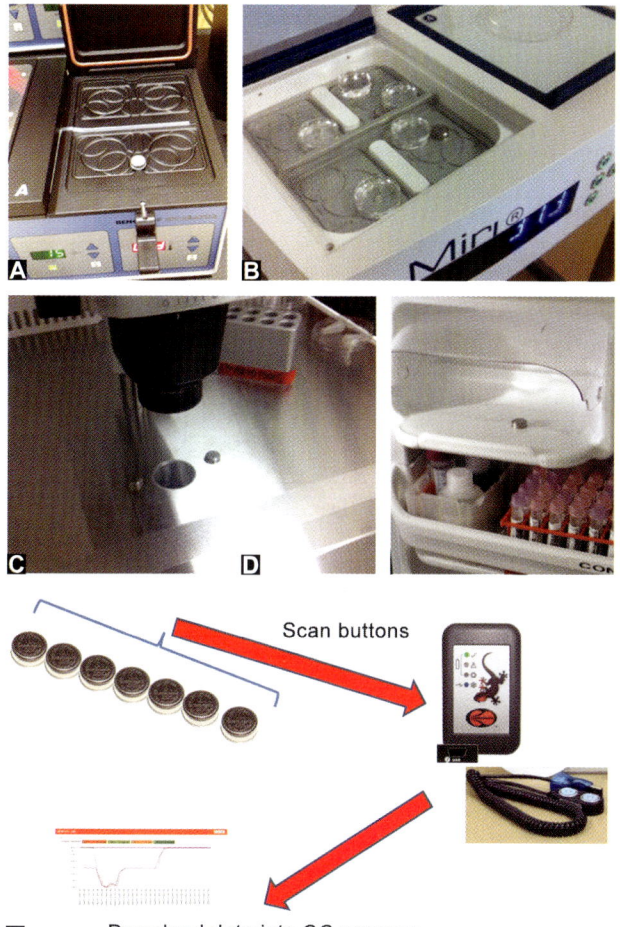

Figs. 1A to E: Thermochron buttons distributed over—(A and B) benchtop incubators, (C) in vitro fertilization (IVF) workstation bench, (D) refrigerator where media is stored, and (E) Thermochron devices.

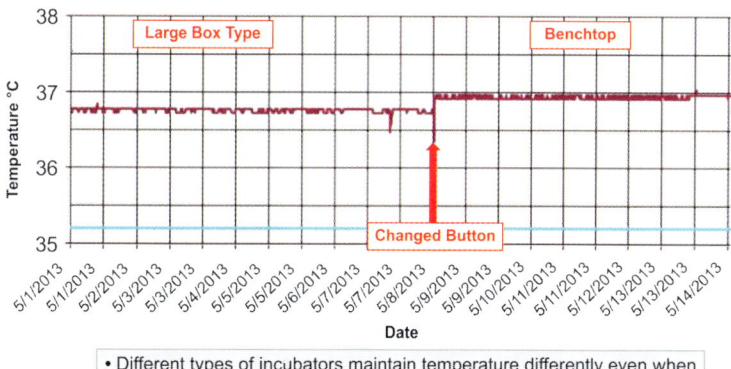

- Different types of incubators maintain temperature differently even when the digital display shows the same value

Fig. 2: Comparing a large to a benchtop incubator.

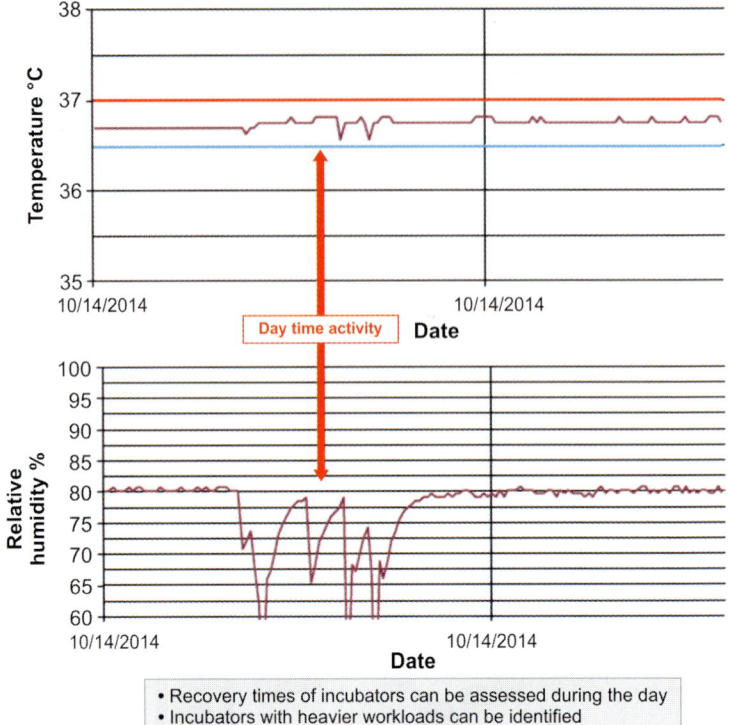

- Recovery times of incubators can be assessed during the day
- Incubators with heavier workloads can be identified

Fig. 3: Data output—continuous monitoring.

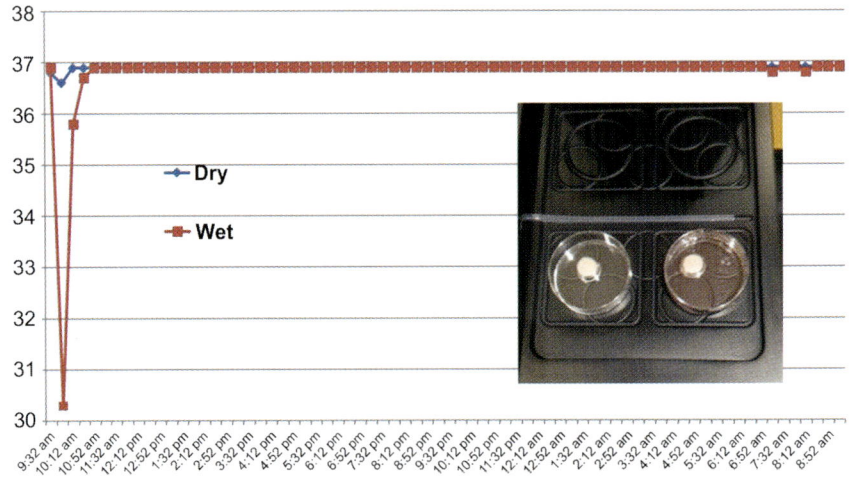

Fig. 4: Thermobutton readings over 24 hours (every 20 minutes) in a benchtop incubator when in media and dry.

incubator can significantly impact mouse blastocyst development and hatching, as well as significantly alter gene expression profiles.[21] One manner in which pHe may be influencing the embryos is likely due, in part, to its impact on intracellular pH (pHi) and cellular resources expended in maintaining intracellular homeostasis. Various commercial media companies recommend differing pHe ranges, most within the range of 7.2–7.4. Historically, CO_2 set points in incubators are adjusted to attempt to create the ideal media pH environment for any development stage of embryos. CO_2 adjustments are generally done by spot checking the pH of equilibrated media once a month or once a week.

In addition to obtaining the ideal pH, maintaining a stable pH environment is important for embryo development. It has been observed that denuded mature oocytes lack robust mechanisms to regulate internal pH, cryopreserved/warmed embryos have a reduced ability to regulate internal pH for several hours, and cleavage stage embryos have reduced ability to regulate internal pH compared to postcompaction embryos. Additionally, changes in pHi of embryos impacts metabolic activity, can impact organelle localization, and can even influence resulting fetal development. Thus, maintaining a stable and appropriate external pH (media pH) is critical.

There are many gadgets for pH measurement for IVF culture systems. A benchtop pH meter can be used for the routine pH measurement with proper calibration buffers. However, it is essential to keep the certificate of analysis of the media being used handy to check the pH of the given media lot each time.

A new technology, SAFE Sens TrakStation (Fig. 5), enables real time noninvasive pH monitoring within an incubator environment. Use of this technology can reveal incubator conditions, which are not ideal for maintaining ideal pH levels (Figs. 6 to 10).

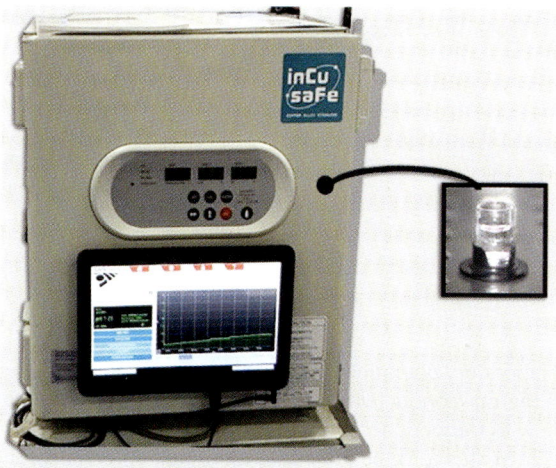

Fig. 5: SAFE Sens TrakStation.

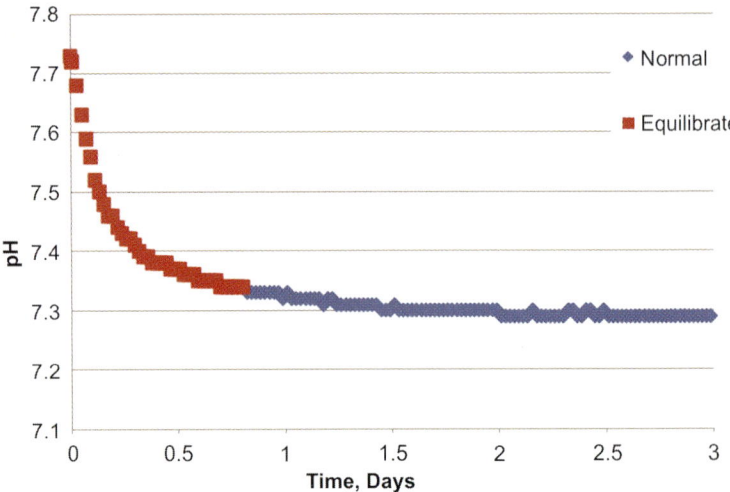

Fig. 6: Normal media potential of hydrogen (pH) equilibration curve. Sufficient time for the initial equilibration of media in a carbon dioxide (CO_2) environment is critical to achieving the desired pH. In many cases, at least 24 hours is needed for pH to reach steady state levels. The equilibration time for pH will vary depending on your culture choices. Oil is essential to slow evaporation of media, but there is a trade-off between speed of reaching pH set point and maintaining pH over a full culture period.

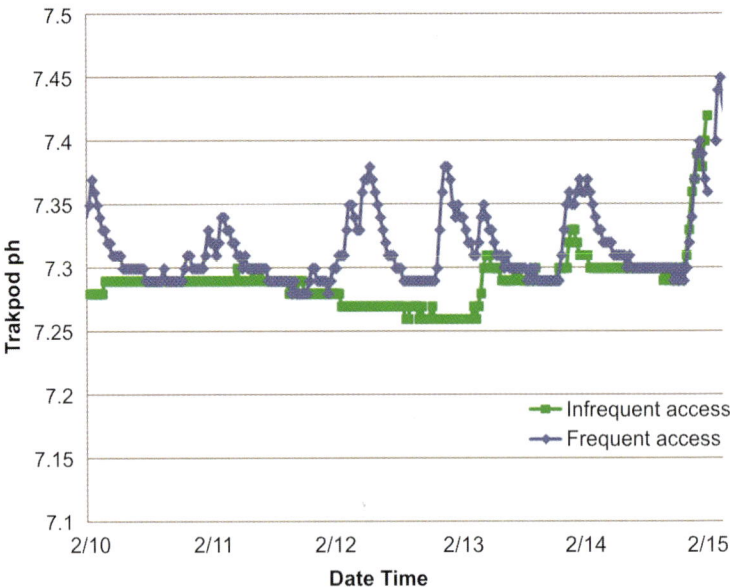

Fig. 7: Effect of laboratory operations on potential of hydrogen (pH) profile for cabinet incubators with thermal conductivity carbon dioxide (CO_2) sensors. Two incubators are monitored. One with frequent access (blue) and one with little access (green) during a week. The pH increases for blue are in the mornings. Afterwards, the environment takes some time to recover and return to the desired pH level. Because the technology used for thermal conductivity CO_2 sensors also depends on temperature and humidity, larger swings in the actual CO_2 can occur.

Recent Advancement in the Maintenance of Laboratory Quality Control

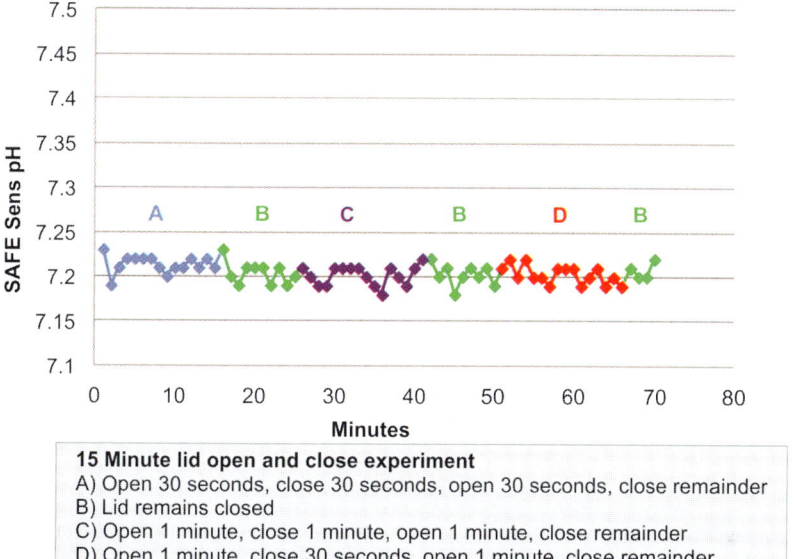

Fig. 8: Effect of benchtop lid openings on potential of hydrogen (pH) in a humidified benchtop incubator (planer BT37). The brief lid openings in benchtop incubators show very small changes in pH, due primarily to the oil overlay of the media slowing shifts in pH values in the media.

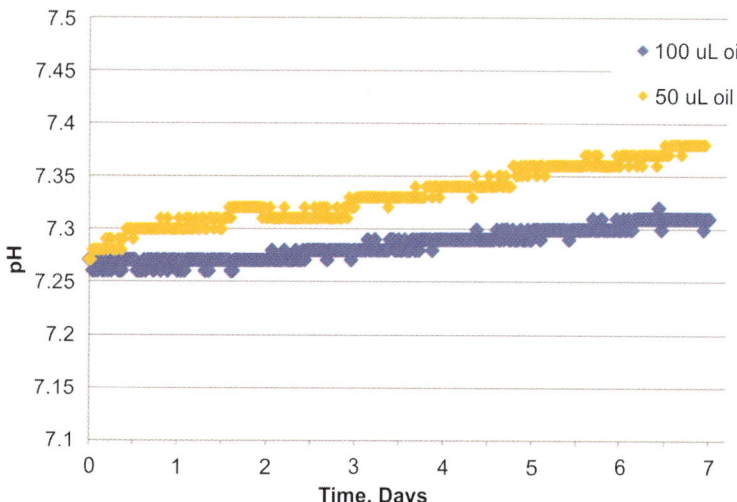

Fig. 9: Effect of laboratory operations on potential of hydrogen (pH) profile for a dry benchtop incubator (Esco Miri). Over the course of a week, the pH in benchtop incubators stays steady. The chamber lids were opened briefly (<5 minutes) in the middle of the pH monitoring time. In dry incubators, evaporation can be a concern. The slight pH increase can be due to evaporation of media and differs based on oil overlay volume.

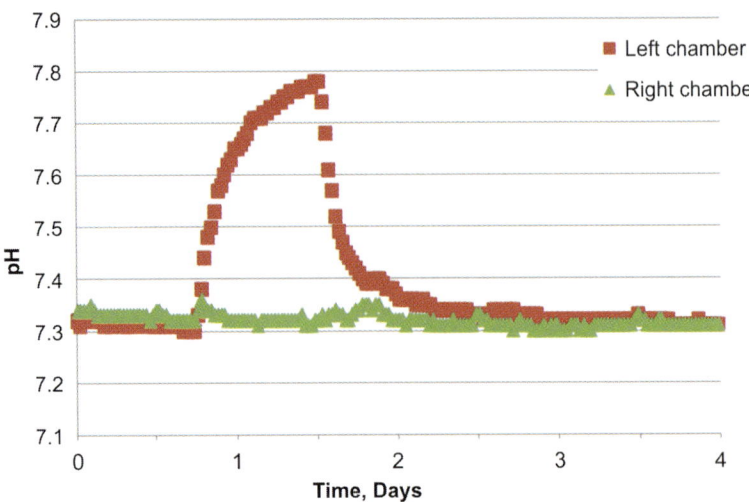

Fig. 10: Profile of a gas line blockage in humidifying bottle tubing (left chamber) as compared to normal function (right chamber). The potential of hydrogen (pH) spikes in the left chamber due to no gas flow to the BT-37 chamber and is resolved in 12 hours. With measurement rather than monitoring, compromised gas line tubing would not be discovered until the next time pH was taken, during an investigation into poor embryo development, or the tubing was manually fixed/replaced.

Many recent studies have suggested an association between poor laboratory air quality conditions and impaired embryo development, and resulting in decreased implantation and pregnancy rates. One the clean room concept is implemented in the IVF program, rigorous QC is required to maintain the clean air. Periodic checks on particle count, volatile organic compounds (VOCs), filter integrity, and microbial count should be undertaken. Though the particle counts and filter integrity tests can be carried by certified vendors, it is ideal to monitor the VOC levels and microbial counts regularly. VOCs can be measured either at ppb (Sparmed VOC meter and GrayWolf VOC meter) or ppm level (should be < 0.5 ppm).

Microbial testing and monitoring should also be part of the routine quality maintenance of the IVF program. Even though regular screening is done on the patient's samples brought into the laboratory environment, the microbial contamination can happen from many other sources. It has been observed that the air handling ducting can become a breeding ground for many molds and even the high-efficiency particulate air (HEPA) filters in the safety hoods and air handling systems can harbor microbes. It is ideal to change the HEPA type of filters (even that of safety hoods) at stipulated intervals, especially in places with high humidity.

Passive microbial air monitoring with the help of settle plates or contact plates is a useful complement to active air sampling methods. Settle plates allow a semiquantitative determination of microbial contaminations in the air. Since they are fairly small, they can also be used conveniently in confined spaces such as laminar air flow hoods. Alternatively, active air monitoring systems are available from many companies.

IoT is the concept of internet-of-things—the interconnection via the internet of computing devices embedded in everyday objects and enabling them to send and receive data. This can be very helpful in QC situations, especially monitoring laboratory conditions for performance-based laboratories such as IVF where the correct temperature, gas concentration, humidity, and VOC content present are critical to human embryo growth.

There are many monitoring systems available in the market (Table 3). Many of these wireless monitoring systems that are easy to install, requires no additional wiring, and can integrate into existing Wi-Fi network infrastructure of the unit. The monitoring software enables organizations to remotely monitor incubators, refrigerators, freezers, and other vital appliances throughout the facility in real time, automates internal monitoring processes, records historical data, and corrective actions associated with all alerts. Users can easily configure the monitoring software to provide automated reports and alarms. Advanced communication functionality of facility monitoring systems (FMS) allows key personnel to view alerts on screen or receive alarm notifications through email or text messaging of incubator temperature, humidity, carbon dioxide and oxygen levels, cryostorage vessels, and fridges.

Cleanroom areas have independent pressure sensors and particle counting duties are performed by a TSI AeroTrak portable particle counter, which feeds data direct to the FMS system in real time.

Typical installations may include the following environmental sensors:
- Temperature
- Relative humidity
- Liquid nitrogen
- Oxygen
- Carbon dioxide
- Room pressure
- Differential pressure

Table 3: Remote monitoring systems.

The XiltriX® laboratory monitoring system	IKS International	The Netherlands
LU 45 (for pathogens) and QA-20 (for VOCs)	NuWave Sensors	Ireland
Log & Guard	Vitrolife	Sweden
Esco Protect Wireless Monitoring System	Esco Global	Denmark
BioEase Inventory and Monitoring Software	Lab IVF	Singapore
Planer Monitoring systems	Planer PLC	UK
Monitoring systems	Mesa labs	USA
TSI FMS system	TSI	USA

(IVF: in vitro fertilization; FMS: facility management system)

- Open/closed doors
- Alarm state (Trigas incubators, time lapse incubators, etc.)
- Airborne particulates.

Volatile organic compounds are known to affect the success rate of assisted reproductive techniques and continuous laboratory VOC monitoring as part of the FMS may be useful. NuWave Sensors' LumAir is a patented rapid microbial detection sensor that facilitates remote monitoring of airborne pathogens (bacteria, yeasts, and molds) and revolutionizes the approach to pathogen detection and control *(www.nuwavesensors.com)*.

CONCLUSION

Quality management is a culture that needs to be implemented at different levels in an organization to yield fruitful results. Introduction of few QC gadgets may not be itself ideal solution to obtain the results. Proper staff training, continuous education, internal and external auditing of the process, implementation of ideal QC strategies, etc. will yield the desired outcomes.

REFERENCES

1. Schenk SL. Das Saugethierei kunstlick befruchtet auberhalb des muttererthieres. Mitt Embr Inst K K Univ Wien. 1880;1:107.
2. Heape W. Preliminary note on the transplantation and growth of mammalian ova within a uterine foster-Mother. Proceed Royal Soc London. 1890;48(292-295):457-8.
3. Rowitz L. Public Health Leadership-putting principles into practice. J Healthcare Quality. 2002;24(3):47.
4. Chua J, Eze U, Goh G. Knowledge sharing and total quality management: A conceptual framework. 2010 IEEE International Conference on Industrial Engineering and Engineering Management. 2010;(DEC):1107-11.
5. Matejka K, Vonne Brooks La, Liz G. The Total Quality Journey: By Invitation Only? Management Decision. 1993;31(5).
6. Sohal AS, Terziovski M. TQM Australian manufacturing: Factors critical to success. Int J Qual Reliab Management. 2000;(17):158-68.
7. Dyer S, Chambers GM, de Mouzon J, et al. International Committee for Monitoring Assisted Reproductive Technologies world report: Assisted Reproductive Technology 2008, 2009 and 2010. Hum Reprod. 2016;31(7):1588-609.
8. Prajogo DI, McDermott CM. The relationship between total quality management practices and organizational culture. Int J Oper Prod Management. 2005;25:1101-22.
9. Kumar M, Sankaran S. Indian culture and the culture for TQM: A comparison. TQM Magazine. 2007;19:176-88.
10. Roldán JL, Leal-Rodríguez AL, Leal AG. The influence of organisational culture on the Total Quality Management programme performance. Sci Direct. 2012;18(3):183-9.

11. Balaban B, Ubaldi FM. Total Quality Management in the ART Laboratory. Global Fertility Academy. [online] Available from *https://media.reachmd.com/uploads/related_-_client_provided_materials/8586_total_quality_management_for_download.pdf.* [Accessed March, 2018].
12. Beer M. Why Total Quality Management Programs Do Not Persist: The Role of Management Quality and Implications for Leading a TQM Transformation. Decision Sci. 2003;34(4):623-42.
13. Matson P. Internal quality control and external quality assurance in the IVF laboratory. Hum Reprod. 1998;13(suppl 4):156-65.
14. Klipfolio.com. (2018). What is a KPI? Definition, Best-Practices, and Examples. [online] Available from *https://www.klipfolio.com/resources/articles/what-is-a-key-performance-indicator.* [Accessed March, 2018].
15. Xix Franco Jr JG, Petersen CG, Mauri AL, et al. Key performance indicators score (KPIs-score) based on clinical and laboratorial parameters can establish benchmarks for internal quality control in an ART program. JBRA Assist Reprod. 2017;21:61-6.
16. ESHRE. The Vienna consensus: report of an expert meeting on the development of art laboratory performance indicators. Reprod Biomed Online. 2017;35(5):494-510.
17. Germond M, Urner F, Chanson A, et al. What is the most relevant standard of success in assisted reproduction?: The cumulated singleton/twin delivery rates per oocyte pick-up: the CUSIDERA and CUTWIDERA. Hum Reprod, 2004;19(11):2442-4.
18. Ethics Committee of the American Society for Reproductive Medicine. Disclosure of medical errors involving gametes and embryos. Fertil Steril. 2011;96(6):1312-4.
19. Bento Fabiola C, Esteves Sandro C. (2016). Establishing a quality management system in a fertility center: experience with ISO 9001. [online] Available from http://*www.scielo.br/scielo.php?script=sci_arttext&pid=S2358-04292016000300002.* [Accessed March, 2018].
20. Koustas G, Sjoblom C. Epigenetic consequences of pH stress in mouse embryos. Hum Reprod. 2011;26:i78.

CHAPTER

19

Troubleshooting in the ART Laboratory from Oocyte Retrieval till Embryo Transfer

Sujatha Ramakrishnan, Amita Subramanian

A problem well put is half solved—John Dewey

■ INTRODUCTION

Troubleshooting is a logical, systematic way of looking at problems often involving process of elimination to determine the source and thereby resolve the problems. Assisted reproductive technology (ART) laboratory is considered to be a high complexity work area where gametes are screened, fertilized and the resultant embryos are transferred back into the uterus or frozen for future purposes. Due to the nature of work performed, presence of sophisticated equipment in the ART laboratory and the biological variations in the samples involved, an ART laboratory is prone to unexpected problems. A thorough knowledge of the processes involved and the working of equipment in the ART laboratory is an absolute necessity for the embryologists and the other personnel associated with the laboratory to face and tackle the problem. Gross issues would result in a complete disaster of ART outcomes and unchecked minor problems would often cause variation in the outcome. An efficient ART laboratory should have all the quality control (QC) and quality assurance in place to avoid unexpected troubles. This chapter is an effort to identify certain issues commonly occurring in the ART laboratory from oocyte retrieval procedure until embryo transfer and the ways to analyze and rectify the issues.

■ OOCYTE RETRIEVAL

Oocyte retrieval is a process of collecting oocytes from the female patient's ovary transvaginally or in some cases transabdominally before they are released from the follicles.[1] The most common problems encountered during this procedure are:

- No oocytes found in the aspirate
- Oocytes with less cumulus, or ruptured zona pellucida
- Presence of blood clots.

In brief, follicular fluid aspirated is poured into 60 mm petri dishes and screened for the presence of oocyte cumulus complexes under a stereo zoom microscope. Presence of immature or postmature cumulus complexes is assessed by looking at the expansion and color of the cumulus coronary cells. Mature oocytes often have expanded fluffy cumulus cells. Postmature oocytes are associated with scanty, clumped cumulus cells, and immature oocytes appear dark with tightly compacted cumulus cells.

When no oocytes are found during screening, the information has to be communicated to the clinician performing oocyte pick-up. Procedure has to be reassessed in terms of suction pressure, diameter of the aspiration needle, leakage in the aspiration system, and presence of granulosa and cumulus cells. If the aspirate is clear without any granulosa cells, it could be an empty follicle. But in case of presence of granulosa cells and absence of oocytes, technical components have to be checked before attributing it to clinical conditions.

If the recovered cumulus oocyte complexes are found with very little surrounding cells the aspiration procedure has to be stopped and the entire system has to be checked. Damage to the oocytes are not just due to increased suction pressure, but a combination of pressure, gauge and length of the needle, length of the aspiration tubing, size of follicles, size of vacuum reservoir in the pump, presence of luer lock fittings which cause turbulence at their boundaries, and clogging of filters in the aspiration pump.[2] Calibration of the pump with every new type of aspiration needle to be used is a must before the actual procedure. Calibration is performed by measuring the flow rate of any fluid in a set time period. It is recommended to have a flow rate of 20–25 mL/min.

Presence of blood clots in the aspirate makes the identification of cumulus oocyte complexes difficult. Hence, heparinized flushing media is recommended for oocyte aspirations. If heparinized media is not available, then it is advised to add 2 µL/mL of heparin to the regular HEPES ((4-(2-hydroxyethyl)-1-piperazineethanesulfonic acid)) media to avoid formation of blood clots.

Cumulus oocyte complexes identified from the follicles aspirated under stereo zoom microscope are washed thoroughly and gently in HEPES buffered media and placed in droplets of culture media. Droplet size, number of combined oral contraceptives (COCs) in each droplet, and the type of dish to be used depends on the individual laboratory protocol. Generally 3–4 COCs are placed in 0.5 mL of culture media. Dishes with COCs are then kept in the incubator at 37°C, 5% CO_2 until further process. It is advisable to segregate the COCs according to the appearance of cumulus cells. After 2–4 hours of culture in the incubator, the COCs are denuded and the oocytes are prepared for intracytoplasmic sperm injection (ICSI). If the patient is scheduled for in vitro fertilization (IVF), the COCs are inseminated with required processed spermatozoa at this stage. Culture media should be checked for the presence of debris, crystals, and bacterial infection before placing the COCs in the dishes.

■ DENUDATION OF OOCYTES

Denudation of cumulus oocyte complexes is performed in a dish which has Hyase and HEPES/MOPS media droplets. Manufacturer's instructions should be followed for equilibration of Hyase. Generally Hyase dishes are equilibrated in incubators without CO_2.

If the corona and cumulus cells are tightly bound, then repeated pipetting of COCs using a pipette of 130–150 μm would help in the removal of the surrounding cells. Pipetting has to be gentle as vigorous handling of COCs can cause the polar body (PB) to move in the perivitelline space (PVS) and trigger parthenogenic activation.[3] Location of PB is used to avoid touching the meiotic spindle which is placed directly beneath the PB in majority of the oocytes.

There is contradictory data on the importance of cumulus cells for the in vitro maturation of oocytes. In stimulated cycles, there is always a possibility of asynchrony between cytoplasmic and nuclear maturation and cumulus cells have shown to offer a metabolic and protective role in oocyte maturation. However, in standardized human menopausal gonadotropin and human chorionic gonadotropin (hCG) protocol, it appears that cumulus cells do not have much of a role in cytoplasmic maturation.[4] As a routine practice, a small amount of cumulus cells are left on the oocytes, which might offer some coculture benefits as cleavage rates were found to be higher in cumulus intact oocytes compared to cumulus denuded oocytes.[5] Care must be taken not to leave most of the cumulus cells for reasons that it might obscure the morphological features of oocyte at the time of ICSI and when culturing in small droplets cumulus cells might use up the nutrients in the media.

Standard concentration of Hyase enzyme used is 80 IU/mL, with an exposure time of 30 seconds. Some studies report better fertilization and cleavage rates, when lower concentration of Hyase was used followed by mechanical denudation an hour later. However, COCs should not be left in Hyase solution for time longer than specified, as it can affect the oocyte quality.[6]

After denudation of COC, the oocytes are cultured in fresh droplets of media until ICSI. Optimal incubation timings to be decided are based on the overall maturity of oocytes retrieved in the program. Literature evidence suggests an incubation of 2 hours between retrieval and denudation for optimal implantation and pregnancy rates. Significant reduction in fertilization rates was observed with increased timing between denudation and ICSI. In cases of hCG-triggered oocytes optimal timing of ICSI is reported to be between 39 and 40.5 hours post hCG trigger.[7]

■ INTRACYTOPLASMIC SPERM INJECTION

It is one of the most technically challenging procedures in the ART armamentarium. Both the equipment and the operator skills play an important role in the successful outcome post ICSI.

Before start of the procedure the micromanipulator is aligned in such a way that both the holding and injection pipettes could be moved in all X, Y, and Z directions without having them removed from the holder. Major problems experienced during ICSI are inability to immobilize spermatozoa and oocyte lysis post ICSI. Spermatozoa are immobilized before ICSI not only to facilitate easy aspiration into the ICSI pipette but also to release factors crucial for oocyte activation. Conventional method involves compressing tail of the spermatozoa against the bottom of the ICSI dish, until a clear kink is visible. It has been proposed that fertilization rates are better with aggressive immobilization of spermatozoa, especially in cases of immature spermatozoa[8] by repeated mechanical rubbing, laser shot[9] or Piezo pulse, though the evidence is contradictory.[10] On a practical note, care should be taken to avoid damage to centrosomes of the spermatozoa and accidental decapitation of the sperm head by aggressive immobilization. Injection capillary should be set in a way to touch the sperm and make a kink on the tail by a single stoke of movement. This is best achieved by aligning the sperm tail at right angle to the injection pipette. ICSI should not be started unless this step is set to perfection. For successful ICSI, the injection pipette is inserted half way into the oocyte and little bit of ooplasm is aspirated into the pipette by exerting a negative pressure. Breakage of ooplasm is confirmed by the sudden rush of ooplasm into the pipette. Aspirated ooplasm along with the immobilized spermatozoa in the pipette is injected back into the oocyte and the injection pipette is carefully withdrawn.

One of the most frustrating mishap post ICSI is the lysis of oocyte. Important points to assess in the event of oocyte degeneration are alignment of injection and holding pipettes. Both the tools should be placed parallel to the bottom of the dish up to the sleeve of the pipette. Injection pipette is set at a lower angle towards the bottom of the dish. Too much of an angle causes oolemma damage during injection procedure. Penetration of the injection pipette should be at the equatorial region of the oocyte in a straight line. Similarly, the holding pipette should be aligned in a way to hold the oocyte in its place without much of a movement during ICSI. One way to check this is by assessing the shape of oocyte on aspiration to the holding pipette. Oocyte should not be contorted or deformed under suction.[11,12]

Diameter and spike of injection pipettes also contribute to oocyte lysis. Pipettes of larger diameter and sharp spike are most likely to damage the oocytes. Spikes can be blunted by repeated rubbing on the holding pipette before injection. Injection pipettes have to be cleaner, especially when injecting spermatozoa from testicular biopsy samples. Debris stuck to the injection pipette may cause leakage of ooplasm post withdrawal from the oocyte. Other causative factor of oocyte lysis post ICSI is the ICSI technique itself, where the injection pipette is withdrawn too faster or too slow. Faster withdrawal of injection pipette results in incomplete ICSI and slower withdrawal results in cytoplasmic leakage and lysis.

Vibrations during ICSI procedure can also cause oocyte damage. So stability of the micromanipulator during the ICSI procedure should be of prime concern. Increase in stage temperature way above 37°C also induces oocyte degeneration. It is mandatory to check the temperature of a media droplet exactly mimicking an ICSI set up to avoid extremes of temperature during ICSI.

Increased oocyte degeneration post ICSI in the hands of properly trained, skilled embryologist is more due to the oocyte quality itself. Immature oocytes, oocytes without a spindle at the time of injection, day 3 follicle-stimulating hormone (FSH) levels, estradiol levels on the day of hCG, and oolemma breakage characteristic at the time of injection have all been correlated to oocyte lysis. However, it is a good practice to constantly examine the technical and operational QC mentioned for increased oocyte degeneration post ICSI since oocyte degeneration is likely to be both a physiological as well as physical phenomenon. In the absence of any of these above-mentioned problems, attention is to be paid to the time taken for denudation, diameter of the oocyte handling pipettes, and osmolarity of culture media droplets.

Fertilization Check

Fertilization is a process of series of events uniting the male and female genomes into a single entity followed by the formation of mitotic spindle which is assessed 16–18 hours postinsemination or 56–58 hours post hCG trigger. Zygotes with two pronuclei (PN) each containing 2–7 nucleoli which are juxtaposed to each other in the center of the ooplasm are considered to be normally fertilized. Abnormal fertilization and fertilization failure can occur in cases after ICSI.

The most commonly occurring configuration indicating abnormal fertilization is one PN and one PB. In these cases, oocytes are activated parthenogenically without the contribution from male gametes. Aggressive sperm immobilization and aspiration of ooplasm into the injection pipette would alleviate oocyte inactivation to a great extent.

One PN and two PBs: This suggests oocyte activation, but failure of sperm head decondensation in IVF and in ICSI cycles it is suggestive of artificial oocyte activation by the ICSI procedure. A second observation at 12–24 hours would help to identify oocytes with asynchronous PN development in single PN zygotes after ICSI, which are less likely to be diploid.[13]

Three PN, one PB: Normal oocyte activation, but the retention of second PB makes this configuration abnormal with two haploid PN from the oocyte origin and the third haploid PN of sperm origin. Subsequent cleavage might result in the formation of triploid embryos, in this case digynic triploidy. Most of the three PN arising from ICSI are digynic origin, since only single sperm is injected into the oocyte.[14]

Three or more PN, two polar bodies: It indicates normal oocyte activation but the chromosome configuration is that of polyspermic fertilization with one haploid nucleus from the oocyte and the remaining nuclei could be of sperm origin suggesting diandry. Most of the three PN zygotes from IVF are diandric. In ICSI, it is suggestive of cytoplasmic injury, fragmentation of nuclei or abnormal chromosomal constitution of the oocytes and sperm. An overall reduction in the size of the PN is observed when there are more than two PN.[15]

But recent evidence shows that a 3PN zygote does not always develop into triploid embryos. Hence if there are only few embryos available, 3PN zygotes can be cultured separately and subjected to genetic analysis and in the event it is normal and can then be transferred into the uterus.[16] With current time lapse imaging, it has been shown that 2PN zygotes may sometimes appear as 3PN few hours later, which could be due to fragmentation of one of its PN.

An increase in the occurrence of abnormally fertilized zygotes warrants troubleshooting. The most likely factors are advanced maternal age, ovarian stimulation in terms of high peak estradiol levels, oocyte yield, dose of gonadotropins and the number of days of stimulation, high sperm concentration in IVF, and poor sperm quality in ICSI.

Failed Fertilization

Total failed fertilization refers to lack of fertilization in all the mature oocytes inseminated or injected and the incidence is about 1–10% in IVF cycles and 2–3% in ICSI cycles.[17] When there is total fertilization failure contributory effects of oocyte quality, maturity, ovarian response to stimulation, sperm quality and origin, and the ICSI procedure itself have to be ruled out. Occasionally, zygotes can be arrested without further progression to embryos and the most common causes are molecular and chromosomal defects. However, gross deviation in culture temperature and osmolality can also cause zygote arrest.

In case of poor fertilization after IVF, a thorough examination of the culture dish is done under inverted microscope at 20× magnification for the presence of bacterial contamination, or change in color of culture media droplets. Sperm motility in the insemination droplet is another indicator of optimal culture conditions. Under normal circumstances, sperm motility is expected to be greater than 60%.

Under normal circumstances, zygotes undergo cell division by mitosis every 18–20 hours. Normal embryos have equal sized blastomeres appropriate for the stage with less extracellular fragments. Earlier studies and prediction by mathematical models suggest that robust embryos continue to grow and result in viable pregnancy in spite of variation in culture conditions. However, embryos with moderate and poor developmental competence will either get arrested or undergo cell death in unfavorable culture environments. Postzygotic chromosomal abnormalities could be due to deficiency in maternal transcript accumulation. Factors such as poor temperature control are known to affect spindle or cytoskeleton in the oocyte or early embryos resulting in poor quality embryos.[18] It has been shown that meiotic spindle disassembles and relocates within the cytoplasm when the temperature is increased from 37°C to 40°C. Multinucleation in embryos could be caused by suboptimal culture conditions with variation in temperature.[19,20] It should be borne in mind that minor variation in culture conditions in terms of pH, temperature, and osmolarity can affect embryo development and should be tightly controlled with diligence.

Culture System

Components of culture system such as culture media, temperature, pH, osmolarity, humidity, culture environment individually or collectively can impact the chromosomal status and the quality of the embryos. Different culture media have been shown to cause difference in rate of cell division. Certain culture media seem to cause early compaction on day 3 (Personal Communication). In humans, an association between culture media, gene expression, and birth weight has been reported. Though it is difficult to elicit a direct relationship of quality of embryos to culture media because of other confounding factors, it is a good practice to keep a complete track of the lot number of culture media, temperature during transportation, and expiry date. Even if the bottle is unopened and within expiry date, aged media has been shown to affect birth weight.[21-23]

Since culture media is an important component of culture system, optimizing is the key to a successful IVF outcome. Culture media should be stored in appropriate conditions. Media should not be exposed to light when stored in refrigerator; clear bottles of media should be covered with aluminum foil or placed in dark containers. Turbidity, if observed, could be due to calcium carbonate and calcium phosphate precipitation. This occurs in cases of altered pH especially in the alkaline range, or because of storage in extreme low temperature. All commercial media undergo rigorous QC at the site of production. However, quality can be compromised during transport and storage. It is advisable to run an in house sperm survival assay with every new lot of media to avoid poor outcome. Lot numbers are to be recorded individually for all the patients. Care should be taken to avoid repeated opening and closing of media bottles. Every time a new bottle is opened, the date of opening should also be recorded.

Instances where embryo quality is deteriorated, it is important to monitor the role of culture oil since oil is susceptible to peroxidation. Improper storage and handling leads to increase in toxic peroxides.[24]

Temperature

Embryo quality and development have been associated with culture temperature. Temperature in the incubator, working stage have been shown to impact, especially the oocyte and early stage embryos. Ambient temperature is known to play an important role in the maintenance of temperature in equipments. Conflicting data exists in the literature on ideal temperature for culturing gametes and embryos.[25] Since temperature in reproductive tract is approximately 1.5°C cooler than core body temperature. However, the best practice now is to culture gametes and embryos at a stable temperature of 37°C.

Drop in temperature occurs when the ambient temperature is set lower than 23°C, on repeated opening and closing of incubators and when the laminar air flow is turned on at high speed. Careful consideration of the above factors would reduce fluctuation in the culture temperature.

pH

The pH of the culture media is determined by the bicarbonate concentration in the media and the concentration of CO_2 in the incubator. Though maintenance of pH between 7.25 and 7.40 in the culture system appears to be straightforward and simple, in practical scenario it is never that easy. The reason for difficulty in maintaining pH is because of its dynamic nature and also due to the lack of availability of user friendly simple equipment to measure pH. However, a tight control of pH over the optimum range is absolutely essential as change in pH has been shown to affect embryo metabolism and development.[26] Exposure to lower pH even for a short period has been correlated to fetal weight and length.[27] Points to be considered for maintenance of optimum pH are:
- pH decreases with increase in CO_2 and vice-versa.
- Embryos should be exposed to non-CO_2 environment for the minimum time possible.
- In cases of expected delay, such as process of denudation, HEPES/MOPS buffered media should be used for handling gametes.
- pH can be measured by standard equipments and regular calibration of the probe is mandatory.

Osmolarity

Osmolarity depends upon the concentration of solutes in the culture media. Disturbance in the balance of the solutes between the intracellular and extracellular regions of gametes and embryos causes movement of fluid across the cell membrane and eventually resulting in shrinkage or swelling. Changes in osmolarity occur, when there is evaporation of culture media droplets. Hence care should be taken during culture dish preparation. The points to be considered are size, shape of the droplets, stage temperature, air flow in the laminar air flow cabinet, and the time taken to aliquot the droplets.[28] In hyperosmotic conditions, cells shrink and if large PVS is noticed in all gametes or embryos, it is important to check osmolarity of the media or re-evaluate dish preparation techniques and change to a fresh bottle of media. Similarly in hypo-osmotic conditions, cells swell and might initially appear as of excellent grade and deteriorate thereon.

Air Quality

The IVF laboratory and its associated areas fall under ISO-8-IS0-5 grade clean rooms where ISO 5 being the most sterile area like laminar air flow cabinet. Air quality in the laboratory is maintained by a series of filters and good laboratory practices. Components of the filtration system should be nontoxic to the embryos. Periodic change of filters and constant monitoring of key performance indicators such as fertilization failure, cleavage arrest, good quality embryos, and embryo developmental rate have to be monitored regularly to avoid detrimental effect of poor air quality in the laboratory.

Careful monitoring of all parameters of culture system should be a day-to-day affair, and in cases of poor embryo quality of development all these parameters such as temperature, pH, osmolarity, and air quality have to be revalidated.

Embryo Transfer

Success after IVF procedure depends on the quality of the embryos transferred and the endometrium. However, embryo transfer technique is a rate-limiting step and can contribute to inefficiency of embryo implantation. Variables important for successful embryo transfer techniques are absence of blood or mucus on the catheter, no retention of embryos in the catheter and no expulsion of embryos and to a great extent depends on ease of transfer. Aspiration of cervical mucus, type of catheter used and loading faulty techniques of embryo transfer catheter adversely affect outcome of embryo transfer.

There are different techniques for loading embryo transfer catheters; emphasis is on low volume with sequences of air and liquid columns. Various schools of thoughts exist on the presence of air column. Loading embryos without air column might cause distribution of embryos over a larger area. However air column is postulated to prevent adherence of embryos to the wall of the catheter and accidental expulsion of embryos during maneuver. Air bubbles also serve as markers on the ultrasound. It has been proposed that fluid volume in the catheter plays an important role in the retention of embryos in the catheter. In our practice, we follow the three drop procedure with two air bubbles separating the drop of medium that contains the embryo, in a total volume of 12–15 μL and the contents are injected gently at the transfer site. Adherent substance like hyaluronan helps in loading the catheter without unwanted air bubbles and eases embryo transfer process. Though exact mechanism is not known, hyaluronan has been shown to improve implantation in many studies.[29,30]

■ CONCLUSION

In vitro fertilization procedures from egg pick up to embryo transfer marks the most crucial set of events leading to the formation of viable embryo outside the body. Development of embryos is subjected to a lot of physiological, physical, and technical risks. An ideal laboratory will have systems in place to prevent detrimental effect on the embryos. Standard operating procedures are to be followed carefully for all the steps from oocyte retrieval to embryo transfer. The processes have to be dissected to finest details and mapped to accurately assess problems occurring at each stage of development. It should be remembered that efforts taken towards troubleshooting is not a one-time phenomenon but an ongoing process.

KEY POINTS

- Troubleshooting involves careful dissection, mapping, and analysis of all the process involved in the in vitro culture of embryos outside the body.
- Culture system is a complex component comprising of media, temperature, pH, and osmolarity and disturbances in one of these can lead to a cascade of events ultimately affecting quality and developmental potential of embryo.
- All equipment involved in the process have to be calibrated and maintained regularly.
- Documentation regarding QC activities like calibration, maintenance details of equipment, temperature and pH measurements, gamete quality, and developmental information has to be maintained with diligence to help in troubleshooting exercise.
- An in-depth knowledge in the biology of gametes and embryos and operation of equipment is necessary to troubleshoot problems.

REFERENCES

1. Antosik P, Jakowski JM, Jeziorkowski M, et al. The influence of vacuum pressure on quality and number of recovered oocytes aspirated from ovarian follicles of swine and cows? Arch Tierz Dummerstorf. 2007;3:260-6.
2. Rose BI. Approaches to oocyte retrieval for advanced reproductive technology cycles planning to utilize in vitro maturation: a review of the many choices to be made. J Assist Reprod Genet. 2014;31:1409-19.
3. Fishel S, Timson J, Lisi F, et al. Evaluation of 225 patients undergoing subzonal insemination for the procurement of fertilization in vitro. Fertil Steril. 1992;57(4):840-9.
4. Kim BK, Lee SC, Kim KJ, et al. In vitro maturation, fertilisation and development of human germinal vesicle oocytes collected from stimulated cycles. Fertil Steril. 2000;74(6):1153-8.
5. Goud PT, Goud AP, Qian C, et al. In-vitro maturation of human germinal vesicle stage oocytes- role of cumulus cells and epidermal growth factor in the culture medium. Hum Reprod. 1998;13(6):1638-44.
6. Moura BR, Gurgel MC, Machado SP, et al. Low concentration of hyaluronidase for oocyte denudation can improve fertilization rates and embryo quality. JBRA Assist Reprod. 2017;21(1):27-30.
7. Catherine Patrat, Aida Kaffel, Lucie Delaroche, et al. Optimal timing for oocyte denudation and intra-cytoplasmic sperm injection. Obstet Gynaecol Int. 2012;403531.
8. Palmero GP, Schlegel PN, Colombero LT, et al. Aggressive sperm immobilization prior to intra cytoplasmic sperm injection with immature spermatozoa improves fertilisation and pregnancy rates. Hum Reprod. 1996;11(5):1023-29.

9. Montag M, Rink K, Delacrétaz G, et al. Laser-induced immobilization and plasma membrane permeabilization in human spermatozoa. Hum Reprod. 2000;15(4): 846-52.
10. Lacham-Kaplan O, Trounson A. Micromanipulation, assisted fertilisation: comparison of different techniques. In: Tesarik J (Ed). Frontiers in Endocrinology, volume 8. Ares-Serono Symposia Publications: Rome; 1994. pp. 287-304.
11. Martin Wilding, Antionio Scotto di Frega, Genc Kabili, et al. Oocyte degeneration after intracytoplasmic sperm injection. J Reprod Stem Cell Biotechnol. 2010;1:196-8.
12. Woodward B. Oocyte degeneration following ICSI. J Reprod Stem cell Biotechnol. 2010;1:199-201.
13. Plachot M, Crozet N. Fertilisation abnormalities in human IVF. Human Reprod. 1992;7:89-94.
14. Palmero GD, Munné S, Colombero LT, et al. Genetics of abnormal human fertilisation. Hum Reprod. 1995;10(Suppl)1:120-7.
15. Palmero GD, Alikani M, Bertoli M, et al. Oolemma characteristics in relation to survival and fertilization patterns of oocytes treated by ICSI. Hum Reprod. 1996;11(1):172-6.
16. Mingzhao Li, Wanqiu Zhao, Xia Xue, et al. Three pronuclei (3PN) incidence factors and clinical outcomes; A retrospective study from the fresh embryo transfer of in vitro fertilisation with donor sperm (IVF-D). Int J Clin Exp Med. 2015;8:13997-4003.
17. Sarikaya E, Eryilmaz OG, Deveer R, et al. Analysis of 232 total fertilisation failure cycles during intracytoplasmic sperm injection. Iran J Reprod Med. 2011;9(2):105-112.
18. Sun XE, Wang WH, Keefe DL. Overheating is detrimental to meiotic spindles within matured human oocytes. Zygote. 2004;12(1):65-70.
19. Hardy K, Winston RM, Handyside AH. Binucleate blastomeres in preimplantation human embryos in vitro; failure of cytokinesis during early cleavage. J Reprod Fertil. 1993;98(2):549-58.
20. Pickering SJ, Taylor A, Johnson MH, et al. An analysis of multinucleate blastomere formation in human embryos. Mol Hum Reprod. 1995;10(7):1912-22.
21. E. C. Nelissen, Van Montfoort AP, Coonen E, et al. Further evidence that culture media affect perinatal outcome: findings after transfer of fresh and cryopreserved embryos. Hum Reprod. 2016;27(7):1966-76.
22. Nelissen EC, Van Montfoort AP, Coonen E, et al. Effect of in vitro culture of human embryos on birthweight of newborns. Hum Reprod. 2010;25:605-12.
23. Kleijkers SH, van Montfoort AP, Smits LJ, et al. Age of G-1 Plus v5 Embryo culture medium is inversely associated with birthweight of the newborn. Hum Reprod. 2015;30(6):1352-7.
24. Otuski J, Nagai Y, Chiba K. Peroxidation of mineral oil used in droplet culture is detrimental to fertilisation and embryo development. Fertil Steril. 2007;88:741-43.
25. Butler JM, Johnson JE, Boone WR, et al. The heat is on: Room temperature affects laboratory equipment—an observational study. J Assist Reprod Genet. 2013;30(10):1389-93.

26. Joe Conaghan. pH control in the embryo culture environment. In: Quinn P (Ed). Culture Media, Solutions, and Systems in Human ART. Cambridge University Press; 2014.
27. Swain JE. Optimizing the culture environment in the IVF laboratory: impact of pH and buffer capacity on gamete and embryo quality. 2010;21(1):6-16.
28. Swain JE, Cabrera L, Xu X, et al. Environmental factors and manual manipulations during preparation influence embryo culture media osmolality. Fertil Steril. 2010;94(2):32.
29. Eytan O, Elad D, Zaretsky U, et al. A glance into the uterus during in vitro stimulation of embryo transfer. Hum Reprod. 2004;19(3):562-9.
30. Lambers MJ, Dogan E, Lens JW, et al. The position of transferred air bubbles after embryo transfer is related to pregnancy rate. Fertil Steril. 2007;88(1):68-73.

CHAPTER 20

Attributes and Responsibilities of an Efficient Embryologist

Rajvi H Mehta

■ INTRODUCTION

The advent of assisted reproductive technologies (ARTs) not only made it possible for infertile couples to become parents, but it revolutionized the field of human reproduction. Along with this, ART gave way to new branches of biology as well as new professions. Clinical embryology is one such new vocation which has emerged in the last two and a half decades. Till then, we had the science of embryology which was the study of fertilization to embryonic to fetal development, which was a part of human anatomy. However, the advent of in vitro fertilization (IVF) and embryo transfer led to term, "clinical embryology" and the profession of "clinical embryologist" which deals with the first 5 days of human development—the in vitro manipulation of human gametes and developments of embryos till the blastocyst stage.

After the birth of Louis Browne, there were very few clinical embryologists in the world and were not even known by that name. There were generally referred to as reproductive biologists. As the number of ART clinics started increasing, people from different educational backgrounds with a base in biology entered the profession. Their educational qualifications could be a doctorate, postgraduate or a graduate from fields such as reproductive biology, zoology, life sciences, microbiology, veterinary sciences, pathology, physicians, pharmacology, dentists, obstetrics, and gynecology. I have also met clinical embryologists who have been orthopedic to ophthalmic surgeons or pulmonologists prior to becoming clinical embryologists! The field was emerging and with no formal courses, individuals with some knowledge of biology ventured into the field. Depending upon their basic education or profession, they initially brought a different perspective and different skill sets. This just shows on the very diverse outlook that embryologists would have!

Most embryologists in the first decade of ART in India were self-trained or learned by observing and assisting their seniors. Some did a course abroad while others attended some short-term training courses. Degree, diploma, and certificate courses in clinical embryology were started by a few universities in the last decade. However, the number of individuals who graduate from these courses is far lesser than the current requirement in the country. Today, many study abroad and return to work in Indian clinics and many still follow the old route of doing short-term training courses, observing their seniors as junior embryologists and train their own selves.

As the demand and supply chain for clinical embryologists is not met, we have many clinical embryologists who work at multiple clinics and are referred to as traveling embryologists, visiting embryologists or freelance embryologists. Therefore, the responsibilities taken up by clinical embryologists may vary from clinic to clinic depending upon the role they play. For example, a freelance embryologist is mainly concerned with the skill sets while the in-house embryologist may not have the highest level of skills but would need to take up many more responsibilities.

However, before enumerating the responsibilities of a clinical embryologist, I would like to write about certain attributes that are absolutely necessary for a clinical embryologist. In my personal opinion, these are equally if not more important than even the skill sets. Skill sets can be acquired by diligent, long hours of sincere hard work and practice, but the qualities of clinical embryologists are either inherent or should be cultivated.

■ BASIC ATTRIBUTES OF A CLINICAL EMBRYOLOGIST

Punctuality: All the ART work is time dependent. Anything done a little too early or a little too late would affect the outcome of ART. For example, delaying the ovum pickup would be a disaster as we would lose oocytes if the follicles rupture; or an early pickup accompanied by early denudation of oocytes for intracytoplasmic sperm injection (ICSI), would leave us with more immature oocytes for ICSI. Punctuality is absolutely necessary for ART and one should not compromise on that. For clinics depending upon freelance embryologists, I would recommend that they should have a backup plan lest the clinical embryologist is not able to make it especially if they are traveling long distances.

Basic knowledge of human reproduction: We have embryologists with different educational backgrounds but I feel that each embryologist should study and have basic knowledge of the following subjects which is relevant to human reproduction. These subjects include:
- Reproductive anatomy and physiology
- Reproductive endocrinology
- Cell biology
- Biochemistry
- Microbiology
- Genetics and molecular biology
- Environmental sciences
- Clinical psychology
- Instrumentation and microscopy
- Statistics and basic computer software.

Assisted reproductive technology necessitates good collaboration between the embryologist and the gynecologist. If the clinical embryologist is not well versed with the subjects listed above then there is no scope for them to interact and discuss with the clinician. We must realize that in the field of ART, there is high failure rate. We can be comfortable in talking about our success and state that we are getting the "same" success rates as the rest of the world. But, deep in our hearts, we should think about the failures and also try to analyze the cause of the failures—only then we will and the science progress. We need to question ourselves whether we can find an answer to why a particular patient did not succeed, analyze our data periodically to check if we see some positive or negative trends; discuss whether we could have done a particular case differently. Such a regular reviewing of the cases between the team is only possible if the clinical embryologist has some basics. Otherwise, as one of my fellow embryologist from the United States, once said that his 16-year-old son with no knowledge of biology did better sperm injections than him but we do not call this 16-year-old boy a clinical embryologist!! In case, there is somebody else with better skill sets then the person should be teamed with another one who has better knowledge, only then the team and the ART clinic would progress.

Continuing education: The art and science of ART is developing very fast. Many studies, trials, and reviews are regularly being published and it is important to be well-read on the field. So, the embryologist should always keep some time aside for acquiring knowledge and being updated in the new developments in the world.

Honesty and ethics: In all medical conditions, patients come to the doctors with lot of hopes. But, in ART they come with hope for themselves and the future generations. All the sperms and eggs look similar but each develops into different human beings. Never ever should one compromise on the ethical front for short-term gains of "pregnancy rates". We are "playing" with the body, mind, emotions of the couples, and their children. Leave alone the legal battles that may come in the future but I simply say, do not do anything that you would not want done to you or your dear ones. Let us practice honestly, conscientiously with the responsibility endowed upon us. Let us not make tall claims or state things that have not been done by us. Some clinical embryologists have told me that they do things that they would not want done because they are compelled to do so. Well, whoever may compel, the act is done by the clinical embryologist. We are responsible for our acts. We should have the courage to say "No" irrespective of the consequences. May sound idealistic but the fact that we are "creating life" endows tons of responsibility and we need to respect the trust that the couple has placed on us!

Conscientiousness: Be conscientious about your work. Let there be minimum errors of technique or judgment. We must realize that we may be doing hundreds of cases but for the patient it is not their first or second or third cycle. We may quote success rates of 40–60% but as far as the couple is concerned, it is either one or zero. They either get a baby or do not get a baby. So, the figures and statistics are for us to audit our own work but we need to be conscientious to minimize errors either technical or mix-up or decision making. I would like to ideally say that we should make zero errors but we are humans so we may make an error but the error should be in the rarest of rare cases.

Patience: A clinical embryologist needs loads of patience. It may take a couple of hours to find the few sperms after testicular sperm aspiration. We cannot get disheartened and just give up. Even while training to do sperm immobilization and injections, it may take time initially but we need the patience required to learn.

Speed: Along with patience one needs to be quick in one's work. The culture media and culture conditions influence the outcome of ART. The same culture medium may give differing results in different hands. For example, pH and osmolality of the culture media are constantly changing. If we keep the media in the outside environment for even 5 minutes, its pH as well as osmolality would increase. Placing back the culture medium into the CO_2 incubator would decrease the pH but the osmolality cannot come back to normal—in case of open culture. Even while doing close-culture under a layer of oil, the evaporation of media and change in osmolality can occur very quickly and that cannot be reversed even after oil is overlaid. The number of embryos that cleave varies with even a .05 alteration in pH. Even if we are working under oil, pH changes occur albeit slowly. Therefore, speed at work is absolutely essential.

Focus: The speed with which we perform our procedures would come with practice and experience. But, even the most experienced embryologist could be "exposing" the media to the outside atmosphere while handling if they are distracted while working. The most common cause of distraction is the mobile or talking to people while at work. Therefore, the use of mobiles and personnel interaction while handling media or gametes should be avoided. Focus at the work in hand should be the mantra.

These are some of the basic attributes required by an embryologist. They need to be in control of their own persona to be able to handle the responsibilities that go with their profession.

■ RESPONSIBILITIES OF AN EMBRYOLOGIST

These can be divided into:
- Skills for performing various techniques associated with clinical embryology
- Laboratory maintenance
- Quality control and assurance
- Inventory management
- Data management
- Internal auditing
- Potential legal issues.

Skills Required by a Clinical Embryologist

A clinical embryologist is expected to be proficient in the following techniques associated with ART:
1. Processing of semen by the swim-up and density gradient techniques
2. Cryopreservation of semen
3. Preparation of dishes for conventional IVF and ICSI
4. Screening of follicular aspirates for the presence of oocytes
5. Handling of oocytes and embryos
6. Conventional IVF and embryo—blastocyst culture
7. Denudation of oocytes for ICSI
8. ICSI
9. Vitrification of oocytes and embryos
10. Blastomere biopsy of embryos or trophectoderm biopsy.

Of these 10 techniques, a junior embryologist should be proficient in the first 6 while the senior should be able to perform the first 9 of these techniques. Biopsy, as of now, can be considered as a superspecialty skill as not many clinics offer this service. It is important to mention here that even if one is a senior embryologist, he needs to be able to perform all the procedures and not merely one skill set.

According to me, an individual with all the skills listed above can be considered a good embryology technician, i.e. the individual is good in performing the techniques associated with ART, but may not essentially be knowledgeable about the science and biology behind them. A skilled embryology technician is a boon for any clinic but possessing skills is not enough to be called an embryologist. Any young, skilled person without any biology background can be trained and may become very good at some of the techniques listed above and need not even possess a basic degree! If such persons serve as embryology technicians in a clinic, they should be supervised by other qualified embryologists who are more knowledgeable.

Laboratory Maintenance

Embryology is a high-skilled job which is dependent on the tools that we use. The laboratory environment also influences the outcome of the procedures performed. It is up to the management to provide good equipment and requisite infrastructure but the clinical embryologist would need to maintain the laboratory.

The laboratory may be designed by the best architects and have the best equipment but it has to be maintained well. One of crucial components in ART is the quality of air. It is in a way a "silent killer". The air can be contaminated by volatile organic compounds (VOCs), particulate matter, and micro-organisms. We do have good air handling units but we need to realize that they ensure that we get clean air into the room. But, air also enters the rooms when personnel walk in and out of the room, when material comes into the room and with the substances that the material and people bring along. So, we should not be "comfortable" and "complacent" once an air-handling unit has been placed. We need to periodically check the quality of air in the room, incubators, and workstations using VOC meters and particulate counters. The filters of the air-handling units should also be checked regularly or they themselves may become a source of contamination! There should also be a restriction on the people entering the laboratory and they should change their attire especially wear sterile disposable shoe covers as they are one of the sources of contamination of the air.

The equipment should be calibrated periodically. One should not merely go by the reading on the temperature and CO_2 on the incubator but also check with external tools. It should be a part of the standard operating protocols to check the temperature and CO_2 logs on the incubator every morning and with the external calibrated thermometer once a day. The VOC, particulate matter (PM), and microbial testing can be done once in 3–6 months.

Cleaning of the laboratory should be supervised. The sweepers or cleaners must be educated on not to use strong detergents or swaps which may be used in the other parts of the hospital.

Quality Control and Assurance

Assisted reproductive technology is flooded with many variables which affect the outcome.
- The quality of sperms, oocytes, and embryos which in turn depends on the age, cause of infertility, type of stimulation protocol that has been used.
- The skills of the embryologist.
- The quality of culture media and culture conditions.

Many of these variables are not in the hands of the staff. But, keeping a check on the quality of materials coming in, the outcomes of the various stages of the ART help in predetermining potential problems. There are some in-house checks on how the laboratory is functioning. One of the simplest is the sperm survival assay. Basically, one tries to see how long the processed sperm survive in the incubator, which reflects whether the incubator is functioning optimally, the media is of acceptably quality and the culture conditions are good. Whenever a new batch of disposables or media or oil comes in—this test should be done. In case, the sperms do not survive, then we can avert a calamity when we actually work with the patients. This along with the information given in the earlier session on laboratory equipment and air quality helps us to keep the laboratory in some kind of "control".

Inventory Management

Many ART clinics these days have a computerized inventory of the media and disposables. However, as clinical embryologists, we need to be sure that whatever media and disposables we would need for a patient are available with us or are on their way. Most clinics use media that is imported, so it does take a while for us to get them when we require. We would also want to get media as quickly as possible after it is manufactured so we should order them in good time but not too early. Even if there is another department handling inventory, we are the ones who finally use the material. There should not be a situation when we want to do vitrification and find we have not enough carriers with us or that we have run out of cooling media. We need to create a checklist of requirements per patient or per batch of patients and ensure that all the material is in place.

Data Management

Data on the history of the patients, date and time of the procedures carried out, the outcomes, and the batches of media and disposables used should be recorded. Specialized ART software is available but we need to enter the data regularly. We should never leave anything to memory. All information, however trivial it may seem, should be recorded. Data entry should not be a one-way process, this data should periodically be analyzed to see trends if any! Sometimes, we suddenly perceive that the pregnancy rates have dropped but a proper analysis of data may not reflect that. On the other hand, we may not be aware that there is a gradual drop in the quality of good-quality embryos. By the time we realize it may be too late. But, if we were to look at the data regularly then we may observe the trend and look for the reasons and put corrective measures in place.

Auditing

A periodic review of the outcomes from the take-home baby rates, clinical pregnancy rates, biochemical pregnancy, implantation rates, blastocyst formation, cleavage rates, fertilization as well as the quality of the embryos is mandatory. If any of these drop-down from the standards in the laboratory then an emergency review by the team should be called to determine changes, if any, have been made in the system. We all "think" that we are doing the best we can but an audit substantiates are "thoughts". This is internal auditing.

It may also help to have a senior experienced embryologist who visits the laboratory to survey the laboratory and procedures. The external eye may catch some issues which we may not. So, the laboratory although standardized should be periodically reviewed for improvements.

Legal and Ethical Issues

The embryologist is the person liable for any mistakes that happen in the laboratory. The highest risk is that of mixing gametes from individuals or transferring "wrong" embryos. To prevent any such error, the simplest thing to do is to work on one case at a time. However, such luxury is not possible in

Attributes and Responsibilities of an Efficient Embryologist

busy clinics. Therefore, here, one can either have bar code readers and have another person witnessing the names and IDs of the patients when doing conventional IVF, ICSI, warming postvitrification, embryo transfer. Clean, organized incubators and workstations also reduce such errors.

It is also the job of the embryologist to check the consent forms for all third party-related work—be it donor oocytes, sperms, embryo donation or surrogacy. After all, the clinical embryologist is the one handling the gametes and if the consents are not signed by the couple and concerned donors then we may land up in a legal tangle. Despite any amount of pressure, the checking of the consent forms should be a part of our duty.

KEY POINTS

- To summarize, a clinical embryologist does a lot of high skill as well as administrative and management roles. A visiting or freelance embryologist focuses mainly on the skill sets but he or she should be teaming up with in-house embryologists in the facility who ensure that all the aspects of maintenance, records are being performed. These need to work as a team.
- Larger clinics can have multiple embryologists playing specific roles and doing different jobs. However, it would be advisable that their roles be changed from time to time so that complacency does not set in. And, they also attain different skills in the various aspects of the procedures.
- Let us take the role of the clinical embryologist—the one who "creates" life with great seriousness and responsibility—with the trust and respect that is laid on us and not that of a glorified technician!

CHAPTER 21

Oocyte-Cumulus Insight

Ratna Chattopadhyay, Parag Nandi

■ INTRODUCTION

For the development of an embryo, may be a good or bad one, oocyte's contribution plays the key role. A poor quality oocyte always develops into a poor quality embryo but a good quality oocyte in the optimum environment should develop into a good quality embryo resulting in a healthy fetus.

We know that the fate of poor quality oocytes is either failed fertilization or abnormal fertilization resulting in polyspermia, arrested cleavage or missed abortion.

Oocyte quality is the reflection of oocyte's intrinsic developmental potential which is determined by some biochemical and molecular states and processes of the surroundings. It helps the oocyte to fertilize and develop into a complete embryo, which on transfer is able to reach to the healthy live birth.

It has been reported that developmental programs of embryos and fetus by environmental features are mediated by the oocyte's intrinsic developmental potential.[1-3] To understand the molecular, cellular, and biochemical processes that control oocyte quality is one of the greatest challenges in the field of reproductive medicine.

Ovarian folliculogenesis, gradual maturation, and development of oocyte require gonadotropin from anterior pituitary but a number of factors from within the follicles are responsible for the successive progress from primary to secondary and then to tertiary follicle.

Ovarian follicular microenvironment and maternal signals required for maturation and development of oocytes are mediated through granulosa and cumulus cells (CCs). These are responsible for gradual acquisition of oocyte competence. During antral follicular formation, which is the end of oocyte growth phase, granulosa cells (GCs) are differentiated into two distinct groups of cell line.

1. Mural granulose cells (MGCs) which are playing steroidogenic role.
2. Cumulus cells which are deeply involved with oocyte competence.

Highly specialized cytoplasmic projections originating from CCs penetrate zona pellucida and form gap junction at their tips with oocyte surface and form the cumulus-oocyte complex (COC).[4]

Passage of different small molecules and signals to and from oocyte and cumulus via gap junction is essential to make both the structures viable and functioning at different stage of development (Fig. 1).[5]

Therefore, the relationship between oocyte and cumulus is bidirectional. We have inadequate knowledge about the nature and extent of these molecules and signals.

Gap junction plays an important role in the symbiosis between oocyte and follicle. Within the follicle, communication with the oocyte is everywhere (Fig. 2).

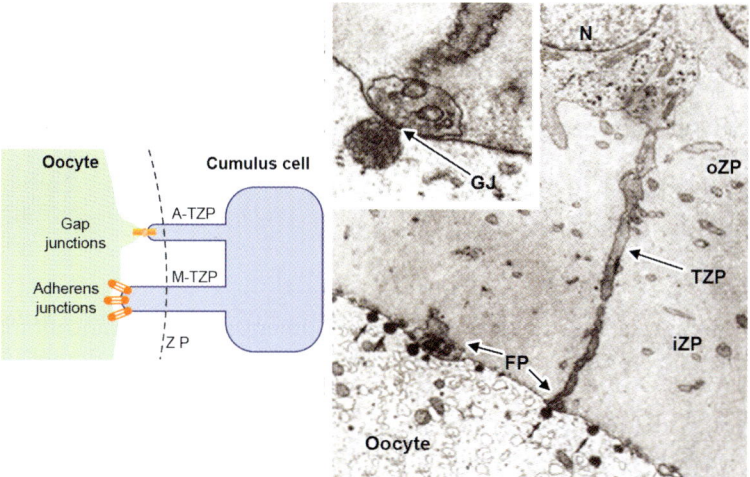

Fig. 1: Cumulus cell-oocyte communication—Gap junctions are key.

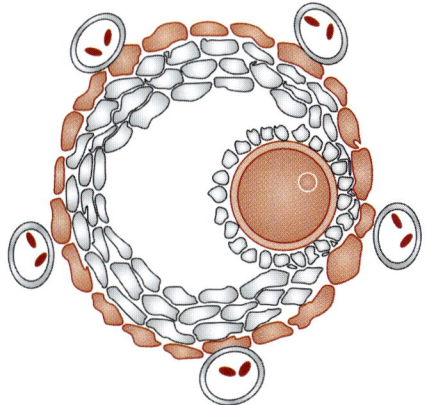

Fig. 2: Communication in the follicle is everywhere.

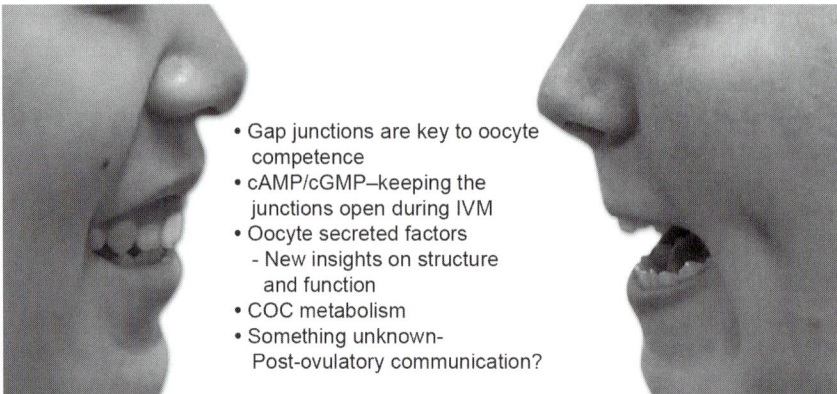

Fig. 3: Cumulus-oocyte communication. It is a conversation……and both sides benefit!
(cAMP: cyclic adenosine monophosphate; cGMP: cyclic guanosine monophosphate; IVM: in vitro maturation; COC: cumulus-oocyte complex)

Communication across:
- Stroma
- Basal lamina
- Mural granulose cells
- Antral fluid
- Cumulus.

Cumulus cells help the oocyte in its development, maturation and ultimately in achieving the competence for healthy embryo formation and normal live birth.

Oocyte cumulus relationship is a conversation by which both the components get benefited (Fig. 3).

ROLE OF CUMULUS CELL

Cumulus cells can be considered as biomarker of oocyte quality, embryo, and pregnancy outcome (Fig. 4).

Cumulus cells coordinate follicular development with oocyte maturation.

During follicular antrum formation granulose cells differentiate into MGCs which line the wall of the follicle having steroidogenic role, and CCs which are closely associated with oocyte and form COC.

During antral follicular development the oocyte gradually and sequentially acquires meiotic and developmental competence through the CCs which in turn support the oocyte for embryo development and this process can be defined as oocyte capacitation.[6]

Oocyte Nutrition and Metabolism

Cumulus cells convert the main bulk of glucose into pyruvate which is the main source of energy for oocyte and zygote. Oocytes are unable for oxidative

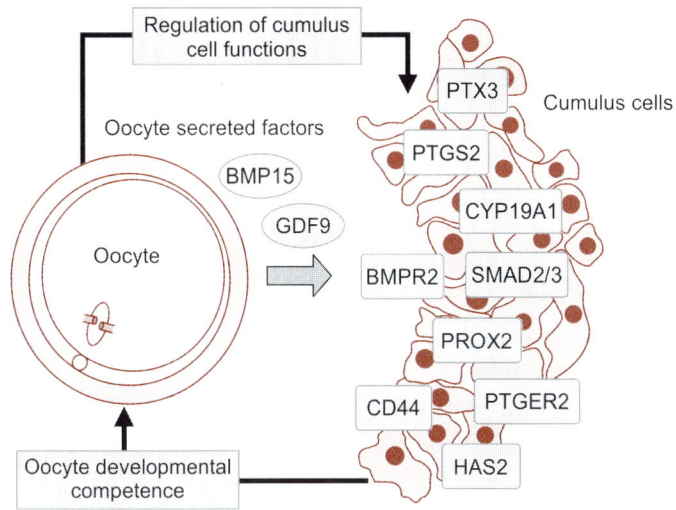

Fig. 4: Cumulus cells as biomarker for oocyte quality, embryo, and pregnancy outcomes.

phosphorylation to produce adenosine tri-phosphate (ATP) and glucose for its own metabolism. Cumulus cell (CC) can uptake and utilize glucose via aerobic glycolysis and provides pyruvate to oocyte and zygote.

Gap junction between CC and oocyte are the main channels allowing the exchange of ions and small molecules like cyclic adenosine monophosphate.[7]

Cyclic adenosine monophosphate inhibits resumption of premature oocyte meiotic progression.

Low-molecular-weight substrates such as amino acid, nucleotides, ribosome, and messenger ribonucleic acid are transported to the oocyte from MCGs and CCs for oocyte nuclear maturation via gap junction.[8]

Expression of some genes like *SLC38A3* for amino acid transportation is limited only to CCs.[9]

Cumulus helps oocyte in fertilization. Higher percentage of fertilization is observed in oocyte cumulus complex (OCC) in vivo than OCC in vitro. It is significantly reduced when oocytes are removed from cumulus but fertilization rate can be improved by replacement of CCs.

Highest nuclear maturation was observed when oocytes were within cumulus complex, no matter whether oocytes were in vivo or in vitro but when oocytes were removed from CCs, first polar body extrusion was significantly disturbed.[10]

Preovulatory Phase

The most critical event at this stage is the resumption of meiosis-I.

Cyclic adenosine monophosphate manufactured by CCs is a key factor for maintaining meiotic arrest.

During luteinizing hormone (LH) surge, CCs allow transmission of maturation including signal to the oocyte and then resumption of meiosis takes place. During LH surge, prior to ovulation, CCs produce hyaluronic acid which helps in CC expansion.[11]

Expression of prostaglandin-endoperoxide synthase (PTGS2) in CCs required for prostaglandin production is induced by growth differentiation factor-9 (GDF9).

After Ovulation

Cumulus cells and its intercellular matrix help in the propagation of COC through the fallopian tube.

Cumulus cells and its matrix also participate in fertilization by influencing sperm binding to, and penetration of zona pellucida.[12] Cumulus cells may secrete chemotactic factors which guide the sperms to the oocyte and this increases the chance of fertilization.[13]

An increase in CCs apoptosis is associated with abnormal oocyte, impaired fertilization, and suboptimal blastocyst formation (Figs. 5A and B).[14]

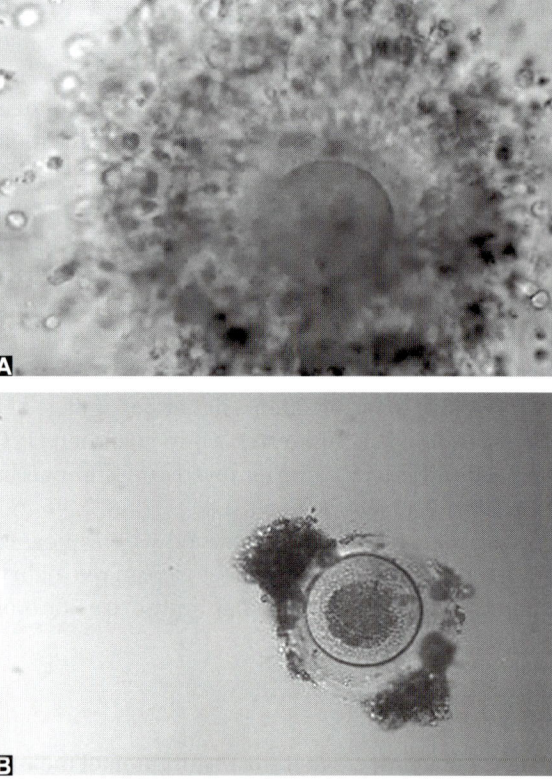

Figs. 5A and B: (A) Normal oocyte with healthy cumulus cells (CCs); (B) Abnormal oocyte with apoptotic CCs.

ROLE OF OOCYTE IN CUMULUS CELLS

Oocyte secretes potent growth factors which are essential for CC differentiation, proliferation, and functioning.[15]

Oocyte-Paracrine Signaling

How oocyte exactly governs folliculogenesis, CC differentiation, and CC function is not yet very clear. But oocyte secretes growth factor, which plays the key role in folliculogenesis, CC differentiation, oocyte development, and capacitation through paracrine signaling. Before the availability of GDF9 and bone morphogenetic protein 15 (BMP15) the members of transforming growth factor (TGF-b) super-family were known to enable FSH induced with hyaluronic acid production, mucification, GCs proliferation, and CC steroidogenesis.[16]

The most important oocyte-secreted factors (OSFs) are GDF9 and BMP15 which play key role in promoting follicular growth beyond primary stage (Fig. 6). Absence of these two growth factors causes impaired folliculogenesis.[17,18] They are the membranes of TGF-β and are required for early folliculogenesis, central regulation for GC/CC, and differentiation and are associated with pathogenesis of ovarian dysfunction (MC Na HY, 2005; MC Na HY 2007).

Role of Oocyte-Secreted Factors on Cumulus Cells

- Stimulation of CC proliferation
- Prevention of CC apoptosis
- Inhibition of luteinization
- Direction to CCs to supply metabolites for its own development
- Mucification and CC expansion.

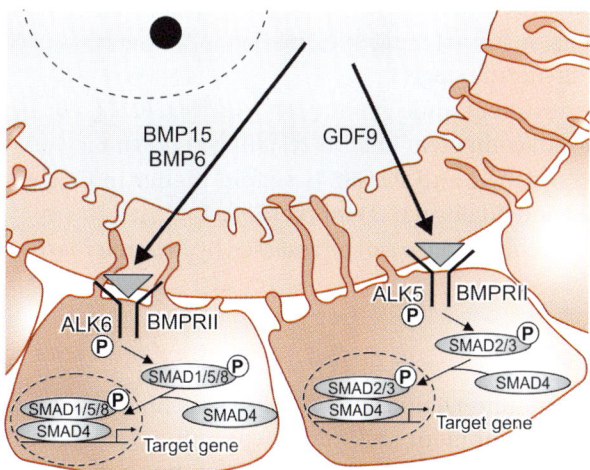

Fig. 6: Bidirectional relationship.

Stimulation of CC Proliferation

In animal model, it has been reported that oocytes are potent stimulators of DNA synthesis and GC proliferation. Various experiments[19,20] via regulation of CCND2, the transcript encoding cyclin D2, etc. showed increase in DNA content and increased number of GCs when cocultured with denuded oocytes.

Prevention of Cumulus Cell Apoptosis

- Microsurgical removal of oocyte to generate oocytectomized complex (OOX) increases CC apoptosis.
- Reverse can be done by exposing oox to OSFs.

Inhibition of Luteinization

- Microsurgical removal of oocytes leads to profuse luteinization of CCs in oox
- Culture of oox with denuded oocytes prevents further luteinization.

Promotion of Mucification and CC Expansion

- Induced by two signaling events
- Stimulation of gonadotropin and epidermal growth factor (EGF)
- Oocyte generates paracrine signals known as-
  - *Cumulus expansion enabling factor signal (CEEFS), which act on CCs and enable them to respond to gonadotropins and EGF to synthesize extracellular matrix.*

Recent Studies on Oocyte Cumulus Insight

- The WNT2/B CATENIN signaling pathway in CCs plays a significant role in human folliculogenesis[21]
- Another gene, maternal antigen expressed in human CCs is essential for oogenesis till morula stage[22]
- Altered expression of some genes *CD44, 3BHSD, FDX1*, etc. in CC/GCs is associated with competent follicles resulting in pregnancy.
- Expression of HAS2 and PTGS2 is sixfold higher in CCs with oocytes developing good quality day 3 embryos (Fig. 7).
- Oocyte follicle competence can be assessed by RNA microarray of CCs and GCs (Fig. 8.).

■ CONCLUSION

Oocyte corona cumulus complex is not only a structural but also a functional unit. For their development and fulfillment of function each component depends on the other. Removal of any one component causes arrest in development and abnormality in function of both oocyte and cumulus.

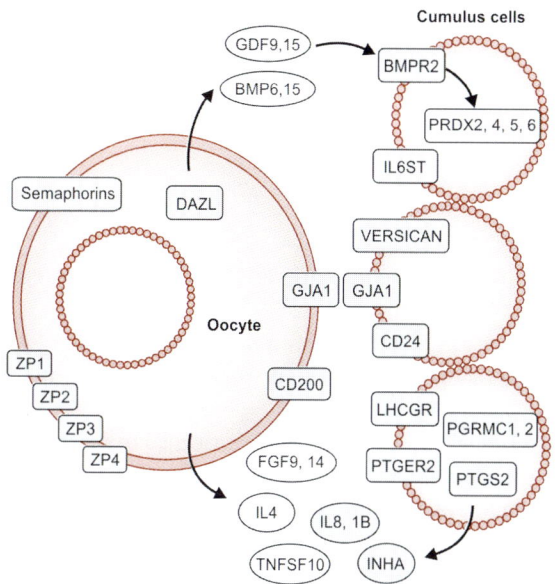

Fig. 7: Expression of gene.

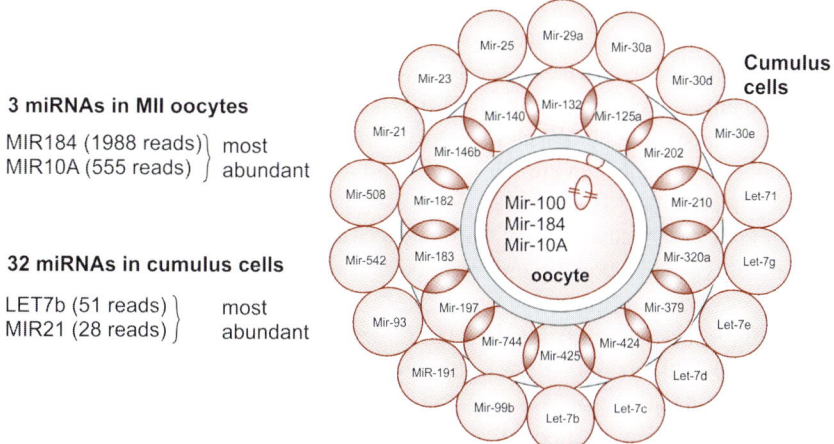

3 miRNAs in MII oocytes

MIR184 (1988 reads) } most
MIR10A (555 reads)   } abundant

32 miRNAs in cumulus cells

LET7b (51 reads) } most
MIR21 (28 reads) } abundant

Fig. 8: MicroRNA (miRNA) expression in cumulus cells and oocyte: Important facts.

Oocyte-cumulus gap junction plays the key role in maintaining their bidirectional relationship. Transmission of oocyte-paracrine signals and different molecules between oocyte and cumulus via gap junction is essential for this symbiotic phenomenon. However the knowledge about these signals and molecules is very limited.

Oocyte is not passive in the follicle, rather it plays the central role in the regulation of folliculogenesis and granulose cell differentiation and their further functioning.

To unravel the mystery in the oocyte cumulus insight, bidirectional communication and research work are mandatory between the basic scientist and the embryologist.

■ REFERENCES

1. Fleming TP, Kwong WY, Porter R, et al. The embryo and its future. Biol Reprod. 2004;71:1046-54.
2. Maloney CA, Rees WD. Gene-nutrient interactions during fetal development. Reproduction 2005;130(4):401-10.
3. Thompson JK, Lane M, Gilcrist RB. Metabolism of bovine cumulus oocyte complex and influence on subsequent development competence. Soc Reprod Fertil Suppl. 2007;64:179-90.
4. Albertini DF, Combellescm, Bonecchi E, et al. Cellular basis for paracrine regulation of ovarian follicle development. Reproduction 2001;121(5):647-653
5. Kidder GM, Mhawi AA. Gap junctions and ovarian folliculogenesis. Reproduction. 2002;123(5):613-20.
6. Hyttel P, Fair T, Callesen H. Oocyte growth, capacitation and final maturation in Cattle. Theriogenology. 1997;47:23-32.
7. Kumar NM, Gilula NB. The gap junction communication channel. Cell. 1996;84:381-99.
8. Feng G, Shi D, Yang S, et al. Co-culture embedded in cumulus clumps promotes maturation of denuded oocytes and reconstructs gap junctions between oocytes and cumulus cells. Zygote. 2013;21(3):231-7.
9. Eppig JJ, Pendola FL, Wigglesworth K, et al. Mouse oocytes regulate metabolic cooperativity between granulosa cells and oocytes: amino acid transport. Biol Reprod. 2005;73:351-7.
10. Zhou CJ, Wu SN, Shen JP, et al. The beneficial effects of cumulus cells and oocyte-cumulus gap junction depends on oocyte maturation and fertilization method in mice. Peer J. 2016;4:e1761.
11. Eppig JJ. Oocyte control of ovarian follicular development and function in mammals. Reproduction. 2001;122:829-38.
12. Hong SJ, Chiu PC, Lee KF, et al. Cumulus cells and their extracellular matrix affect the quality of spermatozoa penetrating the cumulus mass. Fertil Steril. 2009;92(3):971-8.
13. Sun A, Bahet A. Human sperm Chemotaxis: both the oocyte and its surrounding cumulus. Hum Reprod. 2005;20:761-7.
14. Corn CM, Hauser-Kronberger C, Moser M, et al. Predictive value of cumulus cell apoptosis with regard to blastocyst development of corresponding gametes. Fertil Steril. 2005;84(3):627-33.
15. Knight P, Glister C. TGF-beta superfamily members and ovarian follicle development. Reproduction. 2006;132(2):191-206.
16. Vanderhyden BC, Macdonald EA, Nagyova E, et al. Evaluation of members of the TGF-beta superfamily as candidates for the oocyte factors that control mouse cumulus expansion and steroidogenesis. Reprod Suppl. 2003;61:55-70.

17. Galloway SM, McNatty KP, Cambridge LM, et al. Mutations in an oocyte-derived growth factor gene (BMP15) cause increased ovulation rate and infertility in a dosage-sensitive manner. Nat Genet. 2000;25(3):279-83.
18. Dong J, Albertini DF, Nishimori K, et al. Growth differentiation factor-9 is required during early ovarian folliculogenesis. Nature. 1996;383(6600):531-5.
19. Vanderhyden BC, Telfer EE, Eppig JJ. Mouse oocytes promote proliferation of granulosa cells from preantral and antral follicles in vitro. Biol Reprod. 1992;46:1196-204.
20. Gilchrist RB, Ritter LJ, Myllymaa S, et al. Molecular basis of oocyte-paracrine signaling that promotes granulosa cell proliferation. J Cell Sci. 2006;119:3811-21.
21. Wang HX, Tekpetey FR, Kidder GM. Identification of WNT/beta-CATENIN signaling pathway components in human cumulus cells. Mol Hum Reprod. 2009;15(1):11-7.
22. Sena P, Riccio M, Marzona L, et al. Human MATER localization in specific cell domains of oocyte and follicular cells. Reprod Biomed Online. 2009;18(2):226-34.

CHAPTER 22

Time-lapse Videography versus in Time Quick Analysis by an Experienced Embryologist

Varsha Samson Roy, Chaitra K Vannappa

■ INTRODUCTION

The success of assisted reproductive technology (ART) gravitates around identifying that "implantable embryo". Embryologists over the years have relied on conventional morphology to select the best embryo, in spite of its limitations. Over the decades many noninvasive and few invasive methods have been suggested. But inadequate and improperly conducted studies on the benefits of these methods have prevented concluding on the most beneficial one. Time-lapse (TL) technology has been more acceptable due to its noninvasiveness. However, morphological assessment by an embryologist continues to be the most used method for embryo selection. Studies comparing conventional morphology assessment and TL have been conducted to understand their effectiveness in improving the clinical outcome.

■ CONVENTIONAL EMBRYO MORPHOLOGY ASSESSMENT

The ultimate of goal of in vitro fertilization (IVF) is to achieve single live births following each single embryo transfer (SET).[1] In spite of attempts at finding alternatives to identifying the most competent embryo, morphological assessment by an embryologist is still the most commonly used method.

Static conventional morphological assessment lacks the potential to identify a single implantable embryo. Hence, it has been a common practice to replace multiple embryos for transfer. This in turn increases incidence of multiple pregnancy rates. One of the biggest limitations of conventional morphology assessment has been lack of consensus on the grading systems used to analyze the embryos. In 2011, a joint effort by the Alpha Scientists in Reproductive Medicine and ESHRE Special Interest Group[2] in embryology paved the way toward developing common criteria and terminologies for grading of oocytes, zygotes and embryos that would be amenable to the routine application in any IVF laboratory.

It has also been proposed that with the introduction of TL imaging these static morphological scoring systems need to be revised.[3]

Vitrification as a method of cryopreservation gives a good embryo survival rate; especially at the blastocyst stage. Embryos can now be cryopreserved and transferred in subsequent cycles without compromising their ability to implant. Freeze all cycles are being performed with the intention of increasing the success rates. Hence, it has been argued that in such a scenario embryo selection could possibly improve the time to pregnancy.[4]

Current embryo assessment involves two parameters: (1) development rate and (2) morphological features. With each laboratory having their own grading systems, there is lack of uniformity. There also seems to be no uniformity on the timing and number of observations done. Some laboratories preferring to do it the morning of each day, while others preferring an alternate day observation after fertilization check. Standardized timing of observation is critical.[2]

SINGLE STATIC EMBRYO EVALUATION

The evaluation is done under the microscope at distinct time points requiring the embryo to be removed from the incubator for each observation. These events add on to the embryo stress.

Static evaluation of morphology under a microscope apart from providing a single glimpse of the embryo is also limited by substantial intra- and interobserver variation.[5] Conventional embryo assessment will vary according to the embryologists experience and skill. External quality control (QC) programs have been suggested to overcome this bias.[6]

PRONUCLEAR SCORING

The inseminated oocytes are expected to be in the zygote stage of development at 17±1 hours in majority of the oocytes.[2] The zygotes arising from IVF inseminated oocytes are observed to be approximately 1 hour behind the intracytoplasmic sperm injection (ICSI) oocytes. Pronuclear (PN) scoring takes into account the symmetry and alignment of the pronuclei, the number and distribution of the nucleolar precursor bodies (NPBs) and some grading systems also evaluate the appearance of the cytoplasm. In addition, changes in the cytoplasmic appearance and progression to the first division were also considered. Scott and Smith classification[7] and the classification proposed by Tesarik and Greco[8] have been commonly used for zygote scoring. The advantages of Tesarik over the Scott system are the fewer parameters and single observation. To ensure an optimal plane of observation at times the zygotes need to be rolled to identify the equality and number of distribution of the NPBs.[2] In a retrospective study analyzing 446 zygotes, those with a difference of less than three NPBs which were polarized were found to be favorable for implantation.[8]

Pronuclear stage transfers are feasible in scenarios where transfer at embryo stage cannot be done commonly due to religious considerations. Scott et al.[7] reported a 33% delivery rate per oocyte retrieval with zygote transfer. Some studies have found a positive predictive value to PN scoring[7-10] while others did not.[11,12] Positive correlation to blastulation rate and aneuploidy has also been studied.[9,13] PN scoring is a very dynamic process and timing is of extreme importance. It is also highly observer-dependent.

■ CLEAVAGE STAGE MORPHOLOGY

Culturing embryos to a more advanced stage was recommended for better selection to improve the pregnancy rates.[14] Better understanding of the culture conditions and the ability of the culture media to support embryo development has favored embryo selection beyond the blastocyst stage. Embryo development beyond day 3 to the blastocyst stage also reflects gene expression, differentiation and developmental controls.

At 44±1 hours and 68±1 hours, the embryos are expected to be at 4-cell and 8-cell respectively. At 92±2 hours, most of the embryos reach the morula stage. However, this can change with the culture media used. At the cleavage stage, the parameters used for morphological assessment are cell numbers, cell equality and size, percentage of anucleate fragmentation and multinucleation. The localization of the fragmentation can change as this is a dynamic phenomenon and hence should not be included in the morphological assessment.[2] 2-, 4- and 8-cell are symmetrical divisions and the blastomeres should be of even size. For all the other cell stages, the cell cycle is incomplete and hence one should expect a cell size difference. Studies have addressed correlating these different parameters to blastocyst development[15-17] and implantation even with SET.[18,19] A prospective multivariate analysis, which identifies the variable having independent power and finds the correct power balance between independent variables was conducted by Holte et al.[20] Though the entire five variables correlated highly with implantation potential, only blastomere number, mononuclear blastomere and blastomere equality were the significant independent variables.

■ BLASTOCYST STAGE MORPHOLOGY

Extended culture to the blastocyst stage was proposed as a means to select the most developmentally competent embryo. Gardner in 1994[21] suggested using different media during embryo culture to meet the nutritional requirements specific to the evolving embryonic stages. Availability of this stage, specific media have overcome the inability in vitro to produce low number and low viability blastocysts. Delaying embryo selection to the blastocyst stage will also increase the potential for self-selection of the embryos beyond the stage of embryonic genome activation. Obtaining viable and implantable blastocysts also promoted the concept of elective SET thus reducing the multiple order pregnancies. Gardner and Schoolcraft also suggested the widely used blastocyst grading system to select the best blastocysts. This grading system is based on the quality of the inner cell mass, the trophoectodermal cells and the blastocelic expansion. Transferring blastocysts with the highest score of 4AA increases the pregnancy and the implantation rates.[22]

Single embryo transfer with a good blastocyst significantly reduces the multiple pregnancy rates with a comparable pregnancy rate as that of a cleavage stage embryo.[23]

To overcome these fallacies of a single static observation, evaluation of multiple embryo developmental events has been suggested like sequential embryo assessment[24] and graduated embryo score (GES).[25]

SEQUENTIAL EMBRYO MORPHOLOGY ASSESSMENT

Considering that embryo development is a dynamic process, a single observation during these multiple cycles of embryo development does not provide the right information. Hence, it is not surprising that the embryo which morphologically looked poor on a particular day appears to be "good" during the subsequent observation the following day and vice versa. For almost every scoring system, controversial results on its benefits can be found in the literature. Numerous classification systems, confounding laboratory factors, inter- and intrapersonal variations are adverse contributors toward static morphological assessments (Table 1).

Some studies suggest a limited value of single assessment especially on day 1 and day 2.[17] Several studies have demonstrated better implantation rates with sequential observation from zygote stage to cleavage or blastocyst stage.[9,30-32] Embryo selection by sequential embryo evaluation has shown benefits over single static morphological assessment.[31,33,34]

The morphological grading system at different stages of embryo development seems to be having their own merits and demerits. To refine the drawbacks of these single static observational system, a system in which all criteria are used sequentially to predict embryo development have been suggested.[24] According to this study by Neuber et al.,[24] an embryo which showed PN symmetry, PN breakdown and subsequent good quality greater than or equal to 4 and greater than or equal to 7-cell embryos on day 2 and 3 respectively had a 47.9% chance of forming a blastocyst on day 5. In addition to the above criteria, the embryo underwent early cleavage on day 1 then its chance of developing into a good blastocyst on day 5 increased to 54.2%. If the embryo failed to show any of these criteria then it only had a 5.6% chance of forming a good blastocyst. However, this multi-day approach has the limitation of frequent embryo handling and exposure to the potentially embryotoxic conditions outside the incubator.

GRADUATED EMBRYO SCORING SYSTEM

In the GES system,[25] the highest embryo score had 64% blastocyst formation compared to 11% for the lowest embryo score. A multiple-step scoring system suggested by Rienzi et al.[35] reported 77% blastocyst formation on day 5 for

Table 1: Morphological grading systems and their end points.

Author and year	Day/stage of morphological grading	End result compared	Conclusion
Lan et al., 2003[26]	Z score and day 3 morphology	Predicting day 5 embryo viability	Embryos with Z-1 score and grade 1—day 3—could predict best day 5 blastocyst
Tesarik et al., 1999[8]	No. and distribution of nuclear precursor bodies (6 patterns: 0–5)	Clinical pregnancy rate NPB—0 pattern—CPR—50% 1–5 patterns—CPR—9%	PN grading could be a predictor of fate of embryo development
Neuber et al., 2003[24]	PN symmetry, early cleavage, D-2 and D-3 morphology	Blastocyst formation PN symmetry—early cleaving—2 cell, good quality ≥4 cell, ≥7 cell	Sequential assessment of embryos could predict good blastocyst
Nagy et al., 2003[31]	PN, NPB polarization, embryo cleavage, fragmentation	Implantation rate PN morphology and embryo morphology on day 3—21.1%—IR	Combining polarization of NPB and embryo morphology on day 3—marker of implantation
Fisch et al., 2001[25]	GES Nucleolar alignment, cleavage, fragmentation, cell no., morphology	1. Implantation rate GES—>70 vs <65 39% vs 24% 2. Pregnancy rate GES—70 vs <70 PR—59% vs 34%	GES—predict good blastocyst and improve success rate with day 3 transfer
Van et al., 2004[27]	Early cleavage (EC) Cell number Morphology	Blastocyst formation—early cleaving vs non-EC—66% vs 40% Pregnancy rate—Single EC vs non-EC 46% vs 18%	Early cleavage combined with morphology—improves embryo selection for transfer
Heitmann et al., 2013[28]	SART grading—cleavage, morula and blastocyst (good, fair, poor)	IR and LBR Higher LBR, IR—good grade SART embryo	Simple SART grading system can improve embryo selection process and improve IVF outcome
Hardarson et al., 2001[29]	Uneven blastomere cleavage	PR and IR even vs uneven cleaved IR—36.4% vs 23.9% PR—52.9% vs 37.6% Aneuploidy—8.5% vs 29.4% multinuclear rate 2.1% vs 21%	Uneven cleaved embryos have poor pregnancy outcome

embryos with normal PN stage, early cleavage on day 1, 4–5 cells and more than 6 cells respectively on day 2 and 3 with equal blastomere size and less than 10% fragmentation with no multinucleation on day 2 and 3.

The major problem remains the degree of predictability of parameters for non-top quality embryos, rather than the outcome of the best quality embryos.[25] This argument is more valid for early morphological grading systems.

■ TIME-LAPSE IMAGING

The theoretical basis of the benefits of TL is based on the assumption that more number of observations will provide valuable information both on the morphology and the timing of cell cycles. TL allows the digital image capturing at regular specified intervals which increases the quality and quantity of information gathered. Embryo morphokinetic markers are used to identify the implantable embryo.

Time-lapse has been in use for almost 3 decades. Payne and colleagues in 1997[36] were the first to study the initial cytoplasmic events during fertilization of human oocytes using TL cinematography. Since then numerous studies have used this technology to monitor embryo development from fertilization to the blastocyst formation, in an attempt to identify noninvasive prognostic markers to predict embryo development and clinical outcomes.

Commercially TL technology comes with the different design features. Either building an incubator around a microscope (e.g. Stage-top Incubator, Tokaihit, Japan), or inserting a microscope within the incubator (e.g. Primo Vision, Cryo Innovation Ltd), or microscope, camera and incubator all integrated in one equipment (e.g. EmbryoScope, Vitrolife). They allow embryo monitoring without the need of opening incubator doors thus minimizing the environmental fluctuations in temperature, pH and humidity. It has been argued that the studies showing a positive impact of TL cannot attribute it to morphokinetic selection alone as the stable culture conditions could also be influencing the outcome.

A number of algorithms have been proposed for the TL platform (Table 2). Figures 1A to E represent snapshots of the embryos as viewed in the TL imaging system (EmbryoScope). Figures 2A and B illustrate multinucleation at the 2-cell stage and Figures 3A and B depict direct cleavage of the embryo to 3-cell stage. The timing of these key events and their correlation to the embryo development potential, implantation and aneuploidy has been studied as the end points. However, it has been argued that the timing of development which forms the basis of these algorithms depend on various factors like the culture conditions, patient factors and also the treatment protocols. Hence, a single model may not be universally applicable for all patients and under all culture conditions. Hence, the same model may not be transferable from one setting to another.[44] TL also lacks a uniform set of nomenclatures. Some TL systems allow computer-assisted annotations of developmental milestones to reduce inter- and intraobserver variation. They also provide a predictive score which assists

Table 2: Description of the annotations used and their end results.

Author and year	Annotations used	End result — Blastocyst formation	Implantation rate/live birth rate	Aneuploidy	Conclusion
Azzarello et al., 2012[37]	PNB—pronuclei breakdown		Live birth rate 1. Longer in live birth group (24.9 ± 0.6 vs 23.3 ± 0.4 h) 2. Earlier than 20.8 h—no LBR		PNB—lesser than 20 h 45 min did not result in live birth PN morphology does not predict the zygote quality
Chawla et al., 2015[38]	tPB2—timing of second PB appearance tPNa—timing of PN appearance tPnf—timing of pronuclear fading or syngamy			Analyze ploidy status by array CGH (euploid vs aneuploid) 1. tPB2—4 ± 2.2 vs 4.5 ± 1.8 2. tPNA—10.6 ± 3.4 vs 10.8 ± 3.2 3. tNF—24.5 ± 4.3 vs 25.8 ± 5.6, p <0.05	tPNF—significantly lower in aneuploid embryos Time-lapse may play a role in detecting aneuploidy embryos
Chawla et al., 2015[38]	t2—time to 2 cells t3—time to 3 cells t4—time to 4 cells t5—time to 5 cells CC2—t3-t2 CC3—t5-t3 S2—t4-t3			Aneuploidy (euploid vs aneuploid) 1. t2—28.3±7.2 vs 30.6±9.7 2. t3—38.7±7.0 vs 39.7±8.5 3. t5—52.3±8.6 vs 50.1±9.6	Time-lapse may play a role in detecting aneuploidy embryos

Contd...

Contd...

Author and year	Annotations used	End result Blastocyst formation	Implantation rate/live birth rate	Aneuploidy	Conclusion
Meseguer et al., 2011[39]	t3—time to 3 cells t4—time to 4 cells t5—time to 5 cells CC2—t3-t2 S2—t4-t3 Multinucleation at 4-cell stage—more than one nucleus in one or more blastomeres Uneven blastomeres at the 2-cell stage		Implantation rate 1. T5—important p <0.001 t5—48.8–56.6 after ICSI 2. S2—t4-t3 - (≤0.76 h) 3. CC2 = t3-t2 - (≤11.9 h) reduce implantation 4. Multinucleation-4-cell stage—IR 18.1% vs 31.2 in non-MN	4. CC2—10.5±4.2 vs 9.1±4.9 5. CC3—13.5±5.6 vs 10.8±7.0	Implantation rate can be improved by time-lapse
Kirkegaard et al., 2013[40]	PN breakdown Duration of first cytokinesis Division to 2, 3, 4 cell Direct cleavage to 3 cell Multinucleation at the 2-cell stage	Duration of first cytokinesis, t2, t3—predictor of high quality blastocyst formation within first 48 h of culture			Development of high quality blastocyst can be predicted within first 48 h of culture. However, time-lapse parameter could not predict pregnancy

Contd...

Contd...

Author and year	Annotations used	End result		Implantation rate/live birth rate	Aneuploidy	Conclusion
		Blastocyst formation				
Dal Canto et al., 2012[41]	Timing of cleavage to 7 and 8 cell	Blastocyst prediction T7—56.5 ± 8.1 vs 58.8±10.4, p = 0.03 T8—61±9.4 vs 65.2±13 h, p = 0.0008				Early cleaving embryos are more likely to develop into good blastocyst
Campbell et al., 2013[42]	1. tSB—time from insemination to start of first sign of cavitation 2. tB—time of insemination to formation of full blastocyst, the blastocele cavity filled the embryo, the ICM and TE were distinguishable and there was no more than 10% increase in outer diameter of the zona			Implantation rate 1. Low aneuploidy risk—24/33 (72.7%) 2. Medium risk—13/51 (25.5%) 3. High risk—0/4 p <0.0001	Aneuploidy Low aneuploidy risk— tSB <96.2 h tB—<122.9 h	Early blastulation— lower risk of aneuploidy and higher implantation rate
Rubio et al., 2012[43]	Direct cleavage—from zygote to 3-blastomere stage t3-t2 <5 h			Implantation rate, CPR IR—direct cleavage—1.2% vs 20.2% in normal cleavage CPR—direct cleavage—1%		Embryos with direct cleavage had lower implantation rate

Time-lapse Videography versus in Time Quick Analysis

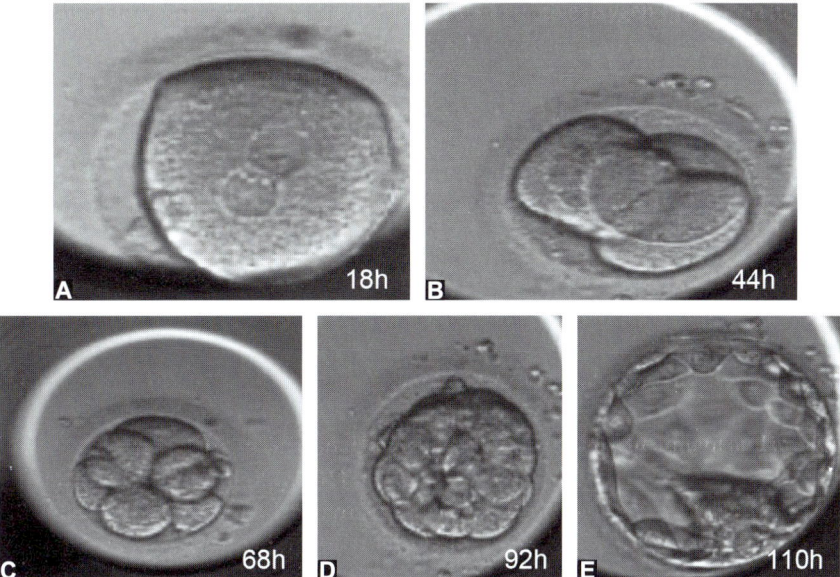

Figs. 1A to E: Snapshot of the embryos developing in the time-lapse imaging system.

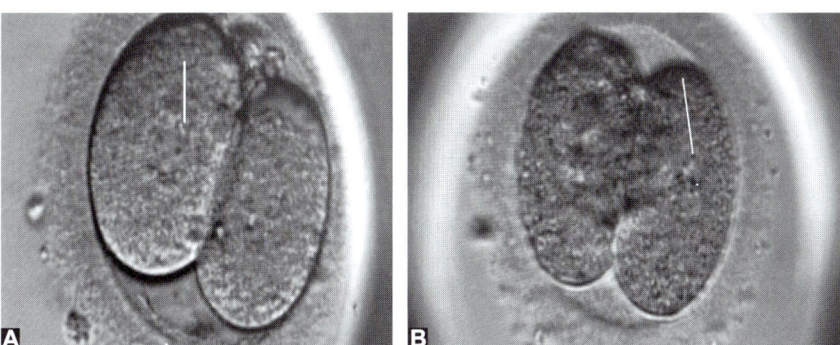

Figs. 2A and B: Multinucleation at the 2-cell stage.

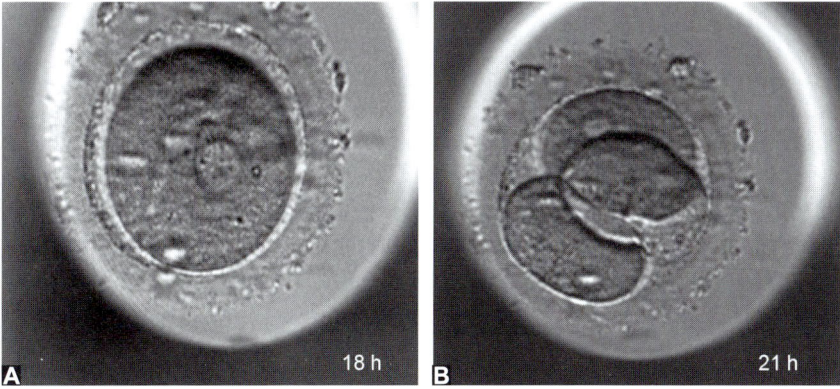

Figs. 3A and B: Depicting direct cleavage of the embryo to 3-cell stage.

in deselecting embryos with poor developmental and implantation potential. The stated benefits of TL can be summarized as follows:[45]

1. Reduces observational dilemma—as it provides more images which are recorded and can be evaluated repeatedly to identify finer details which may be missed or overlooked in a single frame
2. Provides more information on the embryo development
3. Provides unaltered stable culture conditions under strict environmental control
4. Can be used as a tool for QC
5. Allows flexibility in the laboratory workflow
6. Provides a useful tool for communication between the doctors, patients and embryologists.

■ COMPARISON OF TIME-LAPSE VERSUS CONVENTIONAL MORPHOLOGY

Various studies have compared TL imaging with conventional morphology (Table 3). The morphokinetic data on the duration of the first cytokinesis (P1), time between first and second cytokinesis (P2) and between second and third cytokinesis (P3) were used for prediction of the usable blastocyst (one which can be either transferred or frozen).[49] Studies conducted using this Eeva system achieved better prediction of blastocyst formation than by static morphological evaluation alone.

Comparing blastocyst prediction based on day 3 morphology assessment by embryologists of diverse clinical practice and laboratory training with that of an automated TL-generated prediction (Eeva system) model suggested that both these parameters used adjunctively would significantly reduce the variability in blastocyst prediction.[50] Using an automated TL-enabled prognostic test along with morphology can help embryologists with various levels of experience select embryos with high implantation potential.[50] This strategy may improve the success rates of cleavage stage transfers.[49] Studies suggest that using both morphokinetics and morphology together is clinically more useful than using kinetics alone.[51]

During extended culture in vitro, almost 50% of the embryos will arrest its development. The reasons for the high rate of embryo arrest though not fully understood may include chromosomal abnormalities, suboptimal culture conditions and inadequate oocyte maturation. It is important to bear in mind that using blastocyst (usable) formation as the end point has its own limitation as a large population of blastocysts do not implant. No model has yet proven 100% sensitive and specific and hence a prediction model should be used for ranking of the embryos rather than selection to avoid the risk of discarding usable embryos.[52]

Using clinical pregnancy or live birth rate is the most acceptable end point. Direct cleavage from 1 cell to 3 cells, uneven blastomere size at 2-cell,

Table 3: Comparisons of time-lapse (TL) and conventional morphology.

Author and year	Annotations used (TL)	Morphological scoring used	Comments (conclusions)
Conaghan et al., 2013[49]	Key cell divisions in Eeva TL	Day 3 morphology	TL along with morphology could improve IVF outcome in cleavage stage ET
Diamond et al., 2014[50]	Key cell division timings	Day 3 morphology	TL combined with morphology enables better selection of embryos with good implantation potential
Kahraman et al., 2012[46]	t2, t3, t4, t5, t6, t7, t8, t9, tM, tB	Day 2, day 3—cell number, symmetry, fragmentation, multinucleation, compaction, blstocyst grading as per Gardner's criterion	No statistical difference between both the groups for blastocyst development, IR, CPR
Rubio et al., 2014[43]	t2, t3, t4, t5, cc2, s2	Day 2, day 3—cell number, symmetry, fragmentation, multinucleation, compaction Group A—complete TE, high cell no., compact ICM Group B—incomplete TE, several grouped cells Group C—few cells in TE, ICM	TL vs morphology 1. OPR—51.4% vs 41.7% 2. Early pregnancy loss—16.6% vs 25.8% 3. Implantation rate— 44.9 vs 37.1 TL improves reproductive outcome
Kirkegaard et al., 2012[48]	Cytokinesis	Day 2, day 3—cell number, symmetry, fragmentation, multinucleation, compaction, blstocyst grading as per Gardner's criterion	End point—proportion of 4-cell embryos on day 2 Proportion of 7–8 cells on day 3 Proportion of blastocysts on day 5 No difference in the CPR or IR in TL and conventional incubator
Meseguer et al., 2012[47]	t2, t3, t4, t5, t6, t7, t8, t9, tM, tB	Day 2, day 3—cell number, symmetry, fragmentation, multinucleation, compaction, blstocyst grading as per Gardner's criterion	End point—CPR TL embryos had a better CPR (+20.1% per oocyte retrieval, +15.7% per embryo transfer)

multinucleation at the 4-cell stage, reverse cleavage are parameters of an embryo with poor implantation potential.

Traditional morphological assessment has limited success in identifying aneuploid embryos. A TL study[42] analyzing trophoectodermal biopsies evaluated with either array comparative genomic hybridization (array CGH) or single-nucleotide polymorphism (SNP) microarray, revealed a correlation between delay in initiation of blastulation and full blastulation to aneuploidy, but no correlation to any of the early cleavage timings. However, this study was conducted in patients indicated for preimplantation genetic screening (PGS) and has a limited predictive value in the general IVF patients. This model could be useful for ranking the embryos in the high aneuploidy risk PGS population. Other TL models which analyzed chromosomal content at cleavage stage could be limited by the high mosaicism prevalent at this stage.[53] Meseguer and colleagues[39] compared implantation rates between embryos identified to have the highest implantation potential by TL monitoring (TLM) versus those with the best morphology by static grading and embryos selected by a hierarchical TL classification.[47] They reported a 20.1% higher implantation rate in the TL group after adjusting for confounding factors. This relative improvement was reported across 10 clinics and varied from 25% to +50% relative change, which may suggest inconsistencies in how the TLM parameters were measured or used for selection. The main criticism of this latter study was the embryos were cultured in varied culture conditions (EmbryoScope vs standard incubators).

Time-lapse incubator technology has the added advantage of maintaining stability of the culture conditions. It may prove beneficial in a set up with unstable embryology program by stabilizing their performance. Though different parameters for embryo selection have been identified by TL, no single parameter has been found to be consistent in its correlation to the clinical outcome. TL has shown to improve blastocyst prediction and reduce inter- and intraobserver variation compared with conventional morphology.

■ CONCLUSION

Conventional morphology is still the most commonly used method for identifying the best embryos. Its major limitation being nonuniformity in the grading systems practiced by different clinics, limited information, inter- and intraobserver variation, dependent on embryologists skill and experience and increased embryo stress due to removal of the embryo from the incubator for assessment. TL provides the embryo a more stable environment with reduced intra- and interobserver variation. Apart from it being an expensive technology, it still lacks strong convincing evidence to support its use in improving the clinical outcome over morphological assessment. Use of computer-assisted TL prediction models can improve the embryologist's observation and selection of the best embryo.

REFERENCES

1. Cohen J, Alikani M, Bisignano A. Past performance of assisted reproduction technologies as a model to predict future progress: a proposed addendum to Moore's law. Reprod Biomed Online. 2012;25(6):585-90.
2. Alpha Scientists in Reproductive Medicine and ESHRE Special Interest Group of Embryology. The Istanbul consensus workshop on embryo assessment: proceedings of an expert meeting. Hum Reprod. 2011;26:1270-83.
3. Montag M, Liebenthron J, Köster M. Which morphological scoring system is relevant in human embryo development? Placenta. 2011;32:S252-6.
4. Mastenbroek S, van der Veen F, Aflatoonian A, et al. Embryo selection in IVF. Hum Reprod. 2011;26(5):964-6.
5. Arce JC, Ziebe S, Lundin K, et al. Interobserver agreement and intraobserver reproducibility of embryo quality assessments. Hum Reprod. 2006;21(8):2141-8.
6. Castilla JA, de Assín RR, Gonzalvo MC, et al. External quality control for embryology laboratories. Reprod Biomed Online. 2010;20(1):68-74.
7. Scott LA, Smith S. The successful use of pronuclear embryo transfers the day following oocyte retrieval. Hum Reprod. 1998;13(4):1003-13.
8. Tesarik J, Greco E. The probability of abnormal preimplantation development can be predicted by a single static observation on pronuclear stage morphology. Hum Reprod. 1999;14(5):1318-23.
9. Scott L, Alvero R, Leondires M, et al. The morphology of human pronuclear embryos is positively related to blastocyst development and implantation. Hum Reprod. 2000;15(11):2394-403.
10. Scott L. Pronuclear scoring as a predictor of embryo development. Reprod Biomed Online. 2003;6(2):201-14.
11. Salumets A, Hydén-Granskog C, Suikkari AM, et al. The predictive value of pronuclear morphology of zygotes in the assessment of human embryo quality. Hum Reprod. 2001;16(10):2177-81.
12. Weitzman VN, Schnee-Riesz J, Benadiva C, et al. Predictive value of embryo grading for embryos with known outcomes. Fertil Steril. 2010;93(2):658-62.
13. Gianaroli L, Magli MC, Ferraretti AP, et al. Pronuclear morphology and chromosomal abnormalities as scoring criteria for embryo selection. Fertil Steril. 2003;80(2):341-9.
14. Dawson KJ, Conaghan J, Ostera GR, et al. Delaying transfer to the third day post-insemination, to select non-arrested embryos, increases development to the fetal heart stage. Hum Reprod. 1995;10(1):177-82.
15. Nomura M, Iwase A, Furui K, et al. Preferable correlation to blastocyst development and pregnancy rates with a new embryo grading system specific for day 3 embryos. J Assist Reprod Genet. 2007;24(1):23-8.
16. Sjöblom P, Menezes J, Cummins L, et al. Prediction of embryo developmental potential and pregnancy based on early stage morphological characteristics. Fertil Steril. 2006;86(4):848-61.

17. Guerif F, Le Gouge A, Giraudeau B, et al. Limited value of morphological assessment at days 1 and 2 to predict blastocyst development potential: a prospective study based on 4042 embryos. Hum Reprod. 2007;22(7):1973-81.
18. Gerris J, De Neubourg D, Mangelschots K, et al. Prevention of twin pregnancy after in-vitro fertilization or intracytoplasmic sperm injection based on strict embryo criteria: a prospective randomized clinical trial. Hum Reprod. 1999;14(10):2581-7.
19. Thurin A, Hausken J, Hillensjö T, et al. Elective single-embryo transfer versus double-embryo transfer in in vitro fertilization. N Engl J Med. 2004;351(23):2392-402.
20. Holte J, Berglund L, Milton K, et al. Construction of an evidence-based integrated morphology cleavage embryo score for implantation potential of embryos scored and transferred on day 2 after oocyte retrieval. Hum Reprod. 2006;22(2):548-57.
21. Gardner DK, Lane M, Spitzer A, et al. Enhanced rates of cleavage and development for sheep zygotes cultured to the blastocyst stage in vitro in the absence of serum and somatic cells: amino acids, vitamins, and culturing embryos in groups stimulate development. Biol Reprod. 1994;50(2):390-400.
22. Gardner DK, Lane M, Stevens J, et al. Blastocyst score affects implantation and pregnancy outcome: towards a single blastocyst transfer. Fertil Steril. 2000;73(6):1155-8.
23. Zander-Fox DL, Tremellen K, Lane M. Single blastocyst embryo transfer maintains comparable pregnancy rates to double cleavage-stage embryo transfer but results in healthier pregnancy outcomes. Aust N Z J Obstet Gynaecol. 2011;51(5):406-10.
24. Neuber E, Rinaudo P, Trimarchi JR, et al. Sequential assessment of individually cultured human embryos as an indicator of subsequent good quality blastocyst development. Hum Reprod. 2003;18(6):1307-12.
25. Fisch JD, Rodriguez H, Ross R, et al. The graduated embryo score (GES) predicts blastocyst formation and pregnancy rate from cleavage-stage embryos. Hum Reprod. 2001;16(9):1970-5.
26. Lan KC, Huang FJ, Lin YC, et al. The predictive value of using a combined Z-score and day 3 embryo morphology score in the assessment of embryo survival on day 5. Hum Reprod. 2003;18(6):1299-306.
27. Van Montfoort AP, Dumoulin JC, Kester AD, et al. Early cleavage is a valuable addition to existing embryo selection parameters: a study using single embryo transfers. Hum Reprod. 2004;19(9):2103-8.
28. Heitmann RJ, Hill MJ, Richter KS, et al. The simplified SART embryo scoring system is highly correlated to implantation and live birth in single blastocyst transfers. J Assist Reprod Genet. 2013;30(4):563-7.
29. Hardarson T, Hanson C, Sjögren A, et al. Human embryos with unevenly sized blastomeres have lower pregnancy and implantation rates: indications for aneuploidy and multinucleation. Hum Reprod. 2001;16(2):313-8.
30. Scott L, Finn A, O'Leary T, et al. Morphologic parameters of early cleavage-stage embryos that correlate with fetal development and delivery: prospective and applied data for increased pregnancy rates. Hum Reprod. 2007;22:230-40.

31. Nagy ZP, Dozortsev D, Diamond M, et al. Pronuclear morphology evaluation with subsequent evaluation of embryo morphology significantly increases implantation rates. Fertil Steril. 2003;80(1):67-74.
32. Qian YL, Ye YH, Xu CM, et al. Accuracy of a combined score of zygote and embryo morphology for selecting the best embryos for IVF. J Zhejiang Univ Sci B. 2008;9(8):649-55.
33. Finn A, Scott L, O'Leary T, et al. Sequential embryo scoring as a predictor of aneuploidy in poor-prognosis patients. Reprod Biomed Online. 2010;21(3):381-90.
34. Van Loendersloot L, van Wely M, van der Veen F, et al. Selection of embryos for transfer in IVF: ranking embryos based on their implantation potential using morphological scoring. Reprod Biomed Online. 2014;29(2):222-30.
35. Rienzi L, Ubaldi F, Iacobelli M, et al. Significance of morphological attributes of the early embryo. Reprod Biomed Online. 2005;10(5):669-81.
36. Payne D, Flaherty SP, Barry MF, et al. Preliminary observations on polar body extrusion and pronuclear formation in human oocytes using time-lapse video cinematography. Hum Reprod. 1997;12(3):532-41.
37. Azzarello A, Hoest T, Mikkelsen AL. The impact of pronuclei morphology and dynamicity on live birth outcome after time-lapse culture. Hum Reprod. 2012;27(9):2649-57.
38. Chawla M, Fakih M, Shunnar A, et al. Morphokinetic analysis of cleavage stage embryos and its relationship to aneuploidy in a retrospective time-lapse imaging study. J Assist Reprod Genet. 2015;32(1):69-75.
39. Meseguer M, Herrero J, Tejera A, et al. The use of morphokinetics as a predictor of embryo implantation. Hum Reprod. 2011;26(10):2658-71.
40. Kirkegaard K, Kesmodel US, Hindkjær JJ, et al. Time-lapse parameters as predictors of blastocyst development and pregnancy outcome in embryos from good prognosis patients: a prospective cohort study. Hum Reprod. 2013;28(10):2643-51.
41. Dal Canto M, Coticchio G, Renzini MM, et al. Cleavage kinetics analysis of human embryos predicts development to blastocyst and implantation. Reprod Biomed Online. 2012;25(5):474-80.
42. Campbell A, Fishel S, Bowman N, et al. Retrospective analysis of outcomes after IVF using an aneuploidy risk model derived from time-lapse imaging without PGS. Reprod Biomed Online. 2013;27(2):140-6.
43. Rubio I, Galán A, Larreategui Z, et al. Clinical validation of embryo culture and selection by morphokinetic analysis: a randomized, controlled trial of the EmbryoScope. Fertil Steril. 2014;102(5):1287-94.
44. Best L, Campbell A, Duffy S, et al. Does one model fit all? Testing a published embryo selection algorithm on independent time-lapse data. Hum Reprod. 2013;28(Suppl 1):i87-90.
45. Herrero J, Meseguer M. Selection of high potential embryos using time-lapse imaging: the era of morphokinetics. Fertil Steril. 2013;99(4):1030-4.
46. Kahraman S, Çetinkaya M, Pirkevi C, et al. Comparison of blastocyst development and cycle outcome in patients with eSET using either conventional or time lapse

incubators. A prospective study of good prognosis patients. J Reprod Biotechnol Fertil. 2012;3(2):55-61.
47. Meseguer M, Rubio I, Cruz M, et al. Embryo incubation and selection in a time-lapse monitoring system improves pregnancy outcome compared with a standard incubator: a retrospective cohort study. Fertil Steril. 2012;98(6):1481-9.
48. Kirkegaard K, Hindkjaer JJ, Grøndahl ML, et al. A randomized clinical trial comparing embryo culture in a conventional incubator with a time-lapse incubator. J Assist Reprod Genet. 2012;29(6):565-72.
49. Conaghan J, Chen AA, Willman SP, et al. Improving embryo selection using a computer-automated time-lapse image analysis test plus day 3 morphology: results from a prospective multicenter trial. Fertil Steril. 2013;100(2):412-9.
50. Diamond MP, Suraj V, Behnke EJ, et al. Using the Eeva Test™ adjunctively to traditional day 3 morphology is informative for consistent embryo assessment within a panel of embryologists with diverse experience. J Assist Reprod Genet. 2015;32(1):61-8.
51. Ahlstrom A, Park H, Bergh C, et al. Conventional morphology performs better than morphokinetics for prediction of live birth after day 2 transfer. Reprod Biomed online. 2016;33(1):61-70.
52. Kirkegaard K, Ahlström A, Ingerslev HJ, et al. Choosing the best embryo by time lapse versus standard morphology. Fertil Steril. 2015;103(2):323-32.
53. Basile N, Nogales Mdel C, Bronet F, et al. Increasing the probability of selecting chromosomally normal embryos by time-lapse morphokinetics analysis. Fertil Steril. 2014;101(3):699-704.

CHAPTER
23

Noninvasive Method of Embryo Selection

A Suresh Kumar, Ratna Agrawal, Madhuprita Agrawal, Sweta Agrawal

■ NONINVASIVE METHOD OF EMBRYO SELECTION

Infertile couples face many physical, emotional, and financial burdens while they are undergoing in vitro fertilization (IVF) cycles. The aim of IVF cycle is to maximize their chance of delivery in a given cycle to reduce a burden they must shoulder. Despite continuous developments in the field of assisted reproduction, the live birth rate following IVF and intracytoplasmic sperm injection (ICSI) remains low. The most recent statistics of the Society for Assisted Reproductive Technology (SART) of the American Society for Reproductive Medicine (ASRM) show that the live birth rate in women undergoing these procedures in 2011 was 29.2% per retrieval.[1] Modern reproductive medicine is gradually moving from multiple embryo transfer to the transfer of a single embryo due to risking the occurrence of multiple pregnancies.

This concept, however, requires a fast, professional selection of the most viable embryo during the first few days of assisted reproductive technology (ART). Thus the aim of a modern ART is the safe transfer of a healthy, viable, and single embryo. Accurate and rapid methods of quantifying embryo viability are needed to reach this goal.

Various methods for embryo selection have been suggested and practiced. These include invasive and noninvasive methods. Noninvasive methods for embryo selection include:
* Selection on the basis of the morphology of individual embryos at the time of transfer
* Selection on the basis of the morphokinetic changes of individual embryos during early developmental stages observed by time-lapse photography
* Selection on the basis of various biochemical markers measured in the culture medium of individual embryos
* Selection on the basis of the oxygen consumption by individual embryos
* Selection on the basis of oxidative stress to which individual embryos are subjected
* A combination of some of the above methods.

Embryo Selection on the Basis of Morphology

Classically, embryos were and still are selected for transfer on the basis of their morphology based on single time observations. Various scoring systems were developed to evaluate the embryos at various stages of development: (1) in the pronuclear (PN) stage, (2) in the cleavage stage, or (3) in the blastocyst stage.

Scoring at the 2 Pronuclear Stage

In 2000, Scott and coworkers developed a scoring system for embryos in the PN stage. Scoring is performed at 16–18 hours after fertilization and is based on the following criteria: (1) size of the pronuclei and their symmetry, (2) size, number, equality, and distribution of the nucleoli, and (3) the appearance of the cytoplasm (Fig. 1). In a retrospective study, Balaban et al found that embryos that showed an ideal pronuclear pattern (0 PN pattern) cleaved earlier and faster and resulted in better quality cleavage stage embryos and blastocysts. They also found that blastocysts derived from zygotes with a high 2PN stage score have a higher potential for implantation.[2]

However, in 2014, Berger et al challenged these findings and found that PN scoring was not associated with improved cardiopulmonary resuscitation (CPR) in day 3 embryo transfers.

Scoring at the Cleavage Stage

Scoring embryo morphology at the cleavage stage is more commonly used. The scoring systems are largely based on two studies:

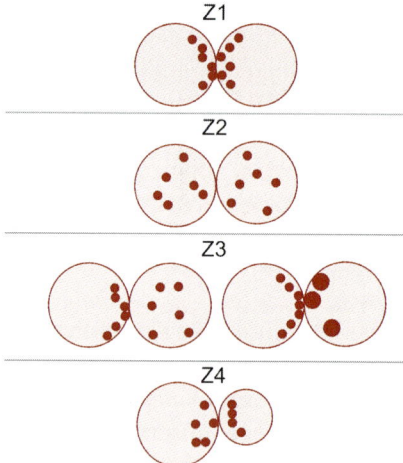

Fig. 1: Embryo scoring at the pronuclear stage (Z1, equal pronuclei, equal number, and size of nucleoli, aligned in both pronuclei at the pronuclear junction, number of nucleoli 3–7; Z2, equal pronuclei, equal number, and size of nucleoli, scattered; Z3-1, Nucleoli aligned in one and scattered in another; Z3-2, unequal number and size of the nucleoli in the two pronuclei; Z4, Unequal size and non alignment of the two pronuclei and unequal size and number of nucleoli.

1. *Giorgetti et al (1995):*[3] The embryos with the best potential for implantation were those:
   - Had cleaved
   - Had no fragmentation
   - Displayed no irregularities
   - Had reached the 4 cell stage by 48 hours after insemination (Fig. 2).
2. *Van Royen et al (1999):* They found that the criteria associated with embryo implantation were:
   - The absence of multi- nucleated blastomeres
   - The presence of 4 or 5 blastomeres on day 2
   - The presence of 7 or more cells on day 3
   - Less than and equal to 20% anucleated fragments.

Graduated Embryo Score: Fish et al (2001) took the matter further and introduced the graduated embryo score (GES) where the embryos are scored on three successive occasions: (1) at 16–18 hours, (2) then at 25–27 hours, and (3) again at 64–67 hours. The total score out of a maximum of 100 is then calculated. In their study, they found that embryos which scored more than 70 had an implantation rate of 39% compared to 24% for embryos that scored less than 65.

Scoring at the Blastocyst Stage

A method for grading embryos at the blastocyst stage was devised. The score is based on three criteria: (1) the blastocyst development and stage status, (2) the inner cell mass quality, and (3) the trophectoderm quality (Fig. 3). They found that when they replaced two top grade blastocysts (> 3AA), the implantation

Optimal cleavage stage development

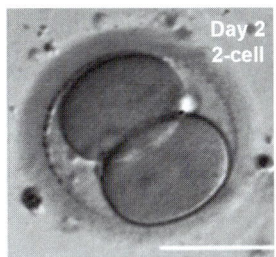
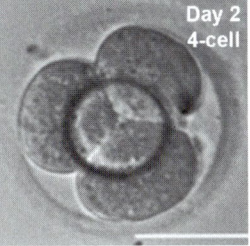
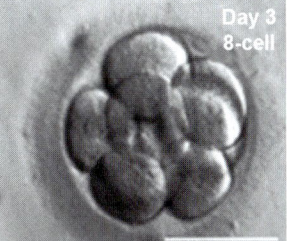

Cleavage stage development with poor quality traits

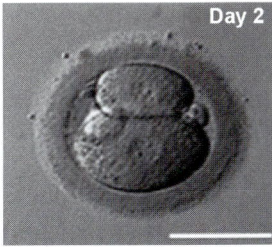
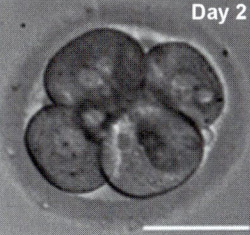
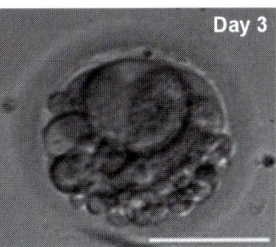

Uneven cleavage — Multinucleated blastomeres — High fragmentation

Fig. 2: Grading the embryo at the cleavage stage.

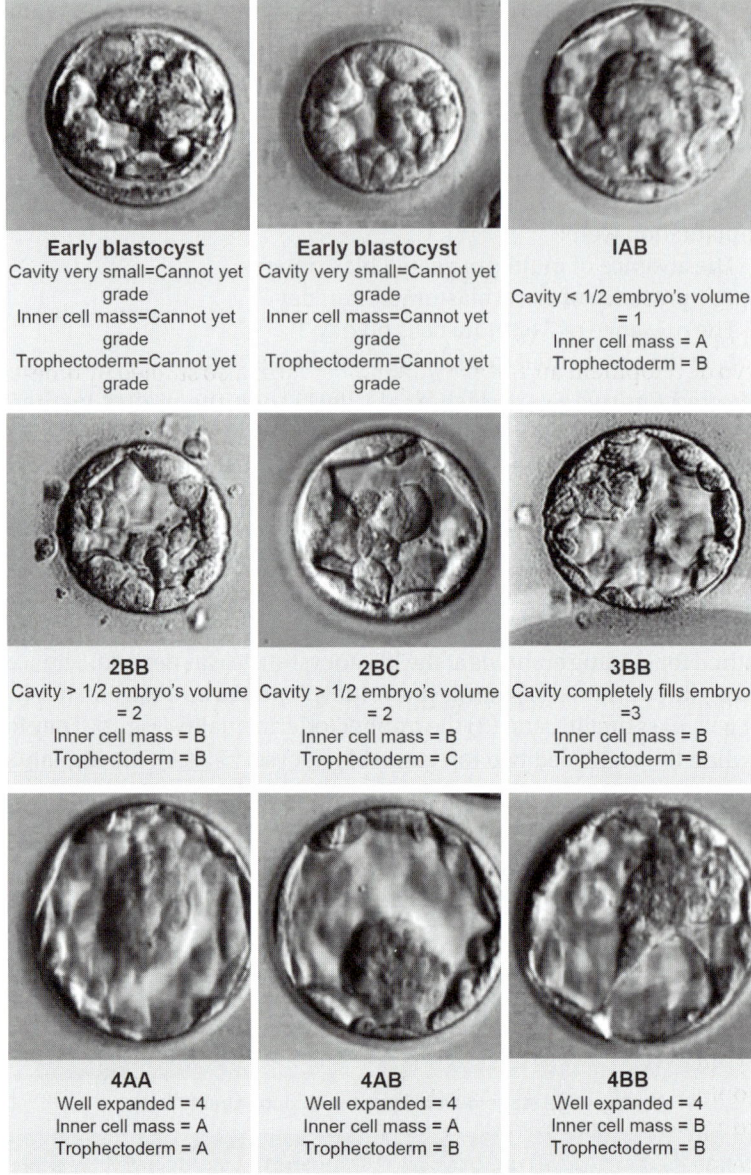

Fig. 3: Scoring the embryo at the blastocyst stage.

and clinical pregnancy rates were 72.8% and 86.8%, 28.1%, and 43.8% when both blastocysts were less than top grade quality (< 3AA).

Blastocyst transfer is now being increasingly used in assisted reproduction as it provides a method of natural selection of embryos when a large number of these are available.[4]

The most recent Cochrane review has shown that there is a small significant difference in live birth rates in favor of blastocyst transfer (day 5-6) compared to cleavage stage transfer (day 2-3).

Embryo Selection on the Basis of Morphokinetics

It has become a new addition for direct morphological assessment of embryo quality. With this technology, the embryos can be monitored without removing them from the incubator. A camera is built into the incubator and takes pictures of the embryos at preset intervals. This type of monitoring allows for the collection of much more information on the timing of the cleavages and the dynamics of the morphologic changes. This software is based upon retrospective studies that identified the morphokinetic changes associated with the best blastocyst formation, the highest implantation, pregnancy, or take home baby outcome. The association between time-lapse markers of embryo development and embryo aneuploidy was also studied by time-lapse systems with contradictory results (Chavez et al, 2012).

The latest Cochrane review shows that the addition of time-lapse monitoring systems did not improve clinical outcomes in all patients.

■ INDIRECT METHODS BASED ON SPENT EMBRYO CULTURE MEDIUM

Various indirect and noninvasive in vitro methods based on analysis of the spent culture medium of the embryo, within the areas of proteomics, metabolomics, and small noncoding ribonucleic acids (RNAs) have been studied.

Some substrates present in the culture medium are consumed by the embryo while others metabolites are secreted. The measurement of some of these products in the culture medium has therefore been suggested as a method for embryo selection.

Proteomics

The proteome represents all proteins translated from the specific gene expression product of a cell at a specific time and condition, whereas the embryonic secretome refers to the proteins produced and secreted by the developing embryo. The secretome profile of embryos is expected to change according to the viability of the embryo.[5]

Several attempts have been made to establish consistent protein biomarkers in embryonic medium. In 2009, Katz-Jaffe et al reviewed finding on potential protein biomarkers in the embryo secretome, including platelet-activating factor, leptin, agrocranin, haptoglobin α-1 fragment, human leukocyte antigen G (HLA-G), and ubiquitin. Although these all appear to promising biomarkers for prediction of transfer success, only HLA-G has been investigated in a clinical setting for its ability to predict pregnancy outcome.

Consequently, the concentration of the soluble moiety of the HLA-G fragment (sHLA-G fragment) was also measured in the spent culture medium as a possible method of embryo selection.

Various studies have shown that the concentration of sHLA-G fragment was significantly higher in the spent culture medium of embryos that implanted versus those that did not.[6]

Multicenter trials have found that HLA-G does not offer any clinical advantages compared with morphological scoring, which seems to be due to variation in HLA-G contents in embryonic media between different ART centers. Prospective randomized trials need to be conducted before this method can be used in a wider clinical context.

More recently, the focus has been on highly multiplexed proteomic methods, such as mass spectrometry (MS). Using such methods, Cortezzi et al (2011)[7] identified 25 proteins in the secretome, of which 15 predicted positive pregnancy outcome and 10 were associated with negative pregnancy outcome. The jumonji protein (JARID2) was the most represented of the proteins that predicted positive pregnancy outcome. Mains et al proved that apolipoprotein A1 is produced by human preimplantation embryos, and correlated the increased levels in spent culture media with higher morphological grade blastocysts. Recently, Dominguez et al analyzed seven proteins in the embryo spent media (SCF, TNFR1, PIGF-1, IFN-a2, IL-6, CXCL13, and GMCSF) with the use of a bead-based multiplexing technology and combined this data with the exact timing (in hours) of cell cycle duration, blastomeric synchrony, and 5-blastomere cleavage with the use of an incubator equipped with time-lapse videography. Finally, only the presence or absence of IL-6 approved to be useful. However, no single biomarker has yet been used in standard clinical practice, mainly due to the differences in culture conditions the complication of the laboratory techniques and the effect of biological variations.

Metabolomics

Metabolomics provides a snapshot of the concentrations of all metabolites in the culture medium as detected by the applied method. The metabolome (small molecule metabolites found within a biological sample) therefore is a good indicator of cellular activity, and may present good biomarkers for viable embryos having a high probability of success after transfer. Metabolomics deals with diverse classes of molecules, such as amino acids, oxidation products, carbohydrates, and carboxylic acids (Nagy et al, 2008).

Embryo Selection on the Basis of the Oxygen Consumption

In 1996, Houghton et al used a noninvasive ultra-micro fluorescence technique to measure oxygen consumption by preimplantation and early postimplantation mouse embryos. Oxygen consumption was detected at all stages of development and remained relatively constant from zygote to morula stages before increasing in the blastocyst stages. In 2000, Trimarchi et al used the self-referencing electrode technique to measure gradients of dissolved oxygen in the culture medium. They found a twofold increase in oxygen consumption at the blastocyst stage. More recently, a respirometric biochip was developed for measuring oxygen consumption and used for embryo assessment.

In 2012, Tejera et al[8] used the Clark O_2 sensor embedded in a time-lapse morphology system to study oxygen consumption by individual human embryos.

These preliminary data require further evaluation by prospective randomized trials and need to be confirm by more studies.

Substrates and Products of Carbohydrate Metabolism

During the first 2 days following fertilization, embryos use pyruvate preferentially as their main source of energy, while after compaction they start to consume glucose as their main source.[9]

In 2001, Gardner et al showed that the utilization of pyruvate and glucose on day 4 was predictive of blastocyst development in human embryos; and was also predictive of pregnancy. Time has come to conduct a prospective randomized study to evaluate the applicability and reliability of this method of embryo selection.

Amino Acid Turnover

Embryos grown in vitro consume some amino acids present in the culture medium and produce (secrete) others. This amino acids turnover was evaluated as a method for embryo selection. In 2002, Houghton et al used high performance liquid chromatography (HPLC) to study the amino acid turnover in the culture medium of individually grown human embryos. They found that embryos that went on to develop top quality blastocysts consumed more leucine and produced more alanine compared to those that did not (Fig. 4). The profiles of alanine, arginine, glycine, methionine, and asparagine flux predicted blastocyst formation in more than 95% of instances. In a subsequent study, Brison et al[10] showed that the turnover of three amino acids, asparagine, glycine, and leucine, was significantly correlated with clinical pregnancy and live birth. It requires randomized trials and need to be confirm by more studies.

Assessment of the Embryo Metabolome

Metabolomic profiling of spent embryo culture (SEC) media has also been proposed as a method for embryo selection. In this method, an overall metabolic footprint of the surrounding medium is determined, rather than measuring specific nutrients and metabolites. Metabolomic profiling of culture medium can be determined by nonoptical spectroscopy such as nuclear magnetic resonance (NMR) and mass spectroscopy (MS) with or without HPLC, which are costly techniques that require trained personnel and expensive equipment.[11]

More commonly, they have been determined using optical spectroscopy such as near infrared (NIR) spectroscopy or Raman spectroscopy, which

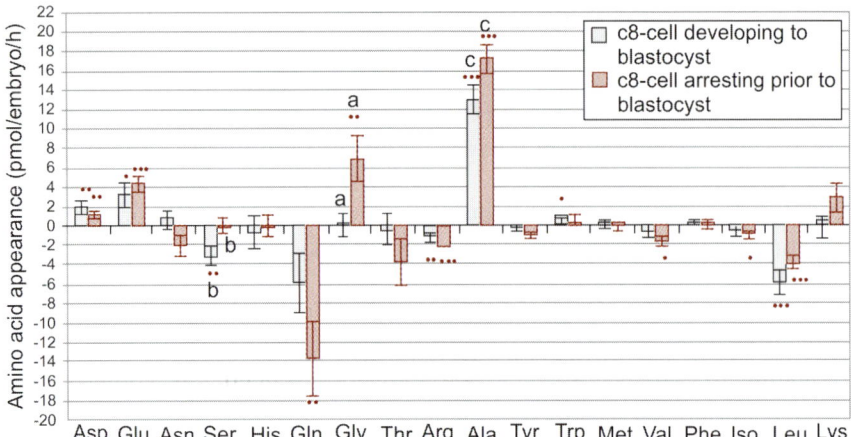

Fig. 4: Amino acid depletion/appearance ± SEM by individual human embryos over the compacting 8-cell to morula transition which subsequently formed blastocysts (n = 23), or which arrested in culture prior to cavitation.

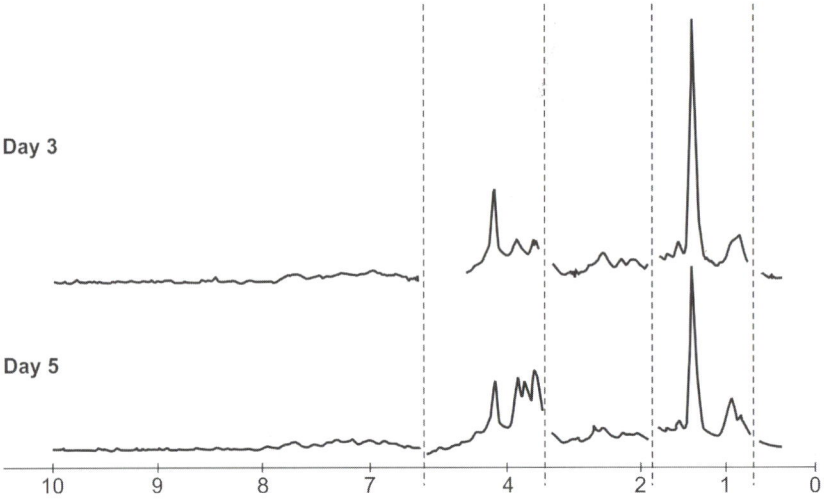

Fig. 5: Spectra of embryo culture media after day 3 and day 5 transfers.
Source: Kirkegaard K, Svane AS, Nielsen JS, et al. Nuclear magnetic resonance metabolomic profiling of Day 3 and 5 embryo culture medium does not predict pregnancy outcome in good prognosis patients: a prospective cohort study on single transferred embryos. Hum Reprod. 2014;29(11):2413-20.

are less expensive, less complex, and do not need sample preparation or separation. The viability score is obtained by comparing regions within the NIR spectrum that discriminate between embryos, which have successfully implanted and those that did not (Fig. 5) (Kirkegaard et al, 2014).

Recently other spectroscopy method, a variant of NIR, namely Fourier transform infrared (FTIR) spectroscopy, which has been used to predict pregnancy viability of bovine embryos. Although there is potential in using

FTIR to predict transfer success, as the method is fast, easy to handle, and inexpensive, it is limited by the relatively small amount of validated data in presently available databases.[12]

ββhCG

In 2011, Butler et al. reported that ββhCG was detectable in the spent culture medium of human embryos from the (2PN) stage through to the blastocyst stage. More recently, Xiao-Yan et al measured ßßHCG in the spent culture media of human embryos using a highly sensitive electrochemiluminescence immunoassay. The authors found a positive correlation between ββhCG concentration and the blastocyst morphological grading, as well as with the implantation rate.[13] These interesting observations need to be confirmed by more studies before being evaluated in prospective randomized trials.

Embryo Selection on the Basis of Oxidative Stress

A relationship between oxidative stress in the culture medium and the growing embryos has been demonstrated. In 1996, Paszkowski and Clarke[14,15] found that impaired embryo development was associated with an increased generation of reactive oxygen species by the embryo and Lipari et al showed that the mean nitric oxide (a pro-oxidant) metabolite levels in the day 5 culture medium were 2.6 times higher in embryos that progressed to the blastocyst stage than in those that did not.

Various systems for the measurement of oxidative stress exist. They include thermochemiluminescence (TCL) analyzer system as well as systems based on electrochemical technology. It requires more studies to be confirmed and required randomized trials.

Small Noncoding Ribonucleic Acid

Recently, a new approach to noninvasive screening of spent embryo medium was suggested. It involves detecting microRNA (miRNA) directly in the spent embryo medium (Lim et al, 2005). Rosenbluth et al (2014)[16] studied 754 human miRNA and found that three (miR-372, miR-191, and miR-645) were differentially expressed on day 5 between the spent culture medium of embryos that had successful pregnancy outcomes and spent culture medium from embryos that did not lead to pregnancy.

However, it is clear that more investigations are needed into more types of miRNA, in larger experimental settings with more samples, and in different laboratories using different types of culture media, so hopefully it will be possible to identify an early, sensitive, and distinctive miRNA profile to select the embryos having the best chance of pregnancy and birth.

Embryo Selection using a Combination of Markers

Combining two or more markers has been tried to increase the predictive value of each marker used alone.[6] Combining sHLA-G prediction with the GES and selecting the best embryo through time-lapse system may increase the clinical and ongoing pregnancies.[6]

CONCLUSION

Embryo selection has been an active research field since the early days of IVF. However, there is no consensus on the best method of embryo selection.

Routinely applied way of the assessment of viability is the morphological evaluation of in vitro fertilized embryos using microscopy. Metabolic and proteomic profiling of SEC media should offer an exceptional opportunity for the assessment of embryo viability. In the future, following time-lapse monitoring and analysis of spent culture media for biomarkers may help to formulate comprehensive and robust algorithms for generating a superior embryo selection diagnostic tool.

KEY POINTS

- Selecting the best embryo is a very important step in IVF treatment process.
- Embryo grading has been proposed as the most appropriate system for selecting the best embryo. The fact that it is based on the assessment of morphological characteristics in an easy and noninvasive way makes it subjective.
- The limitations due to static time-point observation, is now solved with the use of time-lapse microscopy. Time-lapse imaging provides a noninvasive technique of predictive parameters based on developmental kinetics by detecting the dynamics of early embryo development.
- In the field of metabolomics, especially the methods using infrared spectroscopy (NIR and FTIR) might be candidates for clinical applications, as they are rapid and easy to handle.
- Mass spectrometry-based proteomics methods have the advantage of speed compared with traditional immunochemical methods such as enzyme-linked immunosorbent assay (ELISA) and therefore possess a greater potential for application to ART.
- At present no biomarker clearly stands out as a potential early, consistent, and sensitive means of predicting transfer success. However, this will hopefully changed within the next few years as technologies keep improving, and new biological discoveries will help to select the best embryo.

REFERENCES

1. Centers for Disease Control and Prevention. (2014). 2014 Assisted Reproductive Technology National Summary Report. [online] Available from https://*www.cdc.gov/art/reports/2014/national-summary.html* [Accessed March 2018].
2. Balaban B, Urman B, Isiklar A, et al. The effect of pronuclear morphology on embryo quality parameters and blastocyst transfer outcome. Hum Reprod. 2001;16:2357-61.
3. Giorgetti C, Terriou P, Auquier P, et al. Embryo score to predict implantation after in-vitro fertilization: based on 957 single embryo transfers. Hum Reprod. 1995;10:2427-31.

4. Gardner DK, Lane M, Stevens J, et al. Blastocyst score affects implantation and pregnancy outcome: towards a single blastocyst transfer. Fertil Steril. 2000;73: 1155-8.
5. Katz-Jaffe MG, McReynolds S, Gardner DK, et al. The role of proteomics in defining the human embryonic secretome. Mol Hum Reprod. 2009;15:271-7.
6. Kotze D, Kruger TF, Lombard C, et al. The effect of the biochemical marker soluble human leukocyte antigen G on pregnancy outcome in assisted reproductive technology—a multicenter study. Fertil Steril. 2013;100:1303-9.
7. Cortezzi S, Garcia J, Ferreira C, et al. Secretome of the preimplantation human embryo by bottom-up label-free proteomics. Anal Bioanal Chem. 2011;401:1331-9.
8. Tejera A, Herrero J, Viloria T, et al. Time-dependent O_2 consumption patterns determined optimal time ranges for selecting viable human embryos. Fertil Steril. 2012;98:849-57.
9. Leese HJ, Hooper MA, Edwards RG, et al. Uptake of pyruvate by early human embryos determined by a noninvasive technique. Hum Reprod. 1986;1:181-2.
10. Brison DR, Houghton FD, Falconer D, et al. Identification of viable embryos in IVF by noninvasive measurement of amino acid turnover. Hum Reprod. 2004;19:2319-24.
11. Rinaudo P, Shen S, Hua J, et al. H-1 NMR based profiling of spent culture media cannot predict success of implantation for day 3 human embryos. J Assist Reprod Genet. 2012;29:1435-42.
12. Muñoz M, Uyar A, Correia E, et al. Prediction of pregnancy viability in bovine in vitro-produced embryos and recipient plasma with Fourier transform infrared spectroscopy. J Dairy Sci. 2014;97:5497-507.
13. Xiao-Yan C, Jie L, Dang J, et al. A highly sensitive electrochemiluminescence immunoassay for detecting human embryonic human chorionic gonadotropin in spent embryo culture media during IVF-ET cycle. J Assist Reprod Genet. 2013;30:377-82.
14. Paszkowski T, Clarke RN. Antioxidative capacity of preimplantation embryo culture medium declines following the incubation of poor quality embryos. Hum Reprod. 1996;11:2493-5.
15. Bagga S, Bracht J, Hunter S, et al. Regulation by let-7 and lin-4miRNAs Results in Target mRNA Degradation. Cell. 2005;122:553-63.
16. Rosenbluth EM, Shelton DN, Wells LM, et al. Human embryos secrete microRNAs into culture media-a potential biomarker for implantation. Fertil Steril. 2014;101:1493-500.

CHAPTER 24

Embryo Loading: An Important Step in Embryo Transfer Technique

Madhumita Roy Choudhury, Konkon Mitra

■ INTRODUCTION

Embryo transfer (ET) is one of the most critical steps in in vitro fertilization (IVF) process on which the success of IVF depends. Many evidence based researches have been carried out which evaluated the impact of types of catheter used, ultrasound guidance, trial ET, myometrial contraction, ET without trauma on the IVF success rate but less is known about the benefits of specific catheter loading technique. Embryo loading is the final and crucial duty of the embryologist in the laboratory. Therefore it should be carried out in proper way with much attention and effort.

■ MATERIALS REQUIRED FOR ET PROCEDURE

- Pre-equilibrated culture media depending on the development of embryo (cleavage/blastocysts).
- Embryo glue or uterine transfer media (UTM) or media containing GMCSF can be used for putting embryos just 15–20 min prior to ET as it helps in rapid dispersion of embryos in viscous hyaluronic acid rich endometrium. However, there are many reports where the benefit of hyaluronic acid in the transfer media is still unclear.[1-3]
- Sterile, disposable, powder free gloves.
- Sterile pipettes.
- Nontoxic, latex free 1 mL syringe with flat plunger.
- Stereomicroscope with heating stage in laminar flow hood.
- ET catheter.

Choice of suitable catheter is still a matter of debate, SureView soft catheter or EchoTip soft catheter provide better visualization under ultrasound guidance procedure. Soft catheter rather than hard are associated with better pregnancy rate.[4,5]

■ PREPARATION FOR EMBRYO LOADING

- Correct identification of patient and her embryos is vital before ET. It is the duty of embryologist to check the name, medical record number and embryology notes of the patient before ET.
- When the embryos have been identified, scored and selected for transfer, those are placed in fresh, pre-equilibrated media in a single well. The well should be filled up with 0.5 mL of transfer media to avoid air bubble formation during embryo loading in catheter.
- Oil in catheter should be avoided as it may interfere with endometrial receptivity.
- 1 mL syringe is filled up with media and air bubbles if any are ejected out, attached to the catheter and media in the syringe is flushed out through the catheter, discarding the media.
- Sterile, powder free gloves should be worn during loading procedure.

There are several common practices in the area of embryo loading and mainly divided into two categories.
1. Fluid-only method
2. Air fluid methods

Fluid-only Method

1. Flush the catheter with the media in a syringe gently to avoid air bubble formation in the catheter.
2. Place the end of catheter carefully into a drop or well, away from the embryo.
3. Inject a small amount of media to break the boundary of surface tension that may appear at the catheter tip. Aspirate the embryos into the catheter so that the volume to be transferred is 15–20 μL.
4. If the embryos are loaded from the drop under oil then rinse the catheter tip with media.
5. Then keep a small air gap at the catheter tip end.

Merits of Fluid-only Method

It is an easy and simple method. Embryos remain safe and do not have to face any detrimental effect of air.

Demerits of Fluid-only Method

Due to absence of air gap in loading catheter it is difficult to see the position of embryo drop in the uterus.

Air Fluid Methods

The most commonly reported method is medium-air-embryo with media-Air-Media. In a worldwide survey by *www.IVF-worldwide.com*, it has been found that 42% of clinics follow the above method. Another method of loading is media-air-embryo with media-air.

While transferring two or more embryos almost all the clinics load embryos in a same drop.

Merits of Air Fluid Methods

Air gaps in the catheter help to identify the location of the embryo in the uterine cavity. Air buffer zone on either side of the media containing embryos, protect the embryos against spillage.[6] It has been studied that pregnancy and implantation rate were higher when embryos in media are bracketed with air gaps in the catheter (Morano V et al. 2004).

Demerits of Air Fluid Method

Air is nonphysiological factor in uterus, therefore it may be detrimental for the embryos and could also have detrimental effect on implantation rate.

If embryos are not loaded properly, entrapment of embryo in large bubble may prevent proper expulsion of embryo along with the erratic placement in the uterus.

Volume of Transfer Media for Embryo Loading

Several evidence based research studies showed that 15-30 µL of media for loading embryos in the catheter is ideal for ET and it is not responsible for ectopic pregnancy (Montag et al. 2002). Less than 10 µL volume could force the formation of air bubble. Ebnar et al. demonstrated that the presence of air bubbles and extremely low volumes of culture media in catheter (>10 µL) was associated with lower pregnancy rates.[6] Likewise, one study showed that transfer volumes of more than 60 µL may result in expulsion of embryos into the vagina.[7]

Once embryo loading has been done, the catheter with a syringe is handed over to clinician for ET. After the procedure, catheter is checked carefully under the microscope to ensure no embryo is returned or got stuck in the mucus.

If any embryo or embryos have been returned, they should be reloaded in a catheter in the same way and will be transferred again in the uterus.

If difficulties arise during ET procedure causing delay, return the embryos to the culture drop in the incubator, until the clinician is confident that they can be safely transferred to the uterus of the patient.

A systematic review, by Abou Setta et al.,[8] identified two randomized control trials comparing fluid only to air fluid filled catheters and found no significant differences in pregnancy rates between the two methods. Studies showed that different IVF centers follow different technique for embryo loading but with comparable results. Good embryo loading in the catheter should be followed by good ET procedure to get the optimum pregnancy outcome. High success rate always required a close cooperation between the laboratory and clinician.

KEY POINTS

- Embryo loading is the final and crucial duty of the embryologist in the laboratory.
- Choice of suitable catheter is still a matter of debate.
- Soft catheter rather than hard are associated with better pregnancy rate.
- 15–30 µL of media for loading embryos in the catheter is ideal for ET.

REFERENCES

1. Schoolcraft WB, Surrey ES, Gardner DK. Embryo transfer: techniques and variables affecting success. Fertil Steril. 2001;76:863-70.
2. Buckett WM. A meta-analysis of ultrasound-guided versus clinical touch embryo transfer. Fertil Steril. 2003;80:1037-41.
3. Mirkin S, Jones EL, Mayer JF, et al. Impact of transabdominal ultrasound guidance on performance and outcome of transcervical uterine embryo transfer. J Assist Reprod Genet. 2003;20:318-22.
4. Abou Setta AM, Al-Inany HG, Mansour RT, et al. Soft versus firm embryo transfer catheters for assisted reproduction: a systematic review and meta-analysis. Hum Reprod. 2005;20:3114-21.
5. Buckett W. A review and meta-analysis of prospective trials comparing different catheters used for embryo transfer. Fertil Steril. 2006;85:728-34.
6. Ebnar T, Yaman C, Moser M, et al. The ineffective loading process of the embryo transfer catheter alters implantation and pregnancy rates. Fertil Steril. 2001;76:630-2.
7. Poindexter A, Thompson D, Gibbons W, et al. Residual embryos in failed embryo transfer. Fertil Steril. 1986;46:262-7.
8. Abou Setta AM. Air fluid versus fluid-only models of embryo catheter loading: A systematic review and meta-analysis. Reprod Biomed Online. 2007;14:80-4.

CHAPTER
25

Elective Single Embryo Transfer

Gautam Khastgir, Moumita Naha

■ INTRODUCTION

The first successful in vitro fertilization and embryo transfer (IVF-ET) treatment was done in a natural cycle, where only one egg was collected and a single embryo was transferred. However, in order to improve the success rate of IVF-ET, controlled ovarian hyperstimulation (COH) has been practiced to develop multiple oocytes. This has resulted in multiple embryos available for transfer, leading to higher incidence of iatrogenic twins and higher-order multiple pregnancies. In 2001, 24.0% of IVF pregnancies of Europe were twins compared with 1.2% twin pregnancies after natural conception (ESHRE Capri Workshop Group, 2000).[1] The risks related to multiple pregnancies include pregnancy-induced hypertension, gestational diabetes, preterm delivery, low birth weight, higher incidence of birth defects and increase in the relative risk of neurological problems like cerebral palsy. Compared with IVF singletons, IVF twins have a 10-fold increased risk of preterm (< 37 weeks) delivery, a 7-fold increased risk of delivery before 32 weeks' gestation, and a 12-fold and 5-fold increased risk of birth weight less than 2500 g and lower than 1500 g, respectively. The risk of stillbirth is doubled.[2] Single embryo transfer (SET) after IVF has been advocated as the only effective means to avoid multiple pregnancy in IVF cycles.[3] It is defined in the Society for Assisted Reproductive Technologies (SART) reporting guidelines as *an embryo transfer in which more than one high-quality embryo exists but it was decided to transfer only one embryo.* In contrast to the once-believed theory, the numbers of embryos transferred and the incidence of a clinical pregnancy are not proportionally related. Double embryo transfer (DET) was shown to be as effective as multiple SET, but at the same time carried a greater risk of multiple gestations.[4] It has been also proposed that one cycle of elective SET plus one cycle of single cryo-embryo transfer can equalize the difference in pregnancy rates, if any, between SET and DET, but at the same time decrease the twin pregnancy rates.[5] Hence, many reproductive scientists and clinicians from different parts of the world have voiced their opinions and convictions on elective single embryo transfer (eSET), in order to eliminate the problem of iatrogenic twin and higher order multiple pregnancies.

CRITERIA FOR ELECTIVE SINGLE EMBRYO TRANSFER

The essential prerequisites of introducing eSET in an assisted reproductive technology (ART) center are reasonably good ongoing pregnancy rate of the existing treatment protocol along with a compellingly high multiple pregnancy rate, and presence of an efficient cryopreservation program. It is most appropriate for those with a good prognosis: age less than 35 years, more than one top-quality embryo available for transfer, first or second treatment cycle, previous successful IVF, and recipient of embryos from donated eggs. By definition, eSET suggests that there is a choice of selection from among two or more good-quality embryos, with the purpose of transferring only one embryo. However, if only one embryo is available, obviously that is not elective but compulsory SET. Since the majority of these cycles occur in poor prognosis patients, i.e. older women, poor responders to ovarian stimulation, severe male factor subfertility and intrinsic fertilization defects, the only available embryo may be of poor quality resulting in low implantation and live birth rates. Therefore, in such patients, if two or more embryos of suboptimal quality are available, then eSET should be avoided to improve the pregnancy rate as much as possible.

In a subpopulation of women multiple pregnancies substantially increase the risk of premature delivery. Congenital uterine anomaly, previous midtrimester miscarriage due to cervical incompetence, past history of severe prematurity even with singleton pregnancy, previous loss of twin pregnancy, bad obstetrical history and severe systemic disease, i.e. essential hypertension, heart disease, kidney problems and insulin-dependent diabetes constitute absolute contraindication against more than one embryo transfer. This is referred to medically indicated SET. Such contraindications are more relevant both in young women with Turner's syndrome as well as in elderly women, since both groups of patients are at a greater risk of medical complications and also require oocyte donation which has much higher success rate of ART with an increased rate of pregnancy as well as multiples.

Embryo Quality for Elective Single Embryo Transfer

Transfer of blastocyst stage embryos are strongly recommended in eSET because these tend to have higher implantation rate (IR) than those at the cleavage stage.[6,7] However, morphologically high quality cleavage stage embryos may implant at rates of 50% or more.[8,9] Transfer of even two embryos of this quality carries high risk of multiple gestation.

Older women (>35 years) are much less likely to produce embryos able to develop into high-quality blastocysts in vitro. However, developed, those embryos may achieve IRs and pregnancy rate (PR) similar to those of younger patients. Viable PRs of higher than 50% have been reported for single-blastocyst transfers to patients aged 36–42 years and 38–40 years.[10,11]

Morphology as an assessment tool has been the mainstay in the embryo selection process before transfer in ART cycles but it has recognized shortcomings. It is well known that embryos cleaving faster and those of better morphological appearance are more likely to result in a pregnancy. The top-quality embryos have been described as those with less than 20% fragmentation, 4 or 5 blastomere on day 2, 7 or more blastomere on day 3 after insemination, and no multinucleation in any of the blastomere.[12] Such embryos have shown to have an implantation potential of about 40%. The system of morphological assessment of embryos has improved over the period of years and in addition to classical parameters of cell number and fragmentation, the other characteristics including pronuclear morphology, nuclear membrane breakdown and early cleavage to two-cell stage have been found to be of predictive value. The ability to culture and assess blastocyst stage embryos has also significantly improved the ability to select embryos on the basis of their morphology.[13] No single static information gives all the information regarding embryo quality. It is more logical to suggest that a combination of different observation, preferably reflecting different aspects of implantation potential, should be used.

To complement the morphological selection of best quality embryo, noninvasive biochemical assays, such as proteomic and metabolomic analysis of embryo culture media, may eventually prove to be valuable.[14-16] Genomic evaluation through preimplantation genetic screening has the theoretic potential to increase the chance of selecting the most competent embryos and consequently increase the implantation rates; however, prospective trials to date have failed to demonstrate any benefit.[17,18]

Without competent cryopreservation program to store viable embryos for later use, eSET would be difficult to implement. Effective cryopreservation with minimum damage to embryos, in theory, can achieve maximum cumulative birth rates per retrieval when embryos are transferred individually.

■ OUTCOME OF ELECTIVE SINGLE EMBRYO TRANSFER

Nonrandomized Trials

Several nonrandomized trials provide good comparisons of outcomes between eSET and DET at the cleavage and blastocyst stages. A case-control study examining cumulative live birth rates in couples initially receiving a fresh eSET or DET showed that the live birth rate after DET was 31.5%, compared with 26.1% after fresh eSET, with a significantly lower multiple pregnancy rate after eSET (0% vs. 37%). In the subset of women who received another transfer of a single frozen-thawed embryo if they failed to achieve a live birth after fresh eSET, the cumulative live birth rate of 33% was similar to that after fresh

DET.[19] Other observational studies have also found that the cumulative live birth rate after fresh eSET and frozen-thawed embryo (FET) cycles is similar to that following fresh DET. However, in several of these studies, the near elimination of multiples following fresh eSET was lost because of subsequent double FETs.[20,21] On the contrary, when eSET was implemented in majority of frozen cycles, no increase in the cumulative multiple pregnancy rate was seen.[19,22] Another cohort study found no difference in clinical pregnancy (40.7% vs 46.0%) and live birth rates (29.1% vs 35.3%), but a significant reduction in twins (2.3% vs 15.9%, $P < 0.05$) after eSET compared with DET of frozen-thawed blastocyst stage embryos.[23]

Randomized Controlled Trials

Several randomized controlled trials (RCTs) have compared birth rates between eSET and DET.[24-27] The largest and best-controlled among these studies is a double-blinded multicenter trial among 11 clinics in Sweden that randomized 661 patients to either eSET or DET, 98% of them performed with cleavage-stage embryos.[24] Eligibility requirements included age less than 36 years, first or second IVF cycle, and at least two good-quality embryos. Subjects randomized to the eSET group but not achieving a birth from their fresh cycle underwent a subsequent transfer of a single FET. Thus, the maximum possible number of embryos transferred to subjects was identical between treatment groups, with the only difference being whether they were both transferred at the same time while fresh or one at a time in two separate cycles (fresh then frozen, if necessary). Birth rates were significantly lower after fresh transfer of one versus two embryos [28% vs 43%; risk ratio (RR) 0.64; P<.001]. After a single FET following unsuccessful fresh SET, the cumulative birth rates were not statistically different between the treatment groups (39% vs 43%; RR 0.90; P1⁄4.30). Another RCT specifically examined eSET in blastocyst stage embryos, and showed ongoing pregnancy rates for eSET versus DET were 61% versus 76% (RR 0.80; P1⁄4NS).[28]

Two recent meta-analyses compared blastocyst and cleavage stage embryo transfers when equal number of embryo transferred between groups including SET. Both found the live birth rate significantly higher with blastocyst transfer, with odds ratios of 1.39 (95% CI 1.10–1.76, $P = 0.005$)[29] and 1.35 (95% CI 1.05–1.74).[6]

Among the RCTs of cleavage-stage transfers, approximately 30% of all pregnancies and births resulting from DET were twins, whereas only 1–2% of SET were multiples, arising from monozygotic twinning.[24-27] In the RCT of blastocyst transfer, the twin rate was 47% after DET and 0% after eSET.[28]

Thus, both RCTs and these well-controlled nonrandomized comparisons consistently demonstrate that when subsequent FET is factored in, cumulative PRs per oocyte retrieval are similar with eSET or DET with significant reduction in multiple pregnancy rate in eSET group.

■ ECONOMIC ASPECTS OF SINGLE EMBRYO TRANSFER

The prospect of limiting the high costs of multiple IVF treatment cycles may be a powerful incentive for both patients and clinicians to transfer more than one embryo and risk multiple gestation.[6]

There have been several economic and cost-effectiveness studies comparing eSET and DET that generally support eSET, at least in patients with good prognosis.[31,32] Estimated infant and maternal healthcare costs of twin pregnancies are three to five times higher than those of singleton pregnancies, while higher-order multiples cost approximately 20 times more than singletons.[33,34] The increased healthcare costs of multiple births are due to complications during labor and delivery, requirement for cesarean delivery, longer duration of hospital stay, and increased admission to the neonatal intensive care unit.

Increased availability of insurance coverage for infertility treatment could also help to reduce financial disincentives to eSET. Patients having insurance coverage opted for eSET over DET 50% more often than patients without coverage.[30,35]

■ CONCLUSION

In a number of developed countries, the problems associated with multiple pregnancies have been eliminated by legal restrictions on the number of embryos that can be transferred in one ART cycle. In other parts of the world, where no legal bindings exists, the onus is on the individual clinician as well as the patient to limit the number of embryos transferred, so that an acceptable balance can be achieved between the risks associated with multiple pregnancies and a reasonable pregnancy rate with ART. It is expected that the clinics in countries lacking legislation, will be compelled by medicolegal, financial and moral obligations to restrict the number of embryos transferred in order to minimize the risks of multiple pregnancy. The evidence supports successful reduction in the twin rate with eSET in appropriate patients with a minimal reduction in the live birth rate. Economic analyses point to significant cost reductions per live birth after eSET compared with DET. Given the high long-term costs of twins, the significant cost savings resulting from a decrease in the rate of twin pregnancies could be used to fund many cycles of IVF with eSET. In order to promote the uptake of eSET, public funding of IVF should therefore be provided.

■ REFERENCES

1. Andersen AN, Gianaroli L, Felberbaum R, et al. Assisted reproductive technology in Europe, 2001. Results generated from European registers by ESHRE. Hum Reprod. 2005;20:1158-76.
2. Pinborg A, Loft A, Nyboe Andersen A. Neonatal outcome in a Danish national cohort of 8602 children born after in vitro fertilization or intracytoplasmic sperm injection: the role of twin pregnancy. Acta Obstet Gynecol Scand. 2004;83:1071-8.

3. Coetsier T, Dhont M. Avoiding multiple pregnancies in in-vitro fertilization: who's afraid of single embryo transfer? Hum Reprod. 1998;13:2663-4.
4. Veleva Z, Vilska S, Hydén-Granskog C, et al. Elective single embryo transfer in women aged 36–39 years. Hum Reprod. 2006;21:2098-102.
5. Thurin A, Hausken J, Hillensjo T, et al. 2004 Elective single-embryo transfer versus double embryo transfer in in-vitro fertilization. N Eng J Med. 2004;351:2392-402.
6. Blake DA, Farquhar CM, Johnson N, et al. Cleavage stage versus blastocyst stage embryo transfer in assisted conception. Cochrane Database Syst Rev. 2007;(4):CD002118.
7. Zech NH, Lejeune B, Puissant F, et al. Prospective evaluation of the optimal time for selecting a single embryo for transfer: day 3 versus day 5. Fertil Steril. 2007;88:244-6.
8. Van Royen E, Mangelschots K, de Neubourg D, et al. Characterization of a top quality embryo, a step toward single-embryo transfer. Hum Reprod. 1999;14:2345-9.
9. Dennis SJ, Thomas MA, Williams DB, et al. Embryo morphology score on day 3 is predictive of implantation and live birth rates. J Assist Reprod Genet. 2006;23:171-5.
10. Shapiro BS, Richter KS, Harris DC, et al. Influence of patient age on the growth and transfer of blastocyst-stage embryos. Fertil Steril. 2002;77:700-5.
11. Davis LB, Lathi RB, Westphal LM, et al. Elective single blastocyst transfer in women older than 35. Fertil Steril. 2008;89:230-1.
12. Depa-Martynow M, Jedrzejczak P, Pawelczyk L. Pronuclear scoring as a predictor of embryo quality in in vitro fertilization program. Folia Histochem Cytobiol. 2007;45:S85-9.
13. Rehman KS, Bukulmez O, Langley M, et al. Late stages of embryo progression are a much better predictor of clinical pregnancy than early cleavage in intracytoplasmic sperm injection and in vitro fertilization cycles with blastocyst-stage transfer. Fertil Steril. 2007;87(5):1041-52.
14. Katz-Jaffe MG, Gardner DK. Symposium: innovative techniques in human embryo viability assessment. Can proteomics help to shape the future of human assisted conception? Reprod Biomed Online. 2008;17:497-501.
15. Nagy ZP, Sakkas D, Behr B. Symposium: innovative techniques in human embryo viability assessment. Noninvasive assessment of embryo viability by metabolomic profiling of culture media ('metabolomics'). Reprod Biomed Online. 2008;17:502-7.
16. Sturmey RG, Brison DR, Leese HJ. Symposium: innovative techniques in human embryo viability assessment. Assessing embryo viability by measurement of amino acid turnover. Reprod Biomed Online. 2008;17:486-96.
17. Debrock S, Mellote C, Spiessens C, et al. Preimplantation genetic screening for aneuploidy of embryos after in vitro fertilization in women aged at least 35 years. Fertil Steril. 2010;93(2):364-73.
18. Hardarson T, Hanson C, Lundin K, et al. Preimplantation genetic screening in women of advanced maternal age caused a decrease in clinical pregnancy rate: a randomized control trial. Hum Reprod. 2008;23(12):2806-12.
19. Le Lannou D, Griveau JF, Laurent MC, et al. Contribution of embryo cryopreservation to elective single embryo transfer in IVF-ICSI. Reprod Biomed Online. 2006;13:368-75.

20. Kalu E, Thum MY, Abdalla H. Reducing multiple pregnancy in assisted reproduction technology: towards a policy of single blastocyst transfer in younger women. BJOG. 2008;115:1143-50.
21. Henman M, Catt JW, Wood T, et al. Elective transfer of single fresh blastocysts and later transfer of cryostored blastocysts reduces the twin pregnancy rate and can improve the in vitro fertilization live birth rate in younger women. Fertil Steril. 2005;84:1620-7.
22. Lundin K, Bergh C. Cumulative impact of adding frozen-thawed cycles to single versus double fresh embryo transfers. Reprod Biomed Online. 2007;15:76-82.
23. Yanaihara A, Yorimitsu T, Motoyama H, et al. Clinical outcome of frozen blastocyst transfer; single vs. double transfer. J Assist Reprod Genet. 2008;25:531-4.
24. Thurin A, Hausken J, Hillensjo T, et al. Elective single-embryo transfer versus double-embryo transfer in in vitro fertilization. N Engl J Med. 2004;351:2392-402.
25. Van Montfoort AP, Fiddelers AA, Janssen JM, et al. In unselected patients, elective single embryo transfer prevents all multiples, but results in significantly lower pregnancy rates compared with double embryo transfer: a randomized controlled trial. Hum Reprod. 2006;21:338-43.
26. Pandian Z, Bhattacharya S, Ozturk O, et al. Number of embryos for transfer following in-vitro fertilisation or intra-cytoplasmic sperm injection. Cochrane Database Syst Rev. 2009:CD003416.
27. Gelbaya TA, Tsoumpou I, Nardo LG. The likelihood of live birth and multiple birth after single versus double embryo transfer at the cleavage stage: a systematic review and meta-analysis. Fertil Steril. 2010;94:936-45.
28. Gardner DK, Surrey E, Minjarez D, et al. Single blastocyst transfer: a prospective randomized trial. Fertil Steril. 2004;81:551-5.
29. Papanikolaou EG, Kolibianakis EM, Tournaye H, et al. Live birth rates after transfer of equal number of blastocysts or cleavage-stage embryos in IVF. A systematic review and meta-analysis. Hum Reprod. 2008;23:91-9.
30. Stillman RJ, Richter KS, Banks NK, et al. Elective single embryo transfer: a 6-year progressive implementation of 784 single blastocyst transfers and the influence of payment method on patient choice. Fertil Steril. 2009;92:1895-906.
31. Lukassen HG, Braat DD, Wetzels AM, et al. Two cycles with single embryo transfer versus one cycle with double embryo transfer: a randomized controlled trial. Hum Reprod. 2005;20:702-8.
32. Gerris J, De Sutter P, De Neubourg D, et al. A real-life prospective health economic study of elective single embryo transfer versus two-embryo transfer in first IVF/ICSI cycles. Hum Reprod. 2004;19:917-23.
33. Chambers GM, Ledger W. The economic implications of multiple pregnancy following ART. Semin Fetal Neonatal Med. 2014;19(4):254-61.
34. Lemos EV, Zhang D, Van Voorhis BJ, et al. Healthcare expenses associated with multiple vs singleton pregnancies in the United States. Am J Obstet Gynecol. 2013;209(6):586.
35. Ethics Committee of American Society for Reproductive Medicine. Share- d-risk or refund programs in assisted reproduction. Fertil Steril. 2004;82(Suppl 1):S249-50.

CHAPTER
26

Assisted Hatching and its Clinical Application

Shubhangi Gangal

▪ INTRODUCTION

One in four couples around the world is unable to conceive naturally. These couples thus seek help through various assisted reproductive techniques which have become the principle means to resolve long-term infertility. Since the inception of assisted reproduction, Reproductive biologists world over have been trying hard to maximize the take home baby rates by improving the in vitro culture conditions, culturing the embryos to blastocysts in addition to introduction of preimplantation genetic diagnosis in assisted reproduction.[1] Despite these efforts the successes in these procedures are often challenged and still unpredictable. The outcomes of these procedures depend upon the very delicate relationship between the transferred embryo and the endometrium. Even though the ability of an embryo to develop and implant primarily relates to the inherent quality of gametes and intrinsic characteristics of the embryo, such as its chromosomal constitution and the quality of its cytoplasm, some proportion of euploid embryos with full developmental potential still cannot implant due to inability to hatch out of the zona pellucida (ZP).[2-5]

▪ UNDERSTANDING THE ZONA PELLUCIDA AND THE HATCHING PROCESS

The human oocyte and early embryo is surrounded by 13–15 µm thick acellular matrix, the zona pellucida,[6] which is composed of glycoproteins, carbohydrates, and zona pellucida-specific proteins (ZP1, ZP2, ZP3). The ZP is bilayered, the outer is thick, whereas the inner is thin but resilient.[7] ZP begins to form in early antral follicles by the contributions of both oocyte and granulosa cells.

The ZP is of structural and functional importance during fertilization and preimplantation development. The main function of ZP is to induce the acrosome reaction involving the sperm binding to promote the egg fusion.[8,9] The ZP then hardens and becomes impermeable thus preventing polyspermy. After fertilization the other important function of ZP is to protect the embryo, maintain its integrity (before the junctional complexes between blastomeres occur) prior to compaction thus prevent the weakly connected blastomeres from dispersing while migration of embryos through oviductal transport. It also avoids contact with other cells like epithelial lining of the reproductive tract, leucocytes, spermatozoa and other cells of the embryo.[9,10] Thus the ZP protects the embryo. Though zona hardening is a natural process, it has been postulated that additional ZP hardening may occur in both mice and humans as a consequence of in vitro culture.[6,10-13]

Hatching of the embryo is a process, whereby where the ZP ruptures when the embryo reaches the blastocyst stage. The growing embryo physically expands and this embryonic mass reduces the zona thickness in preparation for hatching,[14] at this stage blastocyst also undergoes cycles of contractions and expansions until it becomes almost invisible.[15] Also various combinations of *lysins proteases* are produced by the cleaving embryo (trophectoderm) and/ or the uterus, all assist in zona dissolution.[16-18] As a result the trophectoderm cells interact with endometrial cells and implantation occurs. Elasticity and thinning of the ZP are fundamental for successful hatching. Hatching sites in human embryos is usually close to the inner cell mass.[18-20]

■ WHY AND WHEN ASSISTED HATCHING?

It has been reported that implantation rate per embryo transfer in IVF/ICSI programs is 10–15% for day 2 or day 3 transfers and 23–25% for blastocyst transfers.[20,21]

Assisted hatching (AH) involves the artificial thinning or breaching of the ZP. In order for the embryo implant zona rupture and hatching is a prerequisite. Biochemical modifications of ZP result in zona hardening. Zona hardening (ZH) is induced by several factors like in:

- *Women of advanced maternal age* due to endocrine changes or the absence of lysins as a function of oocyte aging.[22,23,53]
- *Invitro culture conditions*: Some embryos may intrinsically have a thick ZP (>15 Am), or a secondary hardening of the ZP may occur due to sub-optimal culture conditions leading to impairment of zona lysine production, so also prolonged exposure of human embryos to in vitro conditions could lead to the loss of zona elasticity.[24,25] Some embryos may display variation in zona thickness at their early stage of development and since zona thinning is an active process in some instances,[27] the thinning of zona can stop. Some embryos may experience a reduction or even a complete inability to secrete the *hatching factor* (a quantitative impairment), independent of culture conditions or possible uterine lysin, which may inhibit the normal hatching.[25]
- *Cryopreservation*: It has been suggested that the processes of embryo cryopreservation and thawing may lead to changes in the micro architecture of the ZP with associated ZP hardening. These changes theoretically impair the chance of the embryo rupturing from the ZP.[25,26,54]

- *Poorer prognosis groups*: Patient population such as multiple IVF failures due to failed implantation can also benefit from AH.[40]

If due to any of the above reasons, zona fails to rupture and subsequently impairs hatching then it can account for the relatively low implantation rates following assisted reproductive techniques.[28]

Assisted hatching facilitates implantation by allowing earlier embryo–endometrium contact. A two-way transport of metabolites and growth factors across the ZP is made possible. This early contact permits earlier exposure of the embryos to vital growth factors and also opens important routes to convey nutrients from the incubating media. These nutrients enhance embryo development and blastocyst formation.[29]

Since Cohen reported the first pregnancy after AH in 1988, this technique has been used in IVF laboratories for over 30 years with an aim to improve pregnancy rates.[30-32]

METHODS OF ASSISTED HATCHING

The assisted hatching procedure is generally performed prior to embryo transfer (ET) on day 3, 5, or 6 after fertilization. Several methods are used like mechanical incision of the zona[33] chemical zona drilling with acidic medium, chemical zona thinning[35] laser-assisted hatching and, more recently, piezo technology.[37] The mechanical and the chemical methods require extensive technical skill and expertise to produce uniform, well controlled and standardized micro holes using micropipettes mounted on micromanipulators. It is very important to minimize the time the embryo is out from the incubator and to optimize the methodologies to reduce pH and temperature variations that can be detrimental to embryo development.

The Technique of Assisted Hatching Using Partial Zona Dissection

In this method an artificial opening of the ZP of early cleaved embryos is made by holding the embryo by a holding pipette, the ZP is then pierced with a micro needle that is pushed tangentially through the space between the ZP and blastomeres until it pierces through the ZP again. The embryo is released from the holding pipette. The small part of the zona trapped against the micro needle is then rubbed against the holding pipette, thus opening the area between the two sides pierced by the micro needle. The mechanism of partial zona dissection (PZD) is quick to perform, but it produces holes of variable sizes that may not always be optimal.[34,35,38,40] A variation of PZD has been described where a second cut is made in the ZP under the first cut at a right angle, leaving a cross-shaped hole on the surface of the ZP (three-dimensional PZD).[38] This method allows the creation of larger openings while permitting the protection of the embryo by the ZP flaps during embryo transfer.[39] A new technique called *controlled ZP dissection* has been described as a variation of PZD[33] where the embryo is held at the eight o'clock position by a bevel-opened holding pipette, and a thin-angled hatching needle with a blunted tip pierces the ZP at the five o'clock position. The hatching needle is inserted deeply into the holding pipette until the embryo is pushed to the angle of the hatching needle. The curve of the needle is then pressed against the bottom of the dish to cut the pierced ZP. A large slit (two-thirds of the embryo's diameter) created by controlled ZP dissection significantly enhances the rate of complete in vitro hatching of blastocysts compared with 3D-PZD. Embryos are washed before shifting to the transfer dish.

Mechanically Expanding the Zona Pellucida

This technique was inspired by the natural expanding effects of blastocysts on the ZP. This mechanical AH neither thins nor breaches the ZP; rather, it only expands/stretches the ZP via the injected hydrostatic pressure to assist with the embryo hatching process.

Chemical Techniques

Assisted hatching is done using acid Tyrode's. The embryo is secured on a holding pipette and a micro needle is applied to an area of the ZP overlying either empty perivitelline space or extracellular fragments (i.e. a blastomere-free area),[36,48] the micro needle is preloaded with Tyrode's acid before each micromanipulation using mouth-controlled suction. The acidic solution is expelled gently over a small area until the zona is breached. Suction is applied immediately after breaching the ZP to prevent excess acid entering the perivitelline space. This technique requires very quick handling in order to avoid unnecessary exposure of the embryo to the acidic solution. The acid may be detrimental to the blastomeres adjacent to the drilled part of the ZP. The zona dissolves on contact with the acid; hence, the embryo is removed immediately and rinsed several times in culture medium or buffer media to remove any trace of the acid.[13,15,35]

Assisted Hatching by Pronase Thinning of the Zona Pellucida

Pronase solution is commercially available and ready to use. Dilute solution of pronase can be used (10 IU/mL pronase diluted 10x by any culture medium). Embryos are transferred to this solution under oil for 60 seconds for initial stretching and thinning of ZP without complete removal. The embryos are then viewed under inverted microscope to observe expansion. If adequate expansion is not seen then the embryos are further exposed to pronase for additional 30–60 seconds. Later embryos are washed at least twice with culture media and incubated until transfer.[61,62]

Piezo Technology

Recently, piezo technology has been introduced for ZP drilling[37] while a holding pipette holds the embryo; vibratory movements produced by a piezo-electric pulse regulated by a controller are used to carve a limited conical area in the ZP. Five to eight applications in adjacent areas may be used to produce a large hole, which facilitates the complete hatching of blastocyst.

Laser-assisted Hatching

Laser-assisted zona drilling was first reported in 1991 by two groups led by Tadir[41] and Palankar.[42] Depending on the laser equipment, different methods are used, varying in energy, time, and number of pulses needed to open the ZP. Laser is an ideal tool for microsurgical procedures, as the energy can be easily focused on the targeted area producing a controlled and precise hole consistent between operators. All laser systems for IVF work on the same principle, that being to deliver a tightly focused laser beam for a short duration that heats and disintegrates ZP. All commonly available laser systems use lasers that operate in the same part of the light spectrum, near infrared, 1480 nm wavelength. All have the ability to vary the duration of the laser pulse and this directly affects the amount of ZP that will be removed. Different models of laser system available today employ different powers of laser, ranging from ~100 mW up to 400 mW, and some systems even offer variable power.

The laser may be guided through an optical fiber touching the embryo in a *contact mode*. This procedure is performed on a microscope slide, and the embryo is placed on a drop of the medium covered with paraffin oil. The embryo is held with a holding pipette, and the laser is delivered through a microscopic laser glass fiber, fitted to the manipulator by a pipette holder, in direct contact with the ZP. Several pulses are necessary to penetrate the ZP. Because each laser pulse removes only small portions of the ZP, the fiber tip has to be continuously readjusted to guarantee that the laser is in close contact with the remaining zona. The contact approach was used with ultraviolet (UV) wavelength delivered by glass pipette, or infrared (IR) wavelength delivered with a quartz fiber.[41] But the UV radiation can cause harmful mutagenic effects on the embryo. *Noncontact laser* systems allow microscope objective delivered accessibility of laser light to the target. The laser beam is directed using an optical lens tangential to the embryo through the ZP in this noncontact mode using the IR 1.48 μm (1,480 nm) diode laser.[43]

Initially, the laser was used to create a single full thickness hole through the ZP.[44] But now the laser is used to thin an extended area of the ZP. Both light electron microscopy and scanning electron microscopy has revealed no ultra-structural degenerative alterations of the ZP of oocytes and embryos following laser assisted zona drilling.[45] Laser-assisted micro dissection of the ZP can be done with high precision and repeatability with no negative impact on invitro embryo development. The technique is easy to perform, quick and very effective with regard to the overall time requirement and can be performed in a sterile environment without any additional micromanipulations.[46-48] By using the infrared 1.48 μm diode laser it is feasible to open the zona even in largely expanded blastocysts without visible blastocyst damage. The safety of the 1.48 μm diode laser beam has been evaluated in mouse and human oocytes and zygotes.

■ POSSIBLE RISKS OF ASSISTED HATCHING

The assisted hatching procedure may be associated with specific complications independent of the IVF procedure itself, including lethal damage to the embryo and damage to individual blastomeres with reduction of embryo viability. In addition, artificial manipulation of the ZP has been associated with an increased risk of monozygotic twinning.[28,49,50] The higher incidence of monozygotic twins following assisted hatching may result from two reasons. First, a small narrow opening in the zona pellucida, especially that created by PZD, may trap the hatching blastocyst in a figure 8 shape. Subdivision of the blastocyst may lead to the formation of monozygotic twins,[49] the second reason is premature hatching of the blastomeres, which may result in development of another identical embryo.[51]

A hole in the ZP from any technique may deprive the embryo of its protective coat, which shields it from any detrimental factors in the female reproductive tract such as toxins, microorganisms or immune cells. If the holes are small chances that the blastomeres may get trapped during hatching out of ZP and thus resulting in failure to hatch completely cannot be ruled out.[6] Alternatively, blastomeres may be lost through larger holes prior to the formation of tight junctions, possibly causing monozygotic twins, embryonic death or even vesiculation.[13]

■ KEY POINTS

- Assisted hatching is a technique that has been used in IVF laboratories for over 30 years. Although live birth rate data is insufficient,[57] most of the studies have been done patients of prior implantation failure as well as in frozen embryo transfer cycles,[52-54] poor prognosis, including advanced-age patients–women 38 years of age or older,[53] patients with elevated concentrations of follicle-stimulating hormone (FSH), or patients with embryos with thick ZPs; AH seems to increase implantation rate and cumulative pregnancy rate.[58,61]
- Several studies suggest that a larger size of artificial ZP opening/thinning as well as performing AH at a site close to the ICM may be associated with a greater probability for complete hatching.[36]
- The variability of methodologies, study designs, and groups of patients described in the published AH studies make it very difficult to come to a definitive conclusion on the possible effect of AH on clinical outcomes.
- Universal application of AH to all fresh IVF cycles is not recommended in accordance since the existing literature shows no difference in outcomes.[51,55,56]
- Currently, there is insufficient evidence to recommend AH as a routine technique in patients undergoing assisted reproductive techniques.[58]

- More methodical and multicenter trials with proper follow-up needs to be practiced to investigate the role of the various methods of AH. It is unclear whether different methods of AH yield similar outcomes for this too large randomized studies comparing AH methods with regard to embryo implantation and live birth rates are needed, and follow-up of obstetric and postnatal outcomes is recommended.[60,61]
- The variability and possible embryo toxicity are potential problems with the use of AH for ZP drilling. Enzymatic methods to dissolve or thin the ZP seem to be effective and safe. Although the equipment may be expensive, the use of a 1.48 μm diode infrared laser system for ZP drilling offers low potential risk, is quick and relatively simple to perform with high consistency between operators, and appears to be the most suitable method for AH in the IVF laboratory.[59]
- Each IVF center program should assess their own patient characteristics and determine whether or not AH may provide benefit to certain subgroups of their patients. Several studies have been performed to demonstrate the usefulness and efficacy of AH in different groups of patients using the various methods described.

■ REFERENCES

1. Nyboe Andersen A, Gianaroli L, Felberbaum R, et al. Assisted reproductive technology in Europe, 2001. Human Reproduction. 2005;20(5):1158-76.
2. Plachot M. Viability of preimplantation embryos. Bailliere's Clinical Obstetrics and Gynaecology. 1992;6(2):327-38.
3. Cohen J, Alikani M, Liu HC, et al. Rescue of human embryos by micromanipulation. Bailliere's Clinical Obstetrics and Gynaecology. 1994;8(1):95-116.
4. Yaron Y, Botchan B, Amir A et al. Endometrial receptivity in the light of modern assisted reproductive technologies. Fertility and Sterility. 1994;62(2):225-32.
5. Balaban B, Urman B, Alatas C, et al. Comparison of four different techniques of assisted hatching. Human Reproduction. 2002;17(5):1239-43.
6. Cohen J. Assisted hatching of human embryos. J InVitro Fert Embryo Transfer 1991;8(4):179-90.
7. Ducibella T, Kurasawa S, Ramgarajan S, et al. Precocious loss of cortical granules during oocyte meiotic maturation and correlation with an egg-induced modification of the zona pellucida. Dev Biol. 1990;137(1):46-55.
8. Duin M, Polman JE, DeBreet IT, et al. Recombinant human zona pellucida protein zona pellucida3 produced by Chinese hamster ovary cells induces the human sperm acrosome reaction and promotes sperm–egg fusion. Biol Reprod. 1994;51(4):607-17. doi: 10.1095/biolreprod51.4.607.
9. Dean J. Biology of mammalian fertilization: the role of the zona pellucida. J Clin Invest 1992;89(4):1055-9.
10. Modliniski JA. The role of the zona pellucida in the development of mouse eggs in vivo. J Embryol Exp Morphol. 1970;23(3):539-51.
11. Trounson AO, Moore NW. The survival and development of sheep eggs following complete or partial removal of the zona pellucida. J Reprod Fert. 1974;41(1):97-105.
12. De Felici M, Siracusa G. Spontaneous hardening of the zona pellucida of mouse oocytes during in vitro culture. Gamete Res. 1982;6(2):107-13.

13. Cohen J, Elsner C, Kort H, et al. Impairment of the hatching process following IVF in the human and improvement of implantation by assisted hatching using micromanipulation. Hum Reprod. 1990;5:7-13.
14. Cohen J. Assisted hatching of human embryos. J In Vitro Fertil Embryo Transf. 1991;8:179-90. doi: 10.1007/BF01130802.
15. Cole RJ. Cinematographic observation on the blastocyst and zona pellucida of the mouse blastocyst. J Embryol Exp Morphol. 1967;17:481-90.
16. Gordon JW, Dapunt U. A new mouse model for embryos with a hatching deficiency and its use to elucidate the mechanism of blastocyst hatching. Fertil Steril. 1993;59(6):1296-1301.
17. Schiew MC, Araujo E, Asch RH, et al. Enzymatic characterization of zona pellucida hardening in human eggs and embryos. J Assist Reprod Genet. 1995;12(1):2-7. doi: 10.1007/BF02214120.
18. Letterie GS. Assisted hatching: relative techniques and clinical outcomes. Assist Reprod Rev. 1997;8:116-25.
19. Veeck LL, Zaninovic N. Blastocyst hatching. In: Veeck LL, Zaninovic N, (Eds). An Atlas of Human Blastocysts. London: Informa Healthcare; 2003. pp. 159-71.
20. Gonzales DS, Jones JM, Pinyopummintr T, et al. Trophectoderm projections: a potential means for locomotion, attachment and implantation of bovine, equine and human blastocysts. Hum Reprod. 1996;11(12):2739-45.
21. Edwards RG. Clinical approaches to increasing uterine receptivity during human implantation. Hum Reprod. 1995;10(Suppl 2):60-6.
22. Magli MC, Gianaroli L, Ferranetti AP, et al. Rescue of implantation potential in embryos with poor prognosis by assisted zona hatching. Human Reproduction. 1998;13(5):1331-5.
23. Primi MP, Senn A, Montag M, et al. A European multicentre prospective randomized study to assess the use of assisted hatching with a diode laser and the benefit of an immunosuppressive/antibiotic treatment in different patient populations. Human Reproduction. 2004;19(10):2325-33.
24. Drobnis EZ, Andrew JB, Katz DF. Biophysical properties of the zona pellucida measured by capillary suction: is zona hardening a mechanical phenomenon? Journal of Experimental Zoology. 1988;245(2):206-19.
25. Schiewe MC, Hazeleger NL, Sclinenti C, et al. Physiological characterisation of blastocyst hatching mechanisms by use of a mouse anti-hatching mode. Fertil Steril. 1995;63(2):288-94.
26. Gabrielsen A, Agerholm I, Toft B, et al. Assisted hatching improves implantation rates on cryopreserved–thawed embryos. A randomized prospective study. Human Reproduction. 2008;19:2258-62.
27. Wright G, Wiker S, Elsner C, et al. Observations on the morphology of human zygotes, pronuclei and nucleoli and implications for cryopreservation. Hum Reprod. 1990;5(1):109-15.
28. Edwards R, Mettler LE, Walters DW. Identical twins and in vitro fertilisation. J In Vitro Fertil Embryo Transf. 1986;3:114-7. doi: 10.1007/BF01139357.

29. Hershlag A, Feng HL. The effect of pre-freeze assisted hatching on post-thaw survival of mouse embryos. Fertil Steril. 2005;84:1752-4. doi: 10.1016/j.fertnstert.2005.05.065.
30. Cohen J, Malter H, Fehilly C, et al. Implantation of embryos after partial opening of oocyte zona pellucida to facilitate sperm penetration. Lancet. 1998;2(8603):162.
31. Alikani M, Cohen J, Liccardi FL, et al. Micromanipulation: In: Asch RH, Studd JWW (Eds). Annual Progress in Reproductive Medicine. New York: Parthenon; 199. pp. 1-18.
32. Al-Nuaim LA, Jenkins JM. Assisted hatching in assisted reproduction: Review. British Journal of Obstetrics and Gynaecology. 2002;109:856-62.
33. Cohen JH, Mather H, Wright G, et al. Partial zona dissection of human oocytes when failure of zona pellucida penetration is anticipated. Hum Reprod. 1989;4:435-42.
34. Malter HE, Cohen J. Blastocyst formation and hatching in vitro following zona drilling of mouse and human embryos. Gamete Res. 1989;24:67-80. doi: 10.1002/mrd.1120240110.
35. Khalifa EAM, Tucker MJ, Hunt P. Cruciate thinning of the zona pellucida for more successful enhancement of blastocyst hatching in the mouse. Hum Reprod. 1992;7:532-6.
36. Hirotoshi M, Hidehiko M, Noriko F, et al. Relevance of the site of assisted hatching in thawed human blastocysts: a preliminary report. Fertility and Sterility, In Press, Corrected Proof, Available online 2 March 2010.
37. Nakayama T, Fujiwara H, Yamada S, et al. Clinical application of a new assisted hatching method using a piezo-micromanipulator for morphologically low-quality embryos in poor-prognosis infertile patients. Fertil Steril. 1999;71(6):1014-8. doi: 10.1016/S0015-0282(99)00131-4.
38. Cohen J, Feldberg D. Effects of the size and number of zona pellucida openings on hatching and trophoblast outgrowth in the mouse embryo. Mol Reprod Dev. 1991;30(1):70-8.
39. Nijs M, Vanderzwalman P, Bertin G, et al. Pregnancies obtained after zona softening of in vitro cultured or frozen–thawed human embryos. Hum Reprod. 1992;7:82.
40. Cohen J, Alikani M, Trowbridge J, et al. Implantation enhancement by selective assisted hatching using zona drilling of human embryos with poor prognosis. Hum Reprod. 1992;7:685-91.
41. Tadir Y. Ten years of laser-assisted gametes and embryo manipulation. Contemp Ob/Gyn. 1998;9:2-10.
42. Palankar D, Ohad S, Lewis A, et al. Technique for cellular microsurgery using the 193 nm excimer laser. Laser Surg Med. 1991;11(6):580-6.
43. Rink K, Delacretaz G, Salathe RP, et al. Non-contact microdrilling of Mouse zona pellucida with an objective-delivered 1.48um Diode laser. Laser Surg Med. 1996;18:52-62.

44. Blake DA, Forsberg AS, Johansson BR, et al. Laser zona pellucida thinning—alternative approach to assisted hatching. Hum Reprod. 2001;16(9):1959-64.
45. Obruca A, Strohmer H, Blaschitz A, et al. Ultrastructural observations in human oocytes and preimplantation embryos after zona opening using an erbium:yttrium-aluminium Garnet Er: (YAG) laser. Hum Reprod. 1997;12(10):2242-5.
46. Hseih YY, Huang CC, Cheng TC, et al. Laser assisted hatching of embryos is better than the chemical method for enhancing the pregnancy rate in women with advanced age. Fertil Steril. 2002;78(1):179-82. doi: 10.1016/S0015-0282(02)03172-2.
47. Makrakis E, Angeli I, Agapintou K, et al. Laser versus mechanical assisted hatching: a prospective study of clinical outcomes. Fertil Steril. 2006;86(6):1596-600. doi: 10.1016/j.fertnstert.2006.05.031.
48. Lanzendorf SE, Ratts VS, Moley KH, et al. A randomized, prospective study comparing laser-assisted hatching and assisted hatching using acidified medium. Fertil Steril. 2007;87(6):1450-7.
49. Hershlag A, Paine T, Cooper GW, et al. Monozygotic twinning associated with mechanical assisted hatching. Fertil Steril. 1999;71(1):144-6. doi: 10.1016/S0015-0282(98)00402-6.
50. Schieve LA, Meikle SF, Peterson HB, et al. Does assisted hatching pose a risk for monozygotic twinning in pregnancies conceived through in vitro fertilization? Fertil Steril. 2000;74(2):288-94. doi: 10.1016/S0015-0282(00)00602-6.
51. Dale B, Gualtieri R, Talevi R, et al. Intercellular communication in the early human embryo. Mol Reprod Dev. 1991;29(1):22-8. doi: 10.1002/mrd.1080290105.
52. Martins WP, Rocha IA, Ferriani RA, et al. Assisted hatching of human embryos: a systematic review and meta-analysis of randomized controlled trials. Hum Reprod Update. 2011;17:438-53.
53. Hagemann AR, Lanzendorf SE, Jungheim ES, et al. A prospective, randomized, double-blinded study of assisted hatching in women younger than 38 years undergoing invitro fertilization. Fertil Steril. 2010;93(2):586-91.
54. Carroll J, Depypere H, Matthews CD. Freeze-thaw-induced changes of the zona pellucida explains decreased rates of fertilization in frozen-thawed mouse oocytes. J Reprod Fertil. 1990;90(2):547-53.
55. Practice Committee of Society for Assisted Reproductive Technology; Practice Committee of American Society for Reproductive Medicine, The role of assisted hatching in in vitro fertilization: a review of the literature. A Committee opinion. Fertil Steril. 2008;90(5 Suppl):S196-8.
56. Sagoskin AW, Levy MJ, Tucker MJ, et al. Laser assisted hatching in good prognosis patients undergoing in vitro fertilization embryo transfer: a randomized controlled trial. Fertil Steril. 2007;87(2):283-7. doi: 10.1016/j.fertnstert.2006.07.1498.
57. Carney SK, Das S, Blake D, et al. Assisted hatching on assisted conception (IVF and ICSI). Cochrane Database Syst Rev. 2012:12:CD001894.
58. Elhelw BA, Sadek MME, Nomrosy KME. Assisted hatching: routine or selective application in IVF Middle East Fertility Society Journa. 2004;9(3):198-201.

59. Kavoussi SK. Assisted Hatching for In Vitro Fertilization-Embryo Transfer: An Update J IVF Reprod Med Genet 2014, 2:1.
60. Ghobara TS, Cahill DJ, Ford WCL, et al. Effects of assisted hatching method and age on implantation rates of IVF and ICSI. Reprod Biomed Online. 2006;13(2):261-7.
61. Li D, Yang DL, An J, et al; Effect of assisted hatching on pregnancy outcomes: a systematic review and meta-analysis of randomized controlled trials. Scientific Reports. 2016;6:31228.
62. Fong CY, Bongso A, Ng SC, et al. Blastocyst transfer after enzymatic treatment of the zona pellucida:Improving in-vitro fertilization and understanding implantation. Hum Reprod. 1998;13(10):2026-932.

CHAPTER 27

Fertilization Failure: What an Embryologist Should Know?

Vijayakumar Narayanamurthy Chelur

■ INTRODUCTION

With tremendous improvements in assisted reproductive technologies and use of sophisticated facilities for in vitro fertilization (IVF) laboratories, fertilization rates approach 70–80%. However, fertilization failure still exists as a frustrating experience. Not only are the consequences devastating to the patient both financially and emotionally, but it also poses a difficult challenge to the treating team of professionals.

Total fertilization failure (TFF), which is the failure of fertilization in all oocytes, occurs in 5–10% of IVF cycles. The average normal fertilization rate in intracytoplasmic sperm injection (ICSI) is approximately 70%, but TFF still occurs in 2–3% of ICSI cycles. Fertilization failure in IVF is mostly related to sperm abnormalities whereas in ICSI oocyte activation defects are the most frequent cause. If a couple experiences fertilization failure, the likelihood of recurrence in subsequent cycles is approximately 30% suggesting that, to some extent, it is not random and could be predicted. Complete fertilization failure, or poor fertilization, occurs more frequently in unexplained infertile patients undergoing IVF compared with patients with tubal factor infertility.

Fertilization failure may be explained by defects in oocyte, sperm, or the procedure itself. Oocyte immaturity or inherited genetic defects may account for failed fertilization (i) related to oocyte factors—improper zona binding of sperms thus causing no penetration of sperms and/or expulsion of the injected sperm from the oocytes accounts for up to 20% of unfertilized post-ICSI oocytes; (ii) viability, abnormal chromatin status, inability of sperm nucleus to decondense, or inability of sperm to activate oocytes are sperm defects that may account for failed fertilization. Analysis of failed fertilized oocytes, revealed that more than 80% of unfertilized oocytes were arrested at the metaphase II (MII) stage, possibly due to failed oocyte activation.

■ PROCESS OF FERTILIZATION

A human oocyte enters the first meiotic division during embryonic life and arrests in this phase for an extended time. Upon resumption of the first meiotic division, the oocyte is subsequently arrested at the MII where it waits for fertilization. Upon fertilization, spermatozoa overcome the second meiosis arrest by inducing a series of cellular events within the oocyte that are essential for normal development, and are collectively called oocyte activation. These events include an early intercellular rise in calcium concentration from endoplasmic reticulum stores. This increase occurs in 1–3 minutes after fusion of the sperm with oolemma, and it originates at the point of sperm entry. The first calcium transient rise is followed by a series of shorter calcium transient rises of high amplitude, which are known as calcium oscillation. As fertilization progresses, the amplitude and frequency of calcium transient decreases while their duration increases until absolute cessation. Induction of calcium oscillations from intracellular stores in the human oocyte, believed to be triggered by inositol triphosphate, which is catalyzed by sperm-specific phospholipase C named PLCζ, present in the perinuclear theca of sperm. The induced calcium oscillation leads to resumption of meiosis, decondensation of sperm nucleus, maternal ribonucleic acid (RNA) recruitment, formation of male and female pronuclei, initiation of deoxyribonucleic acid (DNA) synthesis, and cleavage.

In addition, the calcium rise induces cortical granule (CG) exocytosis, leading to cortical reaction, which prevents additional sperm from binding and penetrating the zona pellucida. It is of interest to note that a single calcium rise is sufficient for oocyte activation, but calcium oscillations in fertilized eggs are believed to regulate short-term events such as oocyte activation but also long-term developmental events, early gene expression, and possibly methylation status. Indeed, studies have shown that in mice oscillation patterns can be optimized to increase the extent of parthenogenetic development into early fetal stages.

Calcium oscillations are also observed after ICSI. ICSI has allowed researchers to obtain more knowledge about sperm capacitation, oocyte activation, and cytoplasmic factors involved in transformation of the sperm nucleus into a pronucleus. Research thus suggests that a factor or factors present in the spermatozoa—especially in the head region known as PLCζ—are responsible for induced calcium oscillation and subsequent oocyte activation. It is of interest to note that, unlike in IVF, calcium oscillation in ICSI begins after a delay of approximately 30 minutes to several hours.

OOCYTE FACTORS

Meiotic Competence

The administration of human chorionic gonadotropin (hCG) to women undergoing IVF and embryo transfer (ET) results in the meiotic maturation of cumulus-oocyte complexes (COCs). Sometimes oocytes being aspirated for IVF/ET fail to resume meiosis in vivo and even after a subsequent 20 hours incubation in vitro and are thus defined as meiotic competence failure (MCF) oocytes, as compared to the corresponding COC yielding only meiotically competent (MC) oocytes. In a cycle yielding both MC and MCF oocytes, during IVF/ET, incidence of fertilization or cleavage and the number of blastomeres per embryo were significantly reduced concomitant with the increase in percentage of MCF oocytes. When the percentage of MCF oocytes was 25% or more, no pregnancy was achieved.

Follicle to Oocyte Retrieved Ratio

In most TFF cases, studied revealed that though body mass index (BMI), antral follicle count (AFC), and baseline hormone levels were not good predictors, the follicle to oocytes retrieved ratio (<80%) was one of the good predictor of fertilization failure. The less number of oocytes retrieved became all the more prominent, as the total numbers of oocytes retrieved were less than 5 (Flowchart 1).

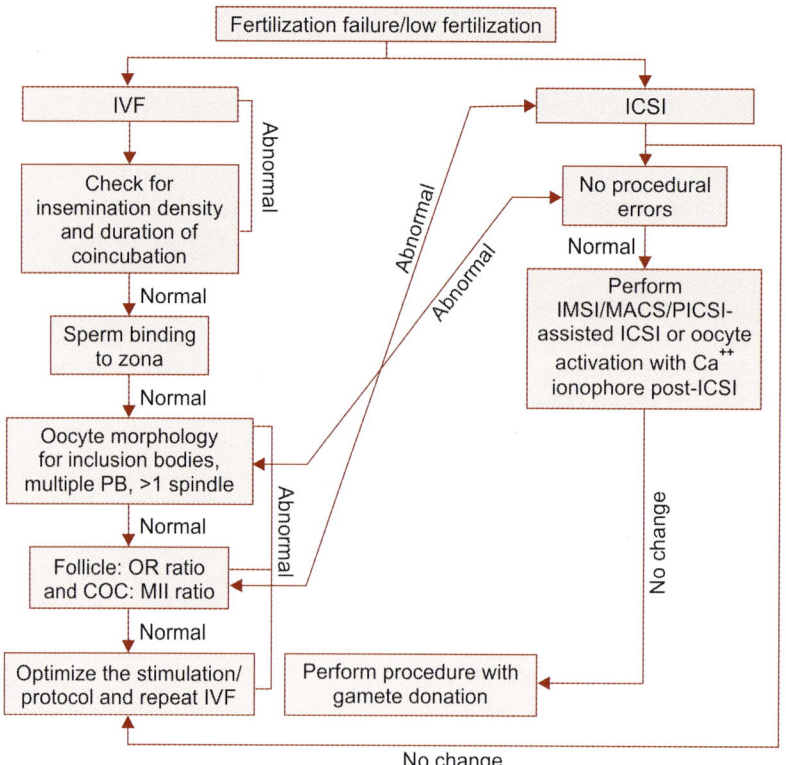

Flowchart 1: Schematic representation of fertilization failure/low fertilization.

(IVF: in vitro fertilization; COC: cumulus-oocyte complex; ICSI: intracytoplasmic sperm injection; IMSI: intracytoplasmic morphologically-selected sperm injection; PICSI: preselective intracytoplasmic sperm injection; MACS: magnetic-activated cell storing)

Morphological Predictors in Oocyte

Significantly lower fertilization rates, embryo cleavage rates, and lower embryo quality were reported for a group of oocytes with cytoplasmic inclusions. The incidence of the oocytes with cytoplasmic inclusions was significantly higher for female factor infertility. The appearance of cytoplasmic inclusions significantly increased in women aged more than 35 years.

Irregular shape of the oocyte, dark zona, or large perivitelline space was not associated with decreased fertilization rate. It concludes that these types of oocyte dysmorphisms are considered as phenotypic deviations rather than abnormalities.

Failed fertilized oocytes of normal fertile (donor) sperm injected oocytes predominantly revealed multiple polar bodies and two disorganized spindle structures, pointing toward these as predictive cytoplasmic defects in the oocytes.

Although meticulous care and continued research is essential for future improvement, failure to fertilize and properly form PN following clinical assisted reproductive technology (ART) is likely to be dependent on historical events in oocyte maturation, not easily explained or prevented through simple modification of contemporary laboratory protocols.

SPERM FACTORS

Sperm Morphology

Data suggests that morphologically abnormal sperm have a negative impact on fertilization and embryo quality, even when ICSI is performed. Morphological quality of spermatozoa used for ICSI plays an important role in fertilization, implantation, and pregnancy. Selection of sperms either by intracytoplasmic morphologically selected sperm injection (IMSI) or by magnetic-activated cell sorting (MACS)/physiological intracytoplasmic sperm injection (PICSI) can improve the embryo morphology and take home baby rate although might not affect the fertilization rates altogether.

Sperm Acrosome and Phospholipase Cζ

Globozoospermia where there is either complete absence/very less acrosome present usually is the sperm type associated with TFF. Most globozoospermic spermatozoa also do lack PLCζ, an important agent to initiate oocyte activation upon injecting the sperm by ICSI. In such cases ICSI with artificial oocyte activation using Ca^{++} ionophore post-ICSI can bring about required change and better fertilization and embryology outcomes.

Sperm Deoxyribonucleic Acid Damage

Due to no conformity or concomitance among the various methods of DNA damage estimation, their predictive cutoff values, and cross-referencing standards being unavailable for diagnostic mode has made very conflicting patterns in the published literature, to draw out a conclusion with respect to predictive value of sperm DNA damage in fertilization failure cases. It is evident by the preimplantation genetic screening (PGS) and preimplantation genetic diagnosis (PGD) data that during the process of embryo development most defects of sperm DNA damages are repaired. Hence, it safely concludes that estimation of DNA damage in sperm during spermiogram is not required as it is not a good predictor of fertilization failure.

■ PROCEDURAL FACTORS

During In Vitro Fertilization

Insemination Concentration/Density

It is normally agreed that the insemination density/concentration must be about 100,000–150,000 normal motile sperms (TMNSC)/mL. High insemination concentration can lead to abnormal fertilization (three PN zygotes) or poor embryo development due to depletion of nutrients by the motile sperms in the insemination well/droplet. Also, it is better to make droplets of 50 µL sperm suspension in fertilization media at recommended concentration and move COCs into them (one/droplet). Upon fertilization check postdenudation and the zygotes can be transferred to cleavage media droplets.

Duration of Coincubation

Whenever reduced fertilization in a tried IVF cycle reported, subsequent cycle with long coincubation of sperms and COCs for 14–16 hours in insemination droplets/wells improves the fertilization outcome. Short coincubation with inseminated sperms can not incorporate the marginal MCF oocytes hence, it is believed that longer coincubation includes those MCF oocytes and hence the fertilization rates might improve. Although might not have any favorable effects on embryo development and implantation.

Meticulous recording of sperm concentration, insemination concentration, insemination density (number of COC/50 µL insemination droplet), time of insemination (hours post-HCG), time of denudation, time of PN check (hours postinsemination), and duration of coincubation. Process and person mapping must be proper.

During Intracytoplasmic Sperm Injection

Failure to Visualize Tail Damage during Immobilization

While immobilizing the sperm the plasma membrane must be disrupted and tail microfilaments must be broken (visualized as a kink in the tail in microphotograph/microvideo graph) to release the PLCζ situated internally to the plasma membrane. The viscous nature of PVP used to reduce the motility of the sperms also inhibits the dissolution of PLCζ in the surrounding media, thus when injected the sperm would be able to activate the oocyte.

Expulsion of Injected Sperm from the Ooplasm

Improper technique used while injecting the oocyte like (i) high speed in moving injecting pipette in/out of ooplasm, (ii) improper oolemma damage, and (iii) improper suction injection technique while injecting pipette and immobilized sperm is within oolemma.

Meticulous recording of duration of COC incubation [hours postovum pickup (OPU)], time and duration of COC denudation (hours post-OPU and HCG), sperm preparation technique, sperm selection criterion/method, time taken for sperm selection (using micromanipulator), time of injection (hours post-HCG), duration of sperm selection and injection process, and time of PN check (hours postinjection). Where possible microvideo graphing must be adopted for review and training. Process and person mapping must be proper.

KEY POINTS

- Diminished ovarian reserve is a risk factor for fertilization failure
- Follicle-oocytes retrieved and oocytes retrieved-mature oocytes are good predictors of fertilization failure
- Fertilization failure in one cycle does not preclude successful fertilization in another cycle
- Sperm motility and morphology are poor predictors of fertilization failure
- Globozoospermia identified during sperm morphology estimation is a good predictor of fertilization failure
- Sperm DNA damage estimation is a poor predictor of fertilization failure
- Training and continuous critical and corrective evaluation of person-process, process-process is the key to avoid procedural errors
- Prognosis may be more encouraging with increasing total number of retrieved oocytes and mature oocytes
- A treatment protocol where the best response is anticipated should be selected for the new cycle.

BIBLIOGRAPHY

1. Bar-Ami S, Zlotkin E, Brandes JM, et al. Failure of meiotic competence in human oocytes. Biol Reprod. 1994;50:1100-7.
2. Ben-Yosef D, Shalgi R. Early ionic events in activation of the mammalian egg. Rev Reprod. 1998;3:96-103.
3. Combelles CM, Morozumi K, Yanagimachi R, et al. Diagnosing cellular defects in an unexplained case of total fertilization failure. Hum Reprod. 2010;25:1666-71.
4. Ducibella T, Huneau D, Angelichio E, et al. Egg-to-embryo transition is driven by differential responses to Ca(2+) oscillation number. Dev Biol. 2002;250:280-91.
5. Kahyaoglu I, Demir B, Turkkanı A, et al. Total fertilization failure: is it the end of the story? J Assist Reprod Genet. 2014;31:1155-60.

6. Lawrence Y, Whitaker M, Swann K. Sperm–egg fusion is the prelude to the initial Ca^{2+} increase at fertilization in the mouse. Development. 1997;124:233-41.
7. McGuinness OM, Moreton RB, Johnson MH, et al. A direct measurement of increased divalent cation influx in fertilised mouse oocytes. Development. 1996;122:2199-206.
8. Nasr-Esfahani MH, Salehi M, Razavi S, et al. Effect of DNA sperm damage and sperm protamine deficiency with fertilization rate and embryo development post-ICSI. Reprod Biomed Online. 2005;11:198-205.
9. Ozil JP. The parthenogenetic development of rabbit oocytes after repetitive pulsatile electrical stimulation. Development. 1990;109:117-27.
10. Ozil JP, Banrezes B, Tóth S, et al. Ca^{2+} oscillatory pattern in fertilized mouse eggs affects gene expression and development to term. Dev Biol. 2006;300:534-44.
11. Raz T, Shalgi R. Early events in mammalian egg activation. Hum Reprod. 1998;13:133-45.
12. Razavi S, Nasr-Esfahani MH, Mardani M, et al. Effect of human sperm chromatin anomalies on fertilization outcome post-ICSI. Andrologia. 2003;35:238-43.
13. Tavalaee M, Razavi S, Nasr-Esfahani MH. Effects of sperm acrosomal integrity and protamine deficiency on in vitro fertilization and pregnancy rate. Iran J Fertil Steril. 2007;1:27-34.
14. Tóth S, Huneau D, Banrezes B, et al. Egg activation is the result of calcium signal summation in the mouse. Reproduction. 2006;131:27-34.
15. Yanagimachi R. Mammalian fertilization. In: Knobil E, Neill J (Eds). The Physiology of Reproduction, 2nd edition. New York: Raven Press; 1994. pp. 189-317.
16. Young C, Grasa P, Coward K, et al. Phospholipase C zeta undergoes dynamic changes in its pattern of localization in sperm during capacitation and the acrosome reaction. Fertil Steril. 2009;91:2230-42.

CHAPTER
28

Oocyte Cryopreservation

Hrishikesh D Pai, Nandita Palshetkar, Rishma Pai

■ INTRODUCTION

Advances in reproductive technologies continue to offer the infertile couple the opportunity to embrace parenthood despite the limitation of infertility. Cryopreservation is one of these advancements in the field of assisted reproduction. It is been rightly described as women's emancipation set in stone.[1] It also serves as a backup method or "insurance" to women who want to postpone their pregnancy. Cryopreservation of oocyte technique yielded successful pregnancies decades ago in Australia, Europe and the United States. However, it took a long time to evolve as a routine procedure. As live birth following oocyte freezing was first reported in 1986,[2] this technique has expanded its role encompassing various medical, legal and social indications. Further, developments in the form of vitrification have provided more reliability compared to an earlier method of slow freezing in terms of actual conception rate. Lilavati Hospital and Research Center is a pioneer Institute in India for *oocyte cryopreservation*, which started in 2007. In this center, we have performed freezing on more than 1,000 oocytes yielding successful pregnancy outcomes using this technique for women with various indications.

■ INDICATIONS

There are several areas where an efficient oocyte cryopreservation program could prove beneficial. Firstly, it can be useful for fertility preservation in females harboring malignant or premalignant conditions, with promising survival chances postchemo or radiotherapy. Also in certain cases, such as breast cancer, where it is not advisable to wait for the next menstrual period to start a stimulation protocol, considering the urgency of cancer therapy. In such case, the random-start ovarian stimulation protocol has been proposed. Further, oocyte freezing is a very good option for these women as embryos can be created at a later stage when they find a suitable partner, or are in remission period. Apart from malignant cases, it is also useful in fertility preservation for women with several genetic conditions, such as *BRCA1* and *BRCA 2* mutation. These women require prophylactic salpingo-oophorectomy at an early age considering their high risk for acquiring ovarian cancer. In addition, other genetic conditions which have been associated with premature ovarian failure, such as Turner's syndrome, fragile X permutation and deletion of X chromosome. Oocyte freezing is a viable option. This technology further has a role in women whose cytotoxic cancer treatment threatens their ovarian reserve, or whose medical pathology presents a similar danger. For example, conditions such as severe endometriosis and severe Crohn's disease.

Successful oocyte freezing/thawing technique has led to the creation of a donor oocyte bank which circumvents the need to match recipient's and donor's cycles. Another group of women who may benefit from oocyte cryopreservation are women who wish to delay the childbirth. Social oocyte freezing provides a good option to women who freeze their eggs at the peak of fertility and creating embryos at a later stage. Oocyte cryopreservation also provides a reasonable option in situations where a husband is unable to give a semen sample, due to an unexpected problem or a failure in yielding sperms during testicular biopsy on the day of oocyte retrieval. A novel indication for oocyte cryopreservation is for women with poor ovarian response. Oocyte pooling and egg banking is a practical option in these women, wherein multiple stimulation cycles are done. All the collected oocytes are thawed together and intracytoplasmic sperm injection (ICSI) is performed creating embryos, hence mimicking a similar situation to a normal responder. It also facilitates performing preimplantation genetic screening (PGS) as there are large a number of embryos. A recent indication is being developed for transgender people, who wish to undergo a sex change from female to male. There are some legal/ethical reasons as well for oocyte freezing. For example, in countries like Italy, as embryo freezing is not yet permitted. Oocyte freezing provides a good option and can be used later.

■ TECHNIQUES OF OOCYTE FREEZING

Cryopreservation refers to the cooling of cells and tissues in live condition at such low temperature, that the entire cell metabolism comes to a standstill. Two techniques commonly used for cryopreservation are slow freezing and vitrification. Slow freezing method (equilibrium method) is freezing method, where extracellular ice formation drives cellular dehydration through an equilibrium process. Vitrification (nonequilibrium method), on the other hand, is a form of rapid cooling which utilizes very high concentrations of cryoprotectant that solidify without forming ice crystals.

The main problem related to slow freezing method noted was its low oocyte survival rate. Evidence showed that meiotic spindle apparatus may be damaged by intracellular ice formation during the freezing or thawing process.[3] However, modifications in the combination and composition of cryoprotectants in slow freeze protocols have improved the survival rate of frozen MII oocytes. The technique of vitrification as a method to cryopreserve oocytes has achieved remarkable success due to its multiple advantages like being rapid, simple, inexpensive, and higher oocyte survival and pregnancy rates. In humans, most studies suggest that post-thaw survival rates of vitrified oocytes are superior to those that have undergone slow-freeze protocols.[4]

A recent Cochrane review has also reported that vitrification was associated with an increased clinical pregnancy rate compared to slow freezing (RR 3.86, 95% CI 1.63–9.11, P = 0.002). The authors concluded that *oocyte vitrification* compared to slow freezing probably increases clinical pregnancy rates in women undergoing assisted reproduction.[5]

■ FACTORS AFFECTING SUCCESS RATE OF OOCYTE CRYOPRESERVATION

Several factors have been attributed to the success of oocyte cryopreservation. Factors can be age, cause of infertility, stimulation protocols, number of oocytes, cryopreservation methods (slow-freezing and vitrification), and devices (cryotop, cryoleaf, cryotip).[6] Age remains one of the most important determination factors of all the causes mentioned earlier. A recent meta-analysis reported live-birth success rates with cryopreserved oocytes show an age-related decline regardless of the freezing technique used, and an aged-based probability of live birth may be calculated for cryopreserved oocytes.[7] Another factor affecting the success is the available number of oocytes for freezing. Study by Rienzi et al. concluded that more than eight vitrified oocytes are required to improve the outcome and delivery rates.[8]

■ ADVANTAGES OF OOCYTE FREEZING

Several advantages related to this technique can be described as follows:
- It simplifies the oocyte donation program as it avoids the need of donor and recipient synchronization and thus avoids the inconvenience and cost
- It also helps in avoiding loss of surplus oocytes in countries, where embryo freezing is not permitted
- Most importantly it empowers women by giving them a way to preserve oocytes against the threat of age or disease and provides a better option for cancer patients than the still experimental ovarian tissue cryopreservation as it is not associated with the risk of reimplantation of malignant cells.

■ PROBLEMS RELATED WITH OOCYTE FREEZING

Despite its advantages, several concerns have been expressed with oocyte freezing. There is a concern related to damage of the meiotic spindle as well as cellular and subcellular alterations that may lead to chromosomal or other cellular anomalies. However, studies are reassuring in this regard. Cobo et al.[9] showed no increase in numerical chromosomal abnormalities in embryos derived from oocytes slow-frozen compared with non-frozen controls.

As stated in the ASRM–SART guideline, "there is not yet sufficient statistics to recommend oocyte cryopreservation for the solitary purpose of circumventing reproductive aging in women because there is no data to support the efficacy, safety, ethics, emotional risks, and cost-effectiveness associated with oocyte cryopreservation for this indication".[10] There is a need for long-term studies on congenital anomalies and health risk associated with egg freezing.

There is also a theoretical concern related to infectious disease due to the use of open vitrification methods. However, infectious transmission has never been observed in reproductive tissues from this technique.[11]

CONCLUSION

Women putting their "eggs on ice" have made several headlines. A recent review in 2016 summarized the history, indications, techniques, and outcome of this technique. It stresses on "the real need to monitor what is being done, and the success rates achieved."[12] It also points out that there is still a need to obtain quantitative as well as qualitative information.

Oocyte cryopreservation has provided high pregnancy and implantation rates, and thus can be considered as an efficient treatment procedure in ART. It has expanded its role from fertility preservation in cancer patients to several nonmedical indications including women with risk of reduced reproductive capacity owing to age-related fertility decline. Further improvements in the form of vitrification technique with successful clinical outcomes are likely to result in an increased utilization of oocyte cryopreservation in clinical practice.

REFERENCES

1. Homburg R, van der Veen F, Silber SJ. Oocyte vitrification--women's emancipation set in stone. Fertil Steril. 2009;91(4 Suppl):1319-20.
2. Chen C. Pregnancy after human oocyte cryopreservation. Lancet. 1986;1:884-6.
3. Bromfield JJ, Coticchio G, Hutt K, et al. Meiotic spindle dynamics in human oocytes following slow-cooling cryopreservation. Hum Reprod. 2009;24:2114-23.
4. Smith GD, Serafini PC, Fioravanti J, et al. Prospective randomized comparison of human oocyte cryopreservation with slow-rate freezing or vitrification. Fertil Steril. 2010;94:2088-95.
5. Glujovsky D, Riestra B, Sueldo C, et al. Vitrification versus slow freezing for women undergoing oocyte cryopreservation. Cochrane Database Syst Rev. 2014;9:CD010047.
6. Cil AP, Seli E. Current trends and progress in clinical applications of oocyte cryopreservation. Curr Opin Obstet Gynecol. 2013;25(3):247-54.
7. Cil AP, Oktay K. Age-based success rates after elective oocyte cryopreservation (EOC): a pooled analysis of 2281 thaw cycles. Fertil Steril. 2011;96(Suppl):S211.
8. Rienzi L, Cobo A, Paffoni A, et al. Consistent and predictable delivery rates after oocyte vitrification: an observational longitudinal cohort multicentric study. Hum Reprod. 2012;27(6):1606-12.

9. Cobo A, Remohí J, Chang CC, et al. Oocyte cryopreservation for donor egg banking. Reprod Biomed Online. 2011;23(3):341-6.
10. Practice Committee of American Society for Reproductive Medicine, Society for Assisted Reproductive Technology Mature oocyte cryopreservation: a guideline. Fertil Steril. 2013;99:37-43.
11. Cobo A, Kuwayama M, Pérez S, et al. Comparison of concomitant outcome achieved with fresh and cryopreserved donor oocytes vitrified by the Cryotop method. Fertil Steril. 2008;89(6):1657-64.
12. Argyle CE, Harper JC, Davies MC. Oocyte cryopreservation: where are we now? Hum Reprod Update. 2016;22(4):440-9.

CHAPTER 29

Embryo Cryopreservation

Hrishikesh D Pai

■ INTRODUCTION

The greatest dream of human mankind is to freeze the life or stay young forever. For some women, childbirth takes a backseat to the pursuit of career, educational or personal goals. For others, in spite of many attempts, unfortunately they are not able to conceive naturally. However, their biological clock keeps on ticking. As the age advances, eggs become older, and their quality diminish. Here comes the need for oocyte or embryo cryopreservation.

Cryopreservation of embryos is the process of preserving an embryo at subzero temperatures, generally at an embryogenesis stage corresponding to preimplantation, that is, from fertilization to the blastocyst stage.[1]

■ HISTORY

Successful freezing of gametes has a track record of more than 60 years. In 1972, Whittingham and coworkers cryopreserved mouse morulae at –196°C in liquid nitrogen followed by a birth of live baby mice. First pregnancy in a human being from a cryopreserved human embryo was reported by Trounson and Mohr in 1983 (although the fetus spontaneously aborted at 10 weeks of gestation). The first term pregnancy resulting in twins live birth was reported by Zeilmaker and colleagues, derived from a frozen embryo, was born in 1984.

With approximately half a million babies born following cryopreservation, this technology has become a well-established procedure that allows a wide expansion of therapeutic strategies when in vitro fertilization is used to treat infertility.

■ INDICATIONS

- Currently, controlled ovulation hyperstimulation protocols, gives human embryos in excess of those needed for fresh transfer. Cryopreservation of the surplus embryos is done in order to decrease risk of multiple pregnancy.
- Postponing the embryo transfer in cases where risk of ovarian hyperstimulation syndrome becomes apparent after oocyte retrieval.

- Postponing the embryo transfer in special cases of poor endometrium or presence of endometrial pathology such as polyp. Embryos can be transferred after rectification of the pathology.
- In oocyte donation or embryo donation cycle synchronization of donor and recipient's cycle is not required with the help of cryopreservation techniques.
- Embryos can be made available for preimplantation genetic screening and can be transferred as per the results.
- In poor responders, it helps in embryo pooling which increases the cumulative pregnancy rate in a female.
- Embryo or oocyte freezing could be done to preserve reproductive potential of a female prior to radiotherapy, chemotherapy or ovariotomy.
- Lastly, if embryos cannot be transferred during fresh cycle due to any medical or technical reasons, they can be cryopreserved and transferred later.

■ TECHNIQUES OF EMBRYO FREEZING

The most important goals for freezing of embryos at –196°C in liquid nitrogen are:
- Arrest of cellular metabolism while maintaining genetic and structural integrity
- Achieve acceptable post-thawing cell survival.
- Technique or protocol must be reliable and consistent.

The two known techniques for embryo freezing are slow freezing and vitrification.

Both methods follow the six basic steps:
1. Initial exposure to cryoprotectant
2. Cooling (rapid/slow) to subzero temperature
3. Low temperature storage
4. Thawing or warming
5. Dilution and removal of the cryoprotectant
6. Return to physiological environment.

The principle behind "slow-freezing method" is extracellular ice formation which drives cellular dehydration by an equilibrium process. The temperature is decreased in a controlled fashion and ice formation (seeding) is introduced around a temperature of –6°C or –7°C and temperature is then decreased further until all biological activity is stopped. Starting temperatures are different for different stages of embryo. It relies on low initial cryoprotectant concentrations. Today, slow-freezing method still has the longest track record and greater "comfort level" among the embryologists.

In contrast "vitrification" is a nonequilibrium cooling method. It utilizes high concentrations of cryoprotectants that solidify to form glass without forming ice crystals. Improvements have been made by using less toxic and more permeable cryoprotectants and by increasing the cooling or warming rates which protect against ice crystal formation. This can be achieved by using novel cryovessels that allow direct contact between liquid nitrogen and the oocyte-containing solution.

Vitrification has shown its popularity in embryo freezing due to its superiority over slow-freezing technology in the form of better survival rate and post-thaw embryonic development in vitro. These results may be due to the fact that vitrification incurs less damage to chromosomal alignment and spindle integrity. With better understanding of biological and physical principles of vitrification, it has led to myriad successful clinical applications in the assisted reproduction technology.

Two important parameters that determine the success of all cryopreservation protocols are:
1. Rate of cells regaining equilibrium in response to cooling
2. Speed of freezing.

Cryoinjury can happen from formation of extracellular or intracellular ice crystals, solution effect injury, osmotic injury, chemical toxicity, and fracture damage. Cryoinjury is dependent upon size and shape of cells, membrane permeability, water content, embryo quality, and stage of development.

■ CRYOPROTECTANTS

Various cryoprotectants used for embryo freezing are:
- Glycerol
- Dimethyl sulfoxide (DMSO)
- Propanediol (PROH)
- Ethylene glycol (EG)
- Nonpermeating compounds.

Monosaccharides like galactose, disaccharides like sucrose and trehalose, polysaccharides like dextran, polymers like polyvinylpyrrolidone and polyvinyl alcohol, and protein like apoprotein.

Cryoprotectant toxicity has been considered as a single most limiting factor for the development of successful cryopreservation protocols. This is particularly true for vitrification that requires initial high concentration of cryoprotectants. For cryopreservation of human embryos, cells are usually exposed to a mixture of both penetrating and nonpenetrating cryoprotectants. The penetrating cryoprotective agents (CPAs) establish equilibrium between the extracellular and intracellular environment and replace intracellular water while the nonpenetrating CPAs cause dehydration through osmosis.

■ EMBRYO VITRIFICATION PROTOCOL

Materials
- Equilibration solution (ES) – HEPES buffered TCM 199 medium + 7.5% (v/v) EG + 7.5% DMSO + 20% SSS

Embryo Cryopreservation

- Vitrification solution (VS) – HEPES buffered TCM 199 medium + 15% (V/V) EG + 15% DMSO + 0.5 M sucrose + 20% SSS
- Wash solution (WS) – HEPES buffered TCM 199 medium + 20% SSS
- Thawing solution (TS) – HEPS buffered TCM 199 medium +1.0 M sucrose + 20% SSS
- Dilution solution (DS) – HEPES buffered TCM 199 medium + 0.5 M sucrose + 20% SSS

Procedure

1. All solutions should be warmed at room temperature. All the solutions should be mixed properly and they should be homogeneous.
2. A culture dish should be prepared with patient identification of 20 μL placements. Also cryotip or cryotop should be labeled with patient identification.
3. Dispense 20 μL drop equilibrium solution inside the culture dish.
4. Select embryo or blastocyst for vitrification. Using a pipette and the least amount of media transfer embryos from culture media to ES drop. The embryos shrink and sink to the bottom of the drop. They will however gradually return to their original size. Embryos are left in ES for 5–15 minutes or until they re-expand to their original size (average 12 minutes).
5. Transfer embryos from ES to VS1 while observing embryos microscopically for 5 seconds.
6. Transfer embryos to VS2 for 5 seconds.
7. Transfer embryos to VS3 for 10 seconds.
8. Finally transfer the embryos to VS4 (Fig. 1).

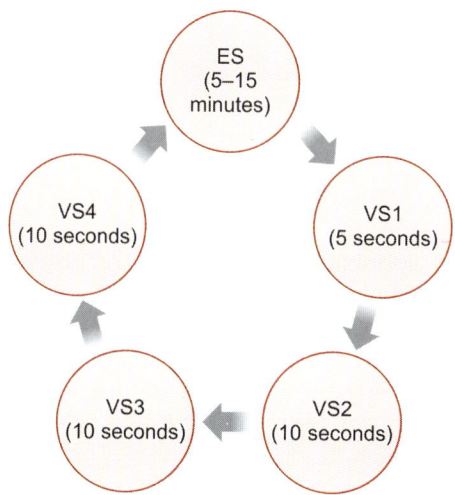

Fig. 1: Embryo vitrification protocol.
(ES: equilibration solution; VS: vitrification solution)

Thawing Protocol (Thawing from Cryotop)

1. All solutions should be warmed to room temperature 24–27°C.
2. Prepare the culture dish with patient identification.
3. The microscope stage is maintained at room temperature.
4. One center well dish with 1 mL thawing media is prepared and placed in the incubator at 37°C for some time before thawing.
5. Three more dishes are prepared with 1 mL each of DS and two with WS1 and WS2. These are kept at 27°C.
6. The cryotop with the patient embryos is located and placed in a container filled with liquid nitrogen next to the thawing stage.
7. The cover of the cryotop is removed under liquid nitrogen and held in the hand such that the tip is under the liquid nitrogen.
8. The thawing solution dish is removed from the incubator and placed on the stage. The cryotop is immediately removed from the liquid nitrogen and tip is plunged into thawing solution.
9. The embryos are located and after a minute they are transferred into the bottom of the dilution solution.
10. After 3 minutes embryos are transferred into the WS1.
11. After 5 minutes embryos are transferred into the WS2.
12. After 5 minutes embryos are transferred into the culture media dish and embryos are graded for recovery.
13. Embryos transfer is done after keeping for 2–3 hours in incubator inside the culture media dish.

DISCUSSION

New Carrier Tools Improving the Outcomes

The rate of cooling can be increased by using the smallest possible volume of cryoprotectant around the embryo and to create a direct contact (without any thermoinsulation layer) between the solution and the liquid nitrogen. Furthermore, when the carrier containing the vitrification solution is immersed in liquid nitrogen, the liquid nitrogen boils and forms a vapor coat around the carrier. The surrounding vapor coat blocks the temperature transfer and this result in reduction of cooling rates. To minimize it, sample size of embryos should be kept minimum.

Seemingly, the simplest and first method to accomplish vitrification was direct drop method. Unfortunately, this technique has disadvantage of using large amount of cryoprotectant and formation of vapor coat. Over a period of time various techniques have been introduced along with new carrier devices. To enumerate, electron microscopic grids, open pulled straw, glass micropipettes, cryoloop, minimum drop size method of Arav, and hemi-straw system were introduced.

Currently, the most commonly used carrier device is cryotop. This is an advanced version of minimum volume cooling technology. It consists of a thin plastic film attached to a handle covered with a cap. This system along with stepwise approach to equilibration and increasing cooling and warming rates has triggered an exponential increase of vitrification.

Concerns Regarding Transmission of Infectious Agents

Embryo freezing can lead to concerns regarding transmission of liquid nitrogen-based diseases. Firstly, semen and embryo collection and their processing are not totally sterile procedures and could be the main source of contamination. Apart from this infectious agent can be transferred via aseptic handling of straws, cryovials, containers, and other tools. To prevent this, aseptic conditions should be maintained in the laboratory. Closed system should always be preferred over open system.

Slow Freezing versus Vitrification

Valozerdi et al. compared the results of slow freezing versus vitrification in terms of survival, postsurvival embryo morphology, and pregnancy outcome in human cleaved embryos. Sample sizes for both the groups were 152 and 153. They found the survival rate of 82.8% vs. 96.9%, postwarm excellent morphology with all blastomeres intact 56.2% vs. 91.8% in slow freezing and vitrification group, respectively. The clinical pregnancy rate (40.5% vs. 21.4%) and the implantation rate (16.6% vs. 6.8%) were also higher in vitrification group.

Another study by Fasano et al. the two freezing methods in 1798 supernumerary embryos. They concluded that vitrification (Irvine and Vitrolife) are more efficient than slow-freezing methods (89.4% and 87.6% vs. 63.8%). However, there is no significant difference between implantation rates.

Several studies by Son WY et al., Keshkintepe et al., and Wilding MG et al. have also confirmed that vitrification is more efficient than slow freezing at different embryonic development stages.

A retrospective study by Basirat et al. on 1,014 intracytoplasmic sperm injection-embryo transfer (ICSI-ET) cycles found that clinical pregnancy rates are comparable and there were no significant differences between biochemical pregnancy rate [23% vs. 18.8%, odd ratio (OR) 1.301; 95% confidence interval (CI) = .95–1.774], gestational sac [95.6% vs. 100% in fresh embryo transfer (FET), OR 0.60; 95% CI 0.54–0.67], and fetal heart activity (87.2% versus 93.6% OR .46; 95% CI .16–1.32) in fresh ET and FET cycles.

Another study by Aflatoonian A on 200 FET and 500 ET cycles have found that FET has similar neonatal outcome in terms of prematurity, low birth weight, stillbirth, neonatal death, and major malformation compared with fresh ET.

Ethical Concerns

The long-term effects of freezing are unknown. Human embryo is being subjected to various injuries during the freezing process with unknown outcomes without being able to give consent for its own treatment. There is one more ethical concern about "orphan embryos". Some countries have come up with some legislation regarding their responsibility and disposal by the parents and the hospital.

■ CONCLUSION

Vitrification is a very promising cryopreservation method with many advantages and an ever-increasing clinical track record. Most important strategy to reduce the injury is to increase the speed of cooling or thermal conduction and to decrease the concentration of cryoprotectant. New carriers have been introduced such as cryotop as well as new medium such as hyaluronan has been introduced to increase cryosurvivability. With the increased use of vitrification technique more clinical data have been accrued regarding safety and efficacy of this method. In the future, standardization of protocols could be possible for different stages of embryos.

CHAPTER
30

Blastocyst Culture and Vitrification: A Step Ahead for Single Embryo Transfer

Vijay Mangoli, Ranjana Mangoli

■ INTRODUCTION

Today, after 4 decades, *in vitro fertilization* (IVF) in human has reached a stage where an impressive fertilization and cleavage rates, in the range of 70–90% can be achieved in most of the cases. Though take home baby rate in combined IVF cycles—without patient selection—remained in the range of 25–35%, large populations of young patients were many times compelled to carry multiple gestations. This situation was mainly on account of transferring more than one embryo with the sole intention of preventing IVF cycle failure. Many fertility experts support this decision citing examples of failed implantation even after transferring 3–4 embryos in multiple cycles.

Though there are many factors responsible for a successful implantation to occur, getting viable embryos for transfer is among most crucial requirements. However, it will be a gross mistake to consider embryo quality as the sole factor responsible for implantation. Uterine receptivity and compatibility has more crucial role to play in a successful implantation. Achache and Revel published an interesting observation in human reproduction update that inadequate uterine receptivity is responsible for approximately two-thirds of implantation failures, whereas the embryo itself is responsible for only one-third of these failures.[1] In IVF, we often experience it when sometimes best quality blastocysts do not implant, and sometimes grade II or even grade III embryos results in healthy babies.

In the above mentioned category of young patients, the only option to minimize multiple pregnancies is to select a single embryo with maximum probability of implantation.

From embryologist point, expecting him to select an implantable embryo among available lot is equivalent to asking him to point a female bird from a flock flying in the sky. Though scientists are trying hard to find a way to evaluate various aspects of embryogenesis that can be correlated to its implantation potential, as of now, there is no established characteristic to confirm it. It is logical to assume that those embryos which displayed consistent morphological normalcy from gamete stage to blastocyst may have better implantation potential. However, as mentioned earlier, unless such implantable embryo is transferred into equally competent uterus, we may not achieve viable pregnancy. Recent advances in the field of assisted reproductive technology (ART) like morphokinetic evaluation and chromosomal analysis supposed to help us in selecting most eligible embryo for transfer.

In IVF procedure, task of an embryologist is to convert maximum retrieved competent oocytes into implantable embryos. It is obvious that more natural environment we provide to the growing embryos in vitro, better will be their performance. It is still unclear whether only those embryos that reach blastocyst in vitro have potential to implant or early stage embryos if transferred in the uterine cavity before blastocyst stage, may acquire implanting ability due to more natural environment.

Dr Edwards had published first hatching human blastocyst in vitro in 1971, much before he and Dr Steptoe created first IVF baby.[2] So, they knew that it is possible to culture human embryos to blastocyst stage in vitro. They were also aware of the fact that it is more physiological to transfer a blastocyst than transferring early cleavage stage embryos. Still they transferred embryos from 2 PN to 4 cell stages during initial phase of IVF. The main reason behind this approach was uncertainty to retain optimum culture conditions to provide supportive microenvironment that can sustain embryonic growth till blastocyst stage. Due to limited availability of human gametes for experimentation, scientists have to depend upon research work carried out on rabbits and mouse for the formulation of culture media. IVF-embryo transfer (ET) in these animals and in cattle yielded a high pregnancy rate of up to 60% after transferring 4–6 stage embryos on day 2 or 3 postinsemination.[3]

Dr Patrick Steptoe and Dr RG Edwards adopted the same trend while treating humans.[4] For years, this pattern resulted in implantation rate restricted to around 15%. The vast difference in pregnancy rates between animals and humans made it clear that species specificity has a greater role to play in embryo culture system and also, the nutritional requirements of human embryos differ significantly among animals. In conventional culture media, comprising mainly of ions, energy substrates, vitamins, nucleic acid precursors, amino acids, and growth factors, a very small population of embryos manage to grow to late embryonic stages, remaining embryos developed fragmentations, blastomere irregularities, and slow growth rate. To avoid disappointment of obtaining unhealthy embryos for transfer beyond day 3 postinsemination, most centers preferred to do ET on day 2 or 3 at 4–6 cell stages.

Physiologically, in vivo, an embryo descends into the uterine cavity at morula stage and after developing into a hatched blastocyst, it starts communicating with the endometrium to initiate implantation. As in IVF procedure, the embryo is transferred into uterus through cervical canal and not from fallopian tube end, it appears more logical to transfer blastocyst stage rather than early cleavage ones. However, all the initial pregnancies of IVF era—including first IVF baby Louise Brown—have resulted from cleavage stage ETs.

Transferring embryos at blastocyst stages has some more advantages as well.
- It is observed that human embryos are more prone to development block at 6–8 cell stages when paternal genome is activated and begins its active participation in embryogenesis. If embryos are allowed to grow beyond this stage, it can be assumed that this block is bypassed
- It also gives sufficient time for "damaged" embryos after intracytoplasmic sperm injection (ICSI) or embryo biopsy to recover before transfer
- Some genetically defective embryos fail to progress beyond day 3 in vitro. So, selecting embryos after this stage eliminates possibility of transferring such embryos
- Even grade I blastocysts may be aneuploid. Embryo biopsy and counting total cell number will provide better selection criteria from given population of blastocysts
- In case if blastocysts have thick zona as a response to in vitro culture conditions, removing zona by enzymatic method further enhances interaction between trophectoderm (TE) and endometrium
- Growing embryos to blastocyst stage, particularly from frozen-thawed embryos provides a period for evaluation of viability of these embryos
- When single blastocyst is transferred, probability of multiple pregnancies is considerably reduced and restricted to mainly monozygotic twinning
- If blastocysts are transferred, the dialog between embryo and uterus begins much earlier than at earlier stage transfer.

Before switching over to blastocyst stage transfer, it is necessary to answer two questions—(1) Is it to improve current pregnancy rate, or (2) To reduce multiple pregnancy rates. If present pregnancy rate is unsatisfactory, then decision to switch over to blastocyst stage may be incorrect. First step would be either to improve cultural conditions or to adapt modified clinical management. Single blastocyst transfer policy, therefore, is adapted mainly to reduce multiple pregnancy rates.

CULTURE MEDIA FOR BLASTOCYST DEVELOPMENT

As more and more information was made available regarding the biochemistry of human follicular, tubal, and uterine environment during embryogenesis, another important aspect came forward that embryo's nutritional requirements changes as they travel from fimbria end of the fallopian tube to the uterus.[5]

Pursuing the aim of getting more blastocysts and largely influenced and impressed by veterinary results, Dr Bolton reported 40% blastocyst formation rate, using Earl's medium supplemented with pyruvate and 10% maternal serum.[6] But the resultant pregnancy rate after transferring these blastocysts remained at only 7%—too low to be considered by IVF community.

So, it was clear that it is not sufficient to just get blastocysts, but it is more important to get viable blastocysts.

On the basis of extensive animal embryology work, Dr David Gardner predicted in 90s—it would seem likely that the optimal development of embryos in vitro could well occur in not one but possibly two or more media, each one reflecting the embryo's requirements as development proceeds.[7]

And then started present era of sequential media where embryo's nutritional requirements are grossly divided into two stages—(1) Up to 6-8 cell stage and (2) Till blastocyst stage.

At present, we know two such major "shifts" in their requirements (Table 1).

Early cleavage embryos, up to 8-cell stage, need glucose in very trace amount and pyruvate in large quantity, whereas later stage embryos have opposite requirements. Early embryos require chelating agent ethylenediaminetetraacetic acid (EDTA) and antioxidant taurine. Late morula and blastocyst stage embryos need vitamin B, and essential as well as nonessential amino acids which acts as building blocks for demanding events of protein synthesis that begins after genomic activation which occurs at around 3 days postinsemination.

Since nutritional requirements of human embryos change day by day from one stage to another, it became essential to expose these embryos to sequential media, containing different nutrients according to their needs.[5]

Initially, a simple medium is used to fertilize the eggs (day 0 to day 1). Then the zygotes are transferred to complex medium (from day 1 to day 3) and then the growing embryos are nourished into a super complex medium (from day 3 to day 5/6).

There are reports of increased blastocyst formation rates using such sequential media.[8]

However, recent publications adapt policy of "let the embryo choose" by culturing them in a single complex medium throughout growth period in vivo citing equal pregnancy rates.[9]

When media based on this concept were marketed and used by many IVF centers all over the world, then there was a flow of publications as a response to blastocyst culture—some in favor of it, and some not so much in favor of it.

Table 1: Nutritional requirements during embryogenesis.

Ingredients	6–8 cell	Blastocyst
Glucose	Trace	++
Na pyruvate	++	+
Ethylenediaminetetraacetic acid (EDTA)	+	–
Vitamin B	–	+
Taurine	+	–
Arginine	–	+
Cystine	–	+
Leucine	–	+
Methionine	–	+

Those who were in favor of it claimed that:
- It is more physiological
- We will have better embryo selection as only competent embryos could reach to blastocyst stage in vitro
- This will increase predictive value of pregnancy
- The duration required starting communication between endometrium and the embryo is reduced considerably
- It will reduce multiple pregnancy rates, as less number of embryos will be transferred
- It is more suitable for preimplantation genetic diagnosis (PGD)/preimplantation genetic screening (PGS) and cryopreservation.

And those who had their doubts and reservations claim:
- This is applicable to only a group of selected patients
- The ET cancellation rate increases because of the "no blastocyst" situation in many cases
- There is increased incidences of "monozygotic twinning" particularly when blastocysts are transferred along with assisted hatching
- It is more feasible to select embryos at much earlier stage like pronuclei or 6–8 cell stage, thereby reducing embryo wastage
- There is no much difference in clinical pregnancy rates between D3 and D5 transfers in nonselected group, with large number of patients.

Whatever may be the option chosen, the fact is—when we do D2 or D3 transfer, we assume that the uterine environment is good enough to take care of these embryos to reach them to blastocyst stage, and when we opt for blastocyst stage transfer, we assume that our cultural conditions are optimum whereas in the heart of hearts we know that both assumptions can be questioned.[10]

In early 80s, when culture conditions were not suitable for acceptable blastocyst rate, Edward and Beard demonstrated that there is a positive correlation between embryonic assessment based on pronuclear orientation and increase in pregnancy rate followed by day 2 or day 3 transfer, hence there is no need for extended culture.[11] This can be challenged by the fact that these observations are made prior to paternal genome activation and thus predict only oocyte quality.

■ MORPHOLOGICAL ASSESSMENT OF BLASTOCYST

Presently, most commonly used noninvasive method of assessment of blastocysts is their morphological evaluation.

Blastocysts can be graded on the basis of four criteria:

1. Its degree of expansion. A fully expanded blastocyst has a diameter of around 200 μm and zona thickness of only 4–5 μm as compared to 120 μm and 12–15 μm of cleavage stage embryos.

2. The cavity size. The blastocoel occupies almost 100% volume. This cavity, which is formed by the coalescence of intercellular spaces and fluid accumulation, enlarges, pushing the zona outward making it thinner and thinner.
3. Trophectoderm composition. It has cohesive layer of many cells having sickle-shaped appearance with clear outline, and
4. Inner cell mass (ICM), which should be well-defined, should occupy around 25% volume of the cavity with many cells tightly packed in it. It is this ICM, which is going to be the offspring, so much depends upon the healthiness of this structure. If a blastocyst splits into two ICMs during hatching, it may result in monozygotic twinning. If it has no ICM or very poorly developed one, it may result in blighted ovum showing an empty sac without any heart beats in it.
5. There are variations in morphology of blastocysts (Figs. 1 to 3).

Over the period, there are many alternatives suggested and introduced in IVF that include—continuous morphological study, using time-lapse imaging, biochemical analysis of follicular fluid, proteomics study involving

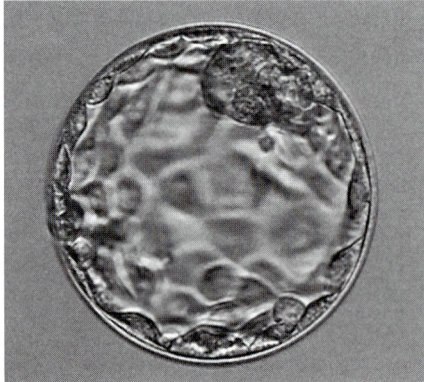

Fig. 1: Grade I blastocyst. Full expansion, defined compacted cells in inner cell mass (ICM), and many trophectoderm cells with sickle cell appearance.

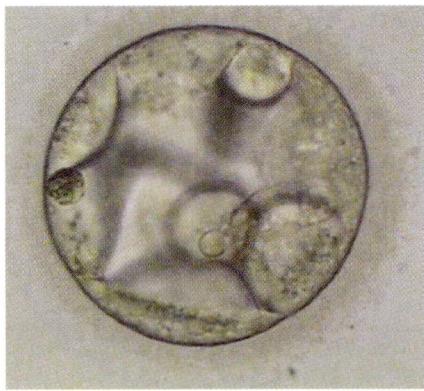

Fig. 2: Grade II blastocyst having multicavities. No defined inner cell mass (ICM).

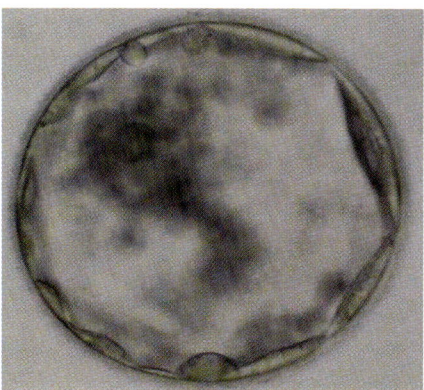

Fig. 3: Grade II blastocyst with unhealthy ICM and TE. (ICM: inner cell mass; TE: trophectoderm)

pyruvate and lactate uptake during embryogenesis, chromosomal analysis of blastomeres or TE for aneuploidy, and known genetic abnormality. However, these evaluating techniques also have flaws. Time-lapse machines can select embryos with consistent optimum growth pattern and suggest them as implantable embryos but they cannot give verdict to discard rest embryos with suboptimum growth pattern as unsuitable for transfer. Biochemical analysis and omics studies are too cumbersome and nonpractical to be incorporated for routine IVF protocols. Regarding PGS, there are papers published reporting births of "normal" babies born after transferring certified aneuploid embryos, when no other option was available and patient gave consent.[12,13]

■ EFFECT OF BLASTOCYST CULTURE ON PREGNANCY RATE

Though number of blastocyst formation per oocytes retrieved increased significantly with current advances, it is interesting to know the effect on qualitative enhancement of blastocysts on actual pregnancy rate.

To confirm the advantage of blastocyst stage transfer, it is necessary to design a randomized trial with patients of same age group, same indication, and same stimulation protocol.

There seems an advantage of blastocyst stage transfer over cleavage stage in fresh cycles, however, same is not applicable to frozen ETs. The American Society for Reproductive Medicine and the 2013 fertility guidelines published by the National Institute for Health and Care Excellence (NICE) have both voiced concern over the use of the blastocyst transfer method for assisted reproduction.[14,15]

Furthermore, the distinct advantage of reducing multiple pregnancies keeping overall pregnancy rate at the higher end will be confirmed only if transfer of single blastocyst results in similar pregnancy rates.

High order monozygotic twinning is common in ETs after assisted hatching at blastocyst stage.[16]

Another very crucial consideration as far as total pregnancy rate is concerned, is taking into account number of gestations resulted after using frozen-thawed cleaved embryos and blastocysts, because for patient it is more important to get highest possibility of cumulative pregnancy rate irrespective of stage at which embryos are transferred. In this regard number of cleaved embryos available for freezing greatly surpasses that of blastocysts out of a given population of zygotes resulted after IVF treatment.

■ BLASTOCYST CRYOPRESERVATION THROUGH VITRIFICATION

In past 10 years, vitrification has changes ART scenario. Comparison between slow cooling and vitrification shows that pregnancy rate postcryopreservation improved from 15% to more than 50%.[17,18]

Main reason for poor survival and viability of blastocysts using slow cooling method was inability to replace high water content effectively with cryoprotectants (CPs) and that of avoiding intra and extracellular ice crystal formation. With development of vitrification, these flaws were effectively bypassed to obtain near 100% survival. Vitrification is so effective that embryos can be repeatedly cryopreserved without compromising viability. This is useful particularly when blastocyst is to be biopsied to rule out aneuploidy or to avoid known genetic disorder.

In poor responders, concept of "pooled IVF"—where collecting four grade I embryos to get least two blastocysts has resulted in significantly improved clinical pregnancy rates.

Vitrification of Blastocyst: Technical Aspects

Though appear simple, it is necessary to perform vitrification using correct CPs, suitable device, and scientific protocol. Blastocyst being a unique entity needs special attention to get optimum outcome. Though the basic principle of vitrification remains same—to dehydrate cell and supercool it using very high cooling rate to avoid crystallization, the protocol must be modified according to cell type, size, membrane structure, and its surface: volume ratio. Among different stages of early embryogenesis, blastocyst has maximum water content hence it should be exposed to permeating CPs like propanediol along with combination of extracellular CP like sucrose or trehalose in a stepwise manner to allow it to complete dehydration and regaining of its original volume before exposing to ultra-high cooling rate in the range of 20,000–25,000°C/min. If performed under optimum conditions, blastocyst vitrification significantly increases cumulative pregnancy rate per embryo transferred thereby reducing multiple pregnancy rates considerably in prone patients (Figs. 4 and 5).

A practical protocol involving combination of morphokinetics, biochemistry, omics, and chromosomal analysis is required to select blastocyst with maximum probability of implantation to reduce multiple gestations without compromising pregnancy outcome.

Blastocyst Culture and Vitrification: A Step Ahead for Single ET

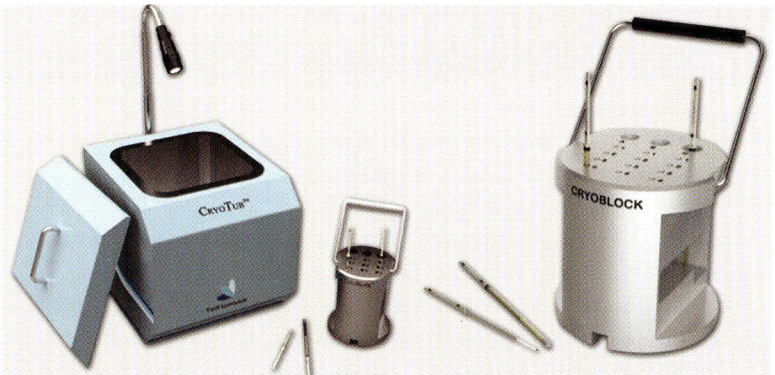

Fig. 4: Scientific device like VitriMate™ gives optimum vitrification outcome.

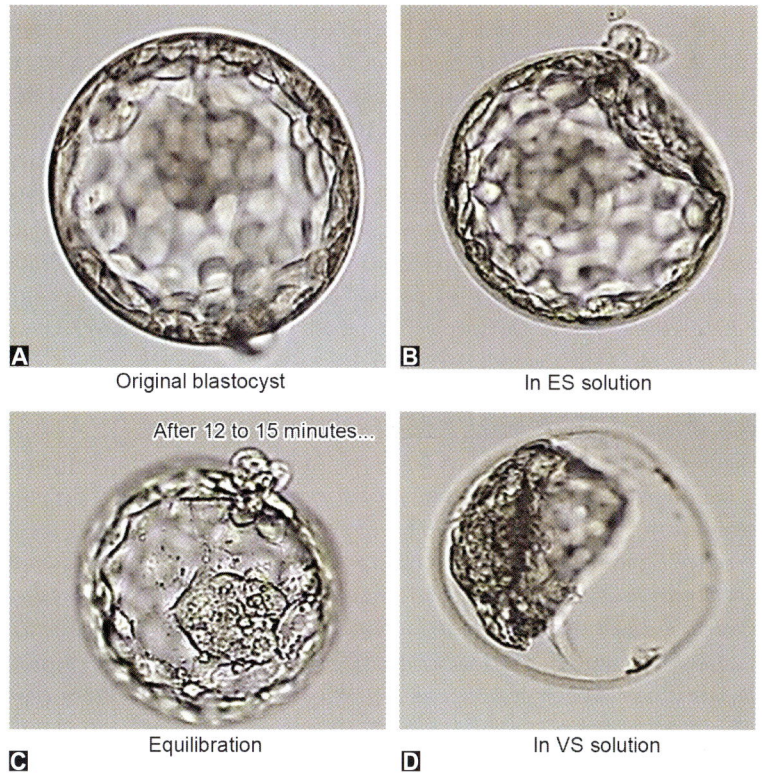

Figs. 5A to D: Stages of dehydration during blastocyst vitrification.

■ KEY POINT

In vitro fertilization (IVF) outcome, multiple pregnancies, embryo selection, blastocyst transfer, vitrification.

REFERENCES

1. Achache H, Revel A. Endometrial receptivity markers, the journey to successful embryo implantation. Hum Reprod Update. 2006;12:731-46.
2. Edwards RG, Surani MA. The primate blastocyst and its environment. Uppsala J Med Sci. 1978;22:39-50.
3. Hafez ES, Sugie T. J Animal Sci. 1963;22:31-5.
4. Steptoe PC, Edwards RG. Laparoscopic recovery of preovulatory human oocytes after priming of ovaries with gonadotrophins. Lancet. 1970;1:683-9.
5. Jones GM, Trounson AO, Gardner DK, et al. Evolution of a culture protocol for successful blastocyst development and pregnancy. Hum Reprod. 1998;13:169-77.
6. Bolton VN, Wren ME, Parsons JH. Pregnancies after in vitro fertilization and transfer of human blastocysts. Fertil Steril. 1991;55:830-2.
7. Gardner DK, Lane M, Calderon I, et al. Environment of the preimplantation human embryo in vivo: metabolite analysis of oviduct and uterine fluids and metabolism of cumulus cells. Fertil Steril. 1996;65:349-53.
8. Wale PL, Gardner DK. The effects of chemical and physical factors on mammalian embryo culture and their importance for the practice of assisted human reproduction. Hum Reprod Update. 2016;22:2-22.
9. Morbeck DE, Baumann NA, Oglesbee D. Composition of single-step media used for human embryo culture. Fertil Steril. 2017;107:1055-60.e1.
10. Mangoli V, Mangoli R. Assisted reproductive technology. In: Rao K (Ed). Principles and Practice of Assisted Reproductive Technology. New Delhi: Jaypee Brothers Medical Publishers (P) Ltd; 2014. pp. 1011-5.
11. Edwards RG, Beard HK. Oocyte polarity and cell determination in early mammalian embryos. Mol Hum Reprod. 1997;3:863-906.
12. Greco E, Minasi MG, Fiorentino F. Healthy babies after intrauterine transfer of mosaic aneuploid blastocysts. N Engl J Med. 2015;373:2089-90.
13. Coulam CB, Branch DW, Clark DA, et al. American Society for Reproductive Immunology report of the committee for establishing criteria for diagnosis of reproductive autoimmune syndrome. Am J Reprod Immunol. 1994;41:121-32.
14. Practice Committees of the American Society for Reproductive Medicine, the Society for Assisted Reproductive Technology. Blastocyst culture and transfer in clinical-assisted reproduction: a committee opinion. Fertil Steril. 2013;99:667-72.
15. National Institute for Health and Clinical Excellence (NICE). Fertility—assessment and treatment for people with fertility problems. London: RCOG Press; 2004.
16. Alikani M, Noyes N, Cohen J, et al. Monozygotic twinning in the human is associated with the zona pellucida architecture. Hum Reprod. 1994;9:1318-21.
17. Practice Committee of American Society for Reproductive Medicine. Smoking and infertility. Fertil Steril. 2008;90(5 Suppl):S254-9.
18. Mains L, Van Voorhis BJ. Optimizing the technique of embryo transfer. Fertil Steril. 2010;94(3):785-90.
19. Mangoli V. Assisted reproductive technology. In: Telang M (Ed). Atlas of Human Assisted Reproductive Technologies. New Delhi: Jaypee Brothers Medical Publishers (P) Ltd; 2007. pp. 151-8.

CHAPTER 31

Criteria to Select Oocytes and Embryos for Cryopreservation

Charulata Chatterjee

■ INTRODUCTION

Cryopreservation—the ability to freeze and thaw with retention of viability—provides flexibility in human infertility therapy when gametes or embryos are handled in vitro because frozen gametes or embryos can be stored indefinitely in liquid nitrogen (LN2) at –196°C.[1]

Successful cryopreservation of oocytes and embryos is essential to maximize the safety and efficacy of ovarian stimulation cycles in an in vitro fertilization (IVF) treatment, but also to enable fertility preservation.

■ CRYOPRESERVATION METHODS

Two cryopreservation methods are routinely used: (1) Slow freezing or (2) Vitrification.

Conventional slow freezing was the first system to be used for embryo cryopreservation. In this system, controlled cooling rates allow extracellular and intracellular water exchange without serious osmotic effects or changes in cell shape.

This technology has been used successfully to cryopreserve embryos of various species.[2] However, unsatisfactory results have been reported for cells more sensitive to chilling, such as oocytes of different species. This can be explained by the decrease in permeability of the cytoplasmic membranes of oocytes during chilling procedure.[3]

Conventional cryopreservation methods consist of several steps:

- *Preequilibration:* Embryos are exposed to a simple salt solution containing a permeable cryoprotectant [1,2-propanediol, dimethyl sulfoxide (DMSO), glycerol, ethylene glycol, etc.] and usually a low concentration of nonpermeable cryoprotectant (sucrose).
- *Cooling:* After a brief time of exposure to allow uptake of cryoprotectant and initial dehydration, the cells are cooled rapidly to a temperature slightly below the melting point of the solution (usually around 7°C).

- *Seeding:* At this point the container with the cells is supercooled in a process known as "seeding" so that ice forms in the extracellular solution.
- *Slow cooling:* Upon ice formation and further cooling at a slow rate (usually 1°C/min to below 30°C), the osmolarity of the extracellular solution increases as water freezes to ice, causing the cells to dehydrate with the increasing tonicity.
- *Plunging/vitrification:* Dehydration continues during slow-cooling until the cells are plunged into LN2, usually at a temperature below 30°C. At this point the intracellular cryoprotectant concentration is high enough so that the remaining intracellular water will vitrify, preventing intracellular ice formation (IIF).
- *Thawing and rehydration:* During thawing, the dehydrated cells are exposed to hypotonic conditions and rehydrate as the cryoprotectant is removed.

Vitrification

Vitrification allows the solidification of the cell(s) and of the extracellular milieu into a glass-like state without the formation of ice. Vitrification uses a high concentration of cryoprotectant and rapid cooling rates to solidify solutions.

Vitrification is a simple technology and it is potentially faster and less expensive than slow freezing. Moreover, it was shown to be more effective than slow freezing for material more sensitive to chilling. It is possible to obtain satisfactory survival rate of in vitro produced oocytes and embryos.

The measure of internal energy in a physical system is temperature. It is this internal energy that allows the molecules in fluids to tumble, twist, dissociate from one another, move from place to place in fluid, and chemically react with other molecules. On reducing the temperature, the energy to drive this molecular motion decreases. In systems such as pure water, temperature reduction below a certain point results in abrupt reorganization of the fluid into an organized solid lattice called crystal. This is referred to as freezing. However, in other systems, temperature reduction just causes more slowing of molecular motion, less molecular mobility, and lowering of chemical reaction rates until a critical temperature is reached below which the system almost completely loses its fluidity. This temperature is known as the "glass transition temperature", and the fluid becomes a "liquid solid" or more formally, a "glass" that is said to have "vitrified".

Success of vitrification depends on type of cryoprotectant, temperature of vitrification solution at exposure, duration exposure to the final cryoprotective agent (CPA) before plunging into liquid N_2, the type of device (influence vapor coat and cooling rate), and quality and developmental stage of embryo.

■ OOCYTE CRYOPRESERVATION

Oocyte cryopreservation has wider clinical implications.

Women who have no partner or are about to lose their ovarian function because of surgery, chemotherapy, or radiotherapy could store their oocytes for future use.[4] It also provides an alternative to embryo preservation to avoid ethical issues and legal restrictions.[5] For patients undergoing IVF, freezing the excess oocytes could avert repeated oocyte retrieval from the patients themselves or be a source for oocyte donation.[6] This is especially important in countries that authorize donation of oocytes, but not embryos, to infertile couples. Other common medical conditions for which oocyte cryopreservation is recommended are polycystic ovarian syndrome, ovarian hyperstimulation, premature menopause risk, poor response to ovarian stimulation, and severe symptomatic endometriosis in young women. In human, the first reported pregnancy from cryopreserved oocytes was reported in 1986.

Cryopreservation of human oocytes has been significantly improved by both the slow-freezing methods with increased sucrose concentration and new vitrification techniques.[7]

The slow-freezing method using a programmed cryomachine is traditionally employed for the cryopreservation of oocytes. These procedures usually take several hours.

Increasing the sucrose concentration in the slow freezing (from 0.1 M to 0.3 M) increased the rate of dehydration and the survival and fertilization rates of metaphase II (MII) oocytes in a dose-dependent manner.[8] Changing the temperature of the equilibration with CPA, ice nucleation (seeding), and plunging embryos into LN2, replacing sodium with choline (low sodium medium), or injecting sucrose directly into the cytoplasm of the oocyte all improved oocyte survival.[9] Oocytes analyzed immediately after thawing displayed severe disorganization or disappearance of the spindle after slow freezing,[10] hence vitrification is a choice of cryofreezing method. The other advantage of vitrification is it is a time-saving and does not require special equipment.[11]

The most widely used vitrification solution consists of a mixture of permeating [2.7 M ethylene glycol (EG) and 2.1 M DMSO] and nonpermeating CPA (0.5 M sucrose). New data obtained with the improved vitrification techniques (i.e. decreased volume of vitrification medium and very rapid cooling speed) show an increase in the post-thaw survival and fertilization rates of vitrified human oocytes which are comparable to the fresh control oocytes. Study on oocyte donation program confirms no detrimental effects of vitrification on subsequent fertilization, development, or implantation.[12]

Among cryopreservation of mature and immature oocytes, mature oocyte freezing is a favored strategy because of high survival rates post-thawing.

Generally oocyte freezing is done 2 hours after an oocyte pickup.

Safety of Oocytes Cryopreservation

Studies indicate that pregnancies and infants conceived after oocyte cryopreservation do not present with increased risk of adverse obstetric outcomes or congenital anomalies.[13]

No increase in the number of abnormal or stray chromosomes has been observed in the thawed oocytes.[14] In addition, no difference was found when comparing the incidence of chromosomal abnormalities in human embryos obtained from fresh and frozen oocytes.[15]

Criteria to Assess Human Oocyte Quality after Cryopreservation

It is well established that the oocyte MII spindle is extremely sensitive to lower temperatures, undergoing depolymerization just a few degrees below the optimal thermal conditions. PolScope is a valid tool to monitor MII spindle during and after the freezing–thawing process. Fluorescence and electron microscopy is another way to check ultrastructure and cortical granule structure. As in routine IVF laboratory it may not be possible in such case of fertilization rate, cleavage rate, embryo development, implantation, and pregnancy rate has to be closely monitored. As despite the promising results, there are still concerns regarding the possibility of chromosomal aneuploidies or other karyotypic abnormalities, organ malformations, or other developmental problems in offspring; therefore, to clarify this very important question.

■ EMBRYO CRYOPRESERVATION

Implantation is "rate-limiting step" and embryo-endometrium asynchrony in controlled ovarian hyperstimulation (COH) cycles impairs implantation and it has been suggested that the asynchrony problem in fresh cycles can be solved by cryopreservation of all embryos and transferring them subsequently in optimal conditions. The first pregnancy and live birth from frozen–thawed embryos was reported in Australia by Trounson and Mohr in 1982.[16]

Selection of embryos can be done on following basis:
Morphological analysis, based on time-lapse imaging and checking lipid composition, and genetic makeup of an embryo. In current practice most of the laboratory select embryos for freezing on morphology basis.

Embryo Selection for Cryofreezing Based on Morphology

Embryos of sufficient morphological quality resulting from assisted reproductive technology (ART) are cryopreserved at either cleavage stage (day 2 or day 3) or at blastocyst stage (day 5 or day 6).

The initial quality of embryos prior to cryopreservation is also a determining factor in their resistance to the freezing process. Embryos quality is rated according to criteria proposed by International Embryologist Society.[17]

For day 2 or 3 embryos grading is done based on blastomere size and equality, degree of fragments, and time frame of embryo development. Heavy fragments indicate chromosomal abnormalities, mosaicism, programmed cell death, and potential for apoptosis.

Early cleavage stage embryos are considered surviving freezing when they keep at least half of their initial blastomeres intact after thawing. The moderate loss of cells did not significantly influence implantation. In one study of over 300 single frozen embryo transfers of day 2 embryos at the 4-cell stage and the embryos lost only a single blastomere during freezing/thawing (25%) similar implantation equivalent with fully intact frozen embryos and also with fresh embryos was obtained.[18] Data obtained from another study with slow cooling that around 75–85% of all cryopreserved cleavage stage embryos survive freezing and that 50–60% of all thawed embryos will be totally preserved by their blastomeres.[19]

For blastocyst inner cell mass (ICM) and trophectoderm (TE) is analyzed.

Advantage of blastocyst freezing is that activation of the embryonic genome occurs after the 8-cell stage is reached. If the activation does not occur, the embryo will not survive further. Therefore, the improvement of human IVF outcomes requires identification of embryos that will progress beyond the 8-cell stage. Blastocyst culture allows for the transfer of embryos that clearly have an activated embryonic genome.

Additional advantages of blastocyst cryofreezing are: At this stage a lower numbers of embryos can be transferred in fresh cycles, hence multiple pregnancy can be avoided, cryopreserved blastocysts showing higher pregnancy rates, and implantation per thawed embryo transferred, blastocyst stage comprised of 50–150 cells, of which about 20–30% make up the ICM, the remainder making up the TE, the higher cell number allows better compensation for cryoinjuries, which results in greater viability and faster recovery. Reexpansion of frozen-thawed blastocysts in vitro is considered to be a very good sign of survival.

Embryo Selection for Cryofreezing Based on Time-lapse Imaging

Time-lapse imaging is an advance method to check embryo morphology. It is a close system which provides optimal conditions for developing embryos in controlled environment.[20] As analysis is done without bringing dish out of incubator, hence media pH, temperature fluctuation, and dish handling risk is minimized but it is an expensive technology.

Embryo Selection for Cryofreezing Based on Lipid Composition

Embryo biochemical information is not indicated in a morphological analysis. Lipid affects cryopresentation outcomes. Cytoplasm of oocyte and embryo differs between species and also embryos from the same cycle. Lipid is evaluated through lethal staining method. Specific gravity device (SGD) estimates lipid status of an embryo based on embryo density. It is an noninvasive method. Total lipid content remains constant up to morula stage and decreases at blastocyst stage.

Increase in lipid composition decreases chances of embryo survival post-thaw because it might aggravates cryoinjury and increase in free radical production.

Embryo Selection for Cryofreezing Based on Genetic Makeup

Genetic selection is done by preimplantation genetic screening (PGS) or preimplantation genetic diagnosis (PGD). PGS is to check euploid embryos whereas PGD is indicated for target-specific hereditary known genetic disease. PGS/PGD increases cost of fertility treatments and only those couple get befitted who are on higher risk of euploid embryos or known genetic disease. The invasive, expensive, and time-consuming nature of PGS/PGD creates a demand for an inexpensive, noninvasive, and quick technique predict genetic properties of embryo which can survive cryofreezing.

■ CRYOPRESERVATION OF OOCYTES VERSUS EMBRYOS

Regardless of the methodology used for cryopreservation, oocytes are much more difficult to cryopreserve than embryos. It may be due to following reasons.

Difference in Size

Because of the large surface area/volume ratio and low water permeability of oocytes, they may retain water when frozen, creating intracellular ice that is extremely damaging to cells and the permeability of the plasma membrane of oocytes and embryos varies among maturational/developmental stages.

Water Content

Oocytes contain more water than embryos and hence more prone to cryoinjury.

Single Cell versus Many Cells

Multicellular embryos can compensate for as much as a 50% loss of their cells as demonstrated by biopsies and live birth after loss of few cells post-thaw of embryos. The oocyte has no such ability and cannot regenerate from a serious cryoinjury.

Continuous research and change in methodology in oocyte freezing now it is considered as a routine part of an IVF laboratory with comparable success rate.

CONCLUSION

The introduction of vitrification over the last decade and its extensive application has improved human oocyte and embryo cryosurvival rates and clinical outcomes after replacement of embryos cryopreserved at different stages of development.

Cryopreservation allows for increased cumulative live-birth rates (LBRs) and offers the possibility to reduce multiple gestations and ovarian hyperstimulation syndrome (OHSS) risk.

Efficient cryopreservation program for oocytes and embryos enhances cumulative LBR per oocyte retrieval cycle, allows systematic application of elective single embryo transfer policy, provides the opportunity to perform cycle segmentation, extends time for embryo evaluation, permits fertility preservation for medical and nonmedical indications, and enables egg banking for donation and/or for oocyte accumulation.

To maximize embryo survival rate and to reduce cryoinjury every laboratory should follow standard operating procedure (SOP) and total quality management system (TQMS).

Take Home Message

- Cryopreservation is a valuable tool to combine a low risk for multiple pregnancies by single embryo transfer with higher cumulative chances to achieve a pregnancy.
- Whether this strategy will benefit from cryopreservation at zygote, early cleavage stage or blastocyst stage needs to be further assessed by studies on cumulative birth rate per oocyte collection.

KEY POINTS

- The methods to cryopreserve mammalian oocytes/embryos can be divided into two categories: (1) Slow freezing and (2) Vitrification. It is evident that vitrification is a viable approach for broad application of cryopreservation in many areas of ART.
- With a better understanding of the physical and biological principles of vitrification, we can achieve more success and higher efficiency.
- Maximizing the survival rate of oocytes/embryos subjected to freezing and thawing requires careful selection of less toxic CPAs, close monitoring of their temperature, time of exposure, concentration, and their stepwise addition and removal from cells.
- Selection of oocytes and embryos to be frozen should be done by prescribed criteria.
- Further studies are needed to ensure the safest and most expeditious development of oocyte/embryo cryopreservation technology and advance vitrification technology to achieve undamaged oocytes/embryos after cryopreservation.

REFERENCES

1. Whittingham DG, Leibo SP, Mazur P. Survival of mouse embryos frozen to −196° and −269°C. Science. 1972;178:411-4.
2. Fuller BJ, Paynter SJ. Cryopreservation of mammalian embryos. Methods Mol Biol. 2007;368:325-9.
3. Ruffing NA, Steponkus PL, Pitt RE, et al. Osmometric behaviour, hydraulic conductivity, and incidence of intracellular ice formation in bovine oocytes at different developmental stages. Cryobiology. 1993;30:562-80.
4. Porcu E, Venturoli S, Damiano G, et al. Healthy twins delivered after oocyte cryopreservation and bilateral ovariectomy for ovarian cancer. Reprod Biomed Online. 2008;17:265-7.
5. Parmegiani L, Cognigni GE, Bernardi S, et al. Freezing within 2 hours from oocyte retrieval increases the efficiency of human oocyte cryopreservation when using a slow freezing/rapid thawing protocol with high sucrose concentration. Hum Reprod. 2008;23:1771-7.
6. Li XH, Chen SU, Zhang X, et al. Cryopreserved oocytes of infertile couples undergoing assisted reproductive technology could be an important source of oocyte donation: a clinical report of successful pregnancies. Hum Reprod. 2005;20:3390-4.
7. Lucena E, Bernal DP, Lucena C, et al. Successful ongoing pregnancies after vitrification of oocytes. Fertil Steril. 2006;85:108-11.
8. Konc J, Kanyo K, Varga E, et al. Births resulting from oocyte cryopreservation using a slow freezing protocol with propanediol and sucrose. Syst Biol Reprod Med. 2008;54:205-10.
9. Stachecki J, Cohen J. An overview of oocyte cryopreservation. Reprod Biol Med Online. 2004;9:152-63.
10. Borini A, Levi Setti PE, Anserini P, et al. Multicenter observational study on slow-cooling oocyte cryopreservation: clinical outcome. Fertil Steril. 2010;94:1662-8.
11. Chian RC, Son WY, Huang JY, et al. High survival rates and pregnancies of human oocytes following vitrification: preliminary report. Fertil Steril. 2005;84:S36.
12. Cobo A, Meseguer M, Remohi J, et al. Use of cryobanked oocytes in an ovum donation programme: a prospective, randomized, controlled, clinical trial. Hum Reprod. 2010;25:2239-46.
13. Noyes N, Porcu E, Borini A. Over 900 oocyte cryopreservation babies born with no apparent increase in congenital anomalies. Reprod Biomed Online. 2009;18:769-76.
14. Gook DA, Osborn SM, Bourne H, et al. Fertilization of human oocytes following cryopreservation: normal karyotypes and absence of stray chromosomes. Hum Reprod. 1994;9:684-91.
15. Cobo A, Rubio C, Gerli S, et al. Use of fluorescence in situ hybridization to assess the chromosomal status of embryos obtained from cryopreserved oocytes. Fertil Steril. 2001;75:354-60.
16. Trounson A, Mohr L. Human pregnancy following cryopreservation, thawing and transfer of an eight-cell embryo. Nature. 1983;305:707-9.

17. Alpha Scientists in Reproductive Medicine and ESHRE Special Interest Group of Embryology. The Istanbul consensus workshop on embryo assessment: proceeding of an expert meeting. Hum Reprod. 2011;26:1270-83.
18. Edgar DH, Gook DA. How should the clinical efficiency of oocyte cryopreservation be measured? Reprod Biomed Online. 2007;14:430-5.
19. Edgar DH, Karani J, Gook DA. Increasing dehydration of human cleavage-stage embryos prior to slow cooling significantly increases cryosurvival. Reprod Biomed Online. 2009;19:521-5.
20. Cruz M, Blanca G, Garrido N, et al. Embryo quality, blastocyst and ongoing pregnancy rates in oocyte donation patients whose embryos were monitored by time-lapse imaging. J Assist Reprod Genet. 2011;28:569-73.

CHAPTER

32

Freeze-All Embryo Versus Freezing on Condition

Rajeev Agarwal, Saroj Agarwal

■ INTRODUCTION

Assisted reproductive technology (ART) has progressed over the last few years, both in terms of techniques and results. The evolution of successful cryopreservation techniques has led to improved pregnancy rates with frozen embryo transfer (FET) over the years.[1] Since vitrification has been introduced as a method for cryopreservation of gametes/embryo in ART it increased the efficacy of freeze-thawing method especially its post-thawing survival rate.

Vitrification method has been an efficient method in providing an excellent solution to postpone embryo transfer (ET) in natural cycles with adequate number and timing for challenges of ART such as polycystic ovarian syndrome (PCOS), advanced female age, low responders, repeated implantation failure (RIF), preimplantation genetic diagnosis/preimplantation genetic screening (PGD/PGS), multiple pregnancy, third-party reproduction, etc.[2]

The first baby born from frozen-thawed embryos was in Australia in 1984 and subsequently in USA in 1986. Due to the limitations of cryopreservation techniques, its low efficiency and low post-thawing survival rate of embryos, less than 1% of all cycles were FET at that time. An increase up to 30% was seen by the year 2004 and this rate has been growing not only due to its better success rate compared to fresh ET but also because of worldwide advocacy of elective single embryo transfer (eSET) over multiple ET. It is estimated now that more than 50% of the children born following ART are from frozen-thawing cycles.[3] An ART program needs an efficient cryopreservation technique for gametes, embryos, and reproductive tissues. It extends time for embryo evaluation, allows systematic application of eSET policy, enables egg banking for donation and/or for oocyte accumulation, permits fertility preservation for medical and nonmedical indications, enhances cumulative live-birth rate per oocyte retrieval cycle, and also provides the opportunity to perform cycle segmentation.[4]

Seeing the low success rate of fresh ET, Edwards and Steptoe discussed the negative effects of superphysiological levels of exogenous and endogenous hormones during ovarian stimulation on endometrium and its receptivity. Therefore, they suggested that freezing all embryos for subsequent transfers of thawed embryos is the best method.[4]

In spite of several advantages and strengths of freeze-all policy, it has some threats especially significantly increased rate of large-for-gestational age (LGA) babies in frozen cycles.[5]

As there are few randomized controlled trials (RCTs) in comparing freeze-all protocols with fresh ET, in different groups of infertile couples it is difficult to compare. The RCTs stated that the benefits of freeze-all strategy are likely for patients with good ovarian response while women with poor response had better results with fresh ET. Obstetric and perinatal outcomes regarding FET are controversial.[6]

In the freeze-all strategy, the entire cohort of embryos is cryopreserved (not just the *second best*), and the best embryos are transferred in a later one cycle into a more physiologic endometrium. In vitro fertilization (IVF) success depends not only on embryo quality, but also on endometrial receptivity and on the embryo-endometrium interaction, these modifications in uterine environment, found during controlled ovarian stimulation (COS), may jeopardize the IVF outcomes after fresh ET, when compared to FET. The deleterious effects of COS over the endometrium could be avoided, by performing delayed FET, and better outcomes could be expected.[7]

Therefore, we must ponder when and for whom is the freeze-all approach most appropriate. We need to think whether this approach represent an opportunity to provide a more physiologically natural environment for the embryo, if so then how can we balance this against the possible unnatural changes that we may be causing to the embryo as a result of freezing. Since, the health of ART born children during the whole length of life is important, caution should be taken in using freeze-all policy universally for all infertile couples. This chapter will go over the different milestones that have led to the establishment of the freeze-all concept, the critical review of published data, and the conclusion whether the shift should be reverted or not.

■ REASONS FOR GOING FOR AN ALL-FREEZE POLICY

Evolution of Better Embryo Freezing Technology

Embryo freezing technology has advanced greatly in recent years. Human embryos were successfully cryopreserved in 1984. Slow freezing has been the method of choice for decades for the cryopreservation of cleavage-stage embryos and blastocysts. Most IVF programs have changed the method of embryo freezing to a technique called "vitrification" over the past 5-6 years. This technique involves exposure of oocytes or embryos to high concentrations of cryoprotectants and ultra-rapid cooling rates causing an instant solidification (vitreous state) that avoids damages to the cell due to ice crystal formation it is here where the major advantage with respect to slow freezing relies. Vitrification has very little (if any) negative impact on the embryo. Given the excellent results provided by this technique, vitrification has become a fundamental tool for the management of our patients. Vitrification according to most studies has led to improved pregnancy and live-birth rates when compared to slow freezing.[8,9] Accumulation of oocytes through vitrification can benefit the low responders by allowing them to achieve similar clinical outcomes as normal responders.[10] Cryopreservation by vitrification or slow freezing when compared by a population-based cohort study in a large data set (over 30,000 cases between the two groups) revealed that transfer cycles with vitrified blastocyst resulted in a significantly higher live delivery rate [adjusted relative risk (ARR) 1.41, 95% confidence interval (CI) 1.34–1.49] compared with slow frozen blastocyst transfer cycles. The lack of information available on clinic-specific cryopreservation protocols and processes for slow freezing/thawing and vitrification/warming of blastocysts and the potential impact on outcome has been a major limitation of these studies.[11] Thus, introducing vitrification has been crucial, and it today represents an excellent tool when it comes to establishing freeze-all policies in our clinics.

Improvements in Stimulation Protocols: Ovarian Hyperstimulation Syndrome-free Clinics

The adverse effect on endometrial receptivity by ovarian stimulation has been cited to be the primary cause for better result with FET.[12] Superovulation may alter the window of implantation and cause advancement in development of endometrium.[13] Ubaldi et al. (1997) performed endometrial biopsies during a fresh cycle and evaluated the histological dating.[14] They reported that when the endometrial advancement was over 3 days, no pregnancy was achieved.

Labarta et al. (2011) and Van Vaerenbergh et al. (2009) found that patients that had endometrial advancement of more than 3 days did not get pregnant, and they correlated these histological findings with the gene expression profile.[15] It is thought that the immune environment and natural killer (NK) cell concentration are altered suggesting that hyperstimulation might be detrimental to implantation, by altering genes that are crucial for the endometrium-embryo interaction. However, all altered findings (histological and gene expression profile) were found in patients with normal to high ovarian response.[14,15] (Kolibianakis et al. 2002; Horcajadas et al. 2005)

Superovulation also causes a high progesterone (P) level at the time of human chorionic gonadotropin (hCG) trigger which is responsible for poor implantation rates, as it causes advancement in endometrial development.[16]

The rise in progesterone is not the only factor causing a lower pregnancy rate. A recent study showed a better pregnancy rate with "freeze-all" policy and FET in cases where progesterone levels were less than 1.5 ng/mL on the day of transfer. When fresh ET was compared with FET in this study, the implantation rate was 19.9% and 26.5%, clinical pregnancy rate was 35.9% and 46.4%, and ongoing pregnancy rate was 31.1% and 39.7%. This shows that even where progesterone levels are normal (P levels ≤1.5 mg/mL), endometrial receptivity may have been impaired by COS. This could also be because of other factors affecting endometrial receptivity, and development of fetus and placenta, leading to poor ongoing pregnancy rates. Besides the already significant reduction of the risk of ovarian hyperstimulation syndrome (OHSS) just by the using a gonadotropin-releasing hormone (GnRH) antagonist by itself,[17] these downregulation protocols allow the implementation of additional measures to further reduce the risk of OHSS, the most notable of which is the replacement of hCG for final oocyte maturation induction by a GnRH agonist.[18,19] This benefit is achieved without hindering the efficacy of the oocyte retrieval procedure when compared with hCG triggering, as shown by the similar yields in terms of oocyte maturation and embryonic development, namely in oocyte donation cycles.[20,21] However, the drastic luteolysis following GnRH agonist triggering is associated with an important luteal phase defect, presumably because of excessive negative steroid feedback resulting in suppressed pituitary luteinizing hormone (LH) release.[22,23] The use of an antagonist protocol followed by a "freeze-all" strategy and transfer of the embryo(s) in a subsequent frozen-thawed cycle seems to be a good option with high cumulative live-birth rates, mainly in patients with a high risk for OHSS.[24-26] This approach resulted in the genesis of the so-called "freeze-all" strategy with the segmentation of ovarian stimulation (using a GnRH antagonist protocol), ovulation triggering (with a GnRH agonist), the elective cryopreservation of all embryos (by vitrification), and a frozen-thawed ET in a subsequent natural or artificial cycle.[27]

Rise in Genetic Screening

Due to the application of PGS for aneuploidy by using array comparative genomic hybridization (aCGH) and next-generation sequencing (NGS) in human IVF, most embryos, especially blastocysts, are cryopreserved after biopsy for PGS. Embryo implantation can be further increased after PGS by transferring normal euploid embryos (Munne S et al. 2009). It is well-known that women of advanced maternal age have a high risk of producing aneuploid embryos, resulting in implantation failure, a higher risk of miscarriage, or birth defects.[11] It has been found that PGS especially benefits women with previous IVF failure(s), repeated miscarriages, and those of advanced maternal ages. Blastocyst biopsy for PGS is thought be to the most efficient approach as multiple cells are biopsied from trophectoderm (TE) cells, which provides more accurate results as compared to cleavage-stage embryo biopsy or polar body biopsy before and after egg fertilization.[28,29]

Preimplantation genetic screening is increasingly being used to improve implantation rates after IVF. Needless to say that a good vitrification program is mandatory and that the logistics of an IVF laboratory will change the more genetic screening we offer to our patients, not only due to biopsy process but due to significant increase in the percentage of patients being vitrified.

Concern on Perinatal and Obstetric Outcomes: Toward Safer Mothers and Offspring

There is a growing body of evidence that highlights concerns about perinatal and obstetric outcomes after ART, particularly following fresh transfers. There is no RCT studying effect of FET and fresh transfers on pregnancy and the baby. However, pooled data from various observational studies have been compiled into systemic reviews and meta-analysis. A recent review of 11 observational studies showed that singleton pregnancies after the transfer of frozen-thawed embryos were associated with better perinatal outcomes compared with those after fresh IVF embryos. Antepartum hemorrhage, preterm birth, small for gestational age, low birth weight (LBW), and perinatal mortality were lower in women who received frozen embryos. Authors concluded that pregnancies with FET had a better perinatal and obstetric outcome than fresh ET.[30]

A Scandinavian study that included three different countries[31] corroborated some of these findings, but also observed that frozen-thawed embryos were at higher risk of post-term birth [adjusted odds ratio (aOR) 1.40, 95% CI 1.27–1.55], LGA (aOR 1.45, 95% CI 1.27–1.64), macrosomia (aOR 1.58, 95% CI 1.39–1.80), and perinatal mortality (aOR 1.49, 95% CI 1.07–2.07), which was in line with other large population-based studies.[31,32]

Finally, this year, a report from a group in Brussels analyzed 1,072 singletons and twins born after embryo vitrification on day 3 and day 5 and concluded that neonatal health parameters, including the prevalence of congenital malformations, were similar to or slightly better than after fresh ET.[1] We could assume that elective FET with first choice embryos could yield even better results, but these studies are yet to be performed. Therefore, published data suggest that it is still unclear if perinatal and obstetric outcomes are better with FETs compared to fresh ones (Table 1).

■ CONCLUSION—CHANGE IN PRACTICE OR NOT?

A change in practice should be based on good evidence and sufficiently powered studies. As of today, the benefits of the freeze-all policy are based mainly on high responder patients, extrapolating these data to the general population should be done by caution. We are entering the era of individualized treatments in IVF, not only from a clinical point of view, but also from the laboratory technologies that we offer our patients, in addition, a fresh look at the new approach should always be able to foresee potential future hazards.[5]

Indications should be clearly specified (Box 1).

Indications for freeze-all, in our center are not only restricted to patients at risk of OHSS but also to any patient with a clear indication, patients with an altered endocrine and cardiovascular profile at the time of transfer (elevated progesterone, hypertension, etc.), patients seeking genetic screening, patients with inadequate uterine cavity for ET (i.e. fluid in cavity), and low responders

Table 1: Perinatal and obstetric outcomes of frozen embryo transfers.

Reduced risks in FET	Increased risks with FET	Unclear
LBW (<2,500 g)	Macrosomia (>4,500 g)	Ectopic pregnancy
SGA (<10%)	Large for GA	Preeclampsia
Placental abruption	Placenta accreta	Congenital abnormalities
Placenta previa	C-section delivery	NICU
Antepartum hemorrhage		VLBW (<1,500 g)
Perinatal mortality		VPTB (<32 weeks)

(FET: frozen embryo transfer; GA: gestational age; LBW: low birth weight; NICU: neonatal intensive care unit; SGA: small for gestational age; VLBW: very low birth weight; VPTB: very preterm birth)

Box 1 Special indications of freeze-all policy in in vitro fertilization patients.

- Ovarian hyperstimulation syndrome (OHSS)
- Low responders
- Genetic screening
- Zika virus (areas affected)
- Hypertension
- Inadequate uterine cavity
- Progesterone level is more than or equal to 1.5 ng/mL on the day of ovulation trigger

who seek a strategy to accumulate oocytes or embryos. Therefore, initiating treatment and freezing all the embryos represents a solution.

Although most obstetrical and perinatal outcomes seem to be better following a FET, other studies have reported that it may, on the other hand, also be associated with an increased incidence of LGA in singletons.[31,32] These results may be a subject for concern and warrant confirmation by larger registry analyses that account for known paternal confounding factors. Whether the potential risk of LGA in FET singletons compared with singletons born after fresh ET is related to the freezing/thawing procedure per se remains unknown, and efforts should be made to evaluate causal pathways between freezing and thawing of embryos and growth potential.

The importance of a good laboratory should be emphasized. Implementation of the freeze-all policy will not work unless high survival rates for oocytes and embryos are guaranteed. The applicability of elective vitrification of all embryos to the whole IVF population can only be a fact whenever good evidence from sufficiently powered studies becomes available, and when laboratories acquire optimal vitrification systems. However, a consensus is currently lacking in this aspect, and as a result, ART centers have developed their own freezing strategies based on their personal experiences and choices. This is a major drawback that limits our ability to effectively compare the different protocols available in order to evaluate the optimal timing for cryopreservation, the best selection criteria for embryo cryopreservation.[28] In this context, perhaps the introduction of automatic systems could help the standardization of results and make the implementation of freeze-all policies easier. It is necessary to assess if the potential effects of a freeze-all policy on perinatal outcomes justify the additional cost and extra workload of elective cryopreservation. A freeze-all policy can be met with considerable resistance from the patients point of view, although there is accumulating evidence to the contrary, patients frequently perceive FET as being inferior in terms of efficacy. Are we ready to handle their expectations?

Physicians play an important role as patient counselors and should adequately inform couples of the potential disadvantages of the temptation to always seek the instant gratification of a quick positive pregnancy test instead of opting for interventions associated with both safer and better long-term outcomes. Thus, for the freeze-all strategy to thrive in the near future, physicians cannot disregard the importance of their own. Therefore, more evidence is needed on the ramifications of freezing embryos. Future studies may confirm the advantages of FET or refuse these finding and support fresh ET. Therefore, clinicians should carefully decide before adopting freeze-all embryos as a beneficent policy for all patients.

Boundless questions still need to be answered to justify the future of the freeze-all policy, therefore, we need to relax and wait for more evidence, prior to shifting our current ART practice.

KEY POINTS

- Freezing-all embryos destined for transfer by avoiding fresh embryo transfer (ET) could improve the safety and effectiveness of IVF and intracytoplasmic sperm injection (ICSI).
- The available evidence does not justify a change in practice at present but strongly supports the need for a large multicenter, randomized trial to evaluate the clinical and cost-effectiveness as well as acceptability of elective cryopreservation versus fresh ET.
- A radical change in strategy will need to accommodate freezing, thawing, and replacement of embryos within the same financial package.
- Compared with slow frozen blastocysts, vitrified blastocysts resulted in significantly higher clinical pregnancy and live delivery rates with similar perinatal outcomes suggesting vitrification is the future of cryopreservation.
- Lastly, the applicability of elective vitrification of all embryos can only be a fact when good evidence from sufficiently powered studies becomes available, and when laboratories acquire optimal vitrification systems. However, a consensus is currently lacking in this aspect, and as a result, ART centers have developed their own freezing strategies based on their personal experiences and choices which is a big limitation.

REFERENCES

1. European IVF-Monitoring Consortium (EIM) for the European Society of Human Reproduction and Embryology (ESHRE), Calhaz-Jorge C, de Geyter C, et al. Assisted reproductive technology in Europe, 2012: results generated from European registers by ESHRE. Hum Reprod. 2016;31:1638-52.
2. Basile N, Garcia-Velasco JA. The state of "freeze-for-all" in human ARTs. J Assist Reprod Genet. 2016;33:1543-50.
3. Evans J, Hannan NJ, Edgell TA, et al. Fresh versus frozen embryo transfer: backing clinical decisions with scientific and clinical evidence. Hum Reprod Update. 2014;20:808-21.
4. Shapiro BS, Garner FC. Recurrent implantation failure is another indication for the freeze-all strategy. Fertil Steril. 2017;108:44.
5. Blockeel C, Drakopoulos P, Santos-Ribeiro S, et al. A fresh look at the freeze-all protocol: a SWOT analysis. Hum Reprod. 2016;31:491-7.
6. Ata B, Seli E. A universal freeze all strategy: why it is not warranted. Curr Opin Obstet Gynecol. 2017;29:136-45.
7. Shapiro BS, Daneshmand ST, Garner FC, et al. Evidence of impaired endometrial receptivity after ovarian stimulation for in vitro fertilization: a prospective randomized trial comparing fresh and frozen-thawed embryo transfer in normal responders. Fertil Steril. 2011;96:344-8.
8. Loutradi KE, Kolibianakis EM, Venetis CA, et al. Cryopreservation of human embryos by vitrification or slow freezing: a systematic review and meta-analysis. Fertil Steril. 2008;90:186-93.
9. Keskintepe YK, Sher G, Machnicka A, et al. Vitrification of human embryos subjected to blastomere biopsy for pre-implantation genetic screening produces higher survival and pregnancy rates than slow freezing. J Assist Reprod Genet. 2009;26:629-35.
10. Rienzi L, Cobo A, Paffoni A, et al. Consistent and predictable delivery rates after oocyte vitrification: an observational longitudinal cohort multicentric study. Hum Reprod. 2012;27:1606-12.
11. Li Z, Wang YA, Ledger W, et al. Clinical outcomes following cryopreservation of blastocysts by vitrification or slow freezing: a population-based cohort study. Hum Reprod. 2014;29:2794-801.
12. Roque M, Lattes K, Serra S, et al. Fresh embryo transfer versus frozen embryo transfer in in vitro fertilization cycles: a systematic review and meta-analysis. Fertil Steril. 2013;99:156-62.
13. Ghumman S. "Freeze all" protocol—has the debate concluded? Fertil Sci Res. 2015;2(2):90-4.
14. Ubaldi F, Bourgain C, Tournaye H, et al. Endometrial evaluation by aspiration biopsy on the day of oocyte retrieval in the embryo transfer cycles in patients with serum progesterone rise during the follicular phase. Fertil Steril. 1997;67:521-6.

15. Labarta E, Martínez-Conejero JA, Alamá P, et al. Endometrial receptivity is affected in women with high circulating progesterone levels at the end of the follicular phase: a functional genomics analysis. Hum Reprod. 2011;26:1813-25.
16. Venetis CA, Kolibianakis EM, Bosdou JK, et al. Progesterone elevation and probability of pregnancy after IVF: a systematic review and meta-analysis of over 60,000 cycles. Hum Reprod Update. 2013;19:433-57.
17. Al-Inany HG, Youssef MA, Aboulghar M, et al. Gonadotrophin-releasing hormone antagonists for assisted reproductive technology. Cochrane Database Syst Rev. 2011;5:CD001750.
18. Kolibianakis EM, Schultze-Mosgau A, Schroer A, et al. A lower ongoing pregnancy rate can be expected when GnRH agonist is used for triggering final oocyte maturation instead of HCG in patients undergoing IVF with GnRH antagonists. Hum Reprod. 2005;20:2887-92.
19. Kolibianakis EM, Tarlatzis B, Devroey P. GnRH antagonists in IVF. Reprod Biomed Online. 2005;10:705-12.
20. Acevedo B, Gomez-Palomares JL, Ricciarelli E, et al. Triggering ovulation with gonadotropin-releasing hormone agonists does not compromise embryo implantation rates. Fertil Steril. 2006;86:1682-7.
21. Galindo A, Bodri D, Guillen JJ, et al. Triggering with HCG or GnRH agonist in GnRH antagonist treated oocyte donation cycles: a randomized clinical trial. Gynecol Endocrinol. 2009;25:60-6.
22. Beckers NG, Macklon NS, Eijkemans MJ, et al. Nonsupplemented luteal phase characteristics after the administration of recombinant human chorionic gonadotropin, recombinant luteinizing hormone, or gonadotropin-releasing hormone (GnRH) agonist to induce final oocyte maturation in in vitro fertilization patients after ovarian stimulation with recombinant follicle-stimulating hormone and GnRH antagonist cotreatment. J Clin Endocrinol Metab. 2003;88:4186-92.
23. Casper RF. Introduction: gonadotropin-releasing hormone agonist triggering of final follicular maturation for in vitro fertilization. Fertil Steril. 2015;103:865-6.
24. Eldar-Geva T, Zylber-Haran E, Babayof R, et al. Similar outcome for cryopreserved embryo transfer following GnRH-antagonist/GnRH agonist, GnRH-antagonist/HCG or long protocol ovarian stimulation. Reprod Biomed Online. 2007;14:148-54.
25. Griesinger G, Berndt H, Schultz L, et al. Cumulative live birth rates after GnRH-agonist triggering of final oocyte maturation in patients at risk of OHSS: a prospective, clinical cohort study. Eur J Obstet Gynecol Reprod Biol. 2010;149: 190-4.
26. Griesinger G, Kolibianakis EM, Venetis C, et al. Oral contraceptive pretreatment significantly reduces ongoing pregnancy likelihood in gonadotropin-releasing hormone antagonist cycles: an updated meta-analysis. Fertil Steril. 2010;94:2382-4.
27. Devroey P, Polyzos NP, Blockeel C. An OHSS-free clinic by segmentation of IVF treatment. Hum Reprod. 2011;26:2593-7.
28. Groenewoud ER, Cantineau AE, Kollen BJ, et al. What is the optimal means of preparing the endometrium in frozen-thawed embryo transfer cycles? A systematic review and meta-analysis. Hum Reprod Update. 2013;19:458-70.

29. Scott BR. Intrapartum management of trial of labour after caesarean delivery: evidence and experience. BJOG. 2014;121:157-62.
30. Pandey S, Shetty A, Hamilton M, et al. Obstetric and perinatal outcomes in singleton pregnancies resulting from IVF/ICSI: a systematic review and meta-analysis. Hum Reprod Update. 2012;18:485-503.
31. Pinborg A, Wennerholm UB, Romundstad LB, et al. Why do singletons conceived after assisted reproduction technology have adverse perinatal outcome? Systematic review and meta-analysis. Hum Reprod Update. 2013;19:87-104.
32. Sazonova A, Kallen K, Thurin-Kjellberg A, et al. Obstetric outcome in singletons after in vitro fertilization with cryopreserved/thawed embryos. Hum Reprod. 2012;27:1343-50.

CHAPTER 33

Ovarian Tissue Freezing

Pankaj Talwar, Pooja Awasthi

■ INTRODUCTION

Advancement in cancer treatment (radiotherapy and chemotherapy) have increased survival rate of the cancer patients. Especially in case of the young cancer patient (survival of childhood cancer) it has been increased up to 90%, however, the adverse effect of anticancer treatment on the reproductive well-being of female patient remains the major focus for various clinicians and researchers.[1] Cancer treatment further impacts the ovarian reserve leading to premature ovarian failure (POF) and premature ovarian insufficiency (POI). (Table 1).[2,3]

Premature ovarian failure—often referred to as primary ovarian insufficiency; implies to the loss of the normal function of ovaries before the age of 40. Premature ovarian insufficiency (POI) is a remarkably heterogeneous gonadal disorder, having a vast spectrum of etiologies, including iatrogenic treatments (chemotherapy, radiotherapy, surgery), inflammatory, infectious, cytogenetic and genetic diseases.

Recently, various innovative technologies have been developed to provide hope of preserving the potential for biological parenthood in patients, in cases of diagnosis of benign, malignant, or genetic diseases where fertility is placed at risk.

The complexity of folliculogenesis along with the ensuing difficulties in oocyte cryopreservation explain why female fertility preservation persists at

Table 1: Number of female germ cells present at the different stages of life.[3]	
Age of the female	Number of oocytes
Fetal mid-gestation	6–7 million germ cells
At the time of birth	1–2 million germ cells
Onset of puberty	3,00,000 germ cells
37–38 years	25,000 follicles
At the time of menopause	1,000 follicles

the pioneering level even though sperm cryobanking has been available for several years.

Based on the age of the patient and the type of disease, the approaches toward fertility preservation vary greatly. Conservative fertility includes sparing treatments that represent the first step of preservation of female fertility. However, the efficiency of administering gonadotropin-releasing hormone (GnRH) agonists for the prevention chemotherapy-induced gonadotoxicity remains controversial. Thus, fertility preservation in most cases will imply more "active" strategies, derived from the assisted reproductive technologies. To deal with this iatrogenic infertility, various fertility preservation techniques like oophoropexy, assisted reproductive technology (ART), oocyte freezing, in vitro maturation (IVM) and follicle culture are available to the reproductive biologist. Ovarian tissue cryopreservation is a technique for preserving gonadal function for cancer patient of reproductive age and can overcome most of the limitations associated with other technologies.

Common alternatives for the preservation of female fertility include:

- Embryo[4]
- Oocyte[5]
- Ovarian tissue cryopreservation.[6]

CANCER TREATMENT AND ITS IMPACT ON OVARIES

Ovarian follicles are vulnerable to agents that lead to DNA damage, including ionizing radiation and chemotherapy, at any age. Such anticancer treatments lead to a reduction in the ovarian follicle reserve in a dose-dependent manner, and can eventually cause amenorrhea and premature ovarian failure.[7]

Alternatively, there could be the occurrence of partial ovarian injury, in which the reduction in primordial follicle stockpiles is manifested by infertility along with a shortened reproductive lifespan despite the resumption of menses following the treatment of cancer.[7] In such instances, the postcancer treatment markers of ovarian reserve [antral follicle count (AFC), follicle-stimulating hormone (FSH), anti-Mullerian hormone (AMH), inhibin B] can often resemble the levels similar to those seen in premenopausal women.[8]

Reproductive Damage due to Radiation

Patients who have cancer, who are scheduled to undergo abdominal, pelvic, and total body irradiation is at risk for infertility, shortened reproductive lifespan, and premature ovarian failure due to the loss of primordial follicles. Older women are at higher risk of ovarian failure as the degree of ovarian damage is determined by the total irradiation dose, location, fractionation schedule, and age at the time of treatment (Table 2).[9,10]

Table 2: Age-related effective sterilizing dose (ESD).[9,10]

Age	Effective sterilizing dose
At birth	20.3 Gy
At 10 years	18.4 Gy
At 20 years	16.5 Gy
At 30 years	14.3 Gy

Table 3: List of drugs used in chemotherapy.[17]

The high-risk chemotherapeutic drugs (Alkylating agents)	The low-risk chemotherapeutic drugs
Busulfan	Cytarabine
Cyclophosphamide (Cytoxan)	5-fluorouracil (5-FU)
Ifosfamide	Gemcitabine
Dacarbazine	Vincristine
Melphalan	Vinblastine
Carboplatin	Bleomycin
Cisplatin	Idarubicin
Chlorambucil	Daunorubicin
Melphalan	Methotrexate
Carmustine (BCNU)	Dactinomycin
Doxorubicin (Adriamycin)	Fludarabine

Reproductive Damage due to Chemotherapy

The severity of the damage to the woman's eggs or fertility by chemotherapy depends on the woman's age, the types of drugs and the drug doses.[7,11,12] Bone marrow or stem cell transplant involves high doses of chemo and sometimes radiation to the whole body before the transplant. In most cases, this permanently stops a woman's ovaries from releasing eggs (Table 3).

Cyclophosphamide is an alkylating agent, acts directly on DNA, crosslinking the N-7 guanine residue and causing DNA strand breaks, leading to abnormal base pairing. Inhibits the cell division and consequently leads to apoptosis. Exposure to cyclophosphamide in pediatric systemic lupus erythematosus is associated with reduced serum AMH.[13]

Anthracycline antibiotic (Doxorubicin) (DXR) is an intercalating agent that blocks DNA replication and leads to double-stranded (ds) DNA breaks; it also induces apoptosis in the stroma and the granulosa cells of growing follicles subsequently.[14,15] DXR is currently considered of low clinical risk for POI even though it has been shown to impact the follicle reserve experimentally.[15-17]

RECOMMENDED GUIDELINES FOR OVARIAN TISSUE BANKING[18]

1. Age of the patient should be under 37 years (may be individualized based on the status of ovarian reserve).
2. Ovarian function: Premenopausal by FSH, AFC or AMH.
3. The communication between the oncologists and patient must be transparent about cancer treatment plan and prognosis.
4. When embryo freezing or oocyte freezing is not indicated: Delaying cancer treatment is not acceptable, hormonal stimulation is not permitted, ART is not allowed
5. Prepubertal girls can also be privileged with the technique who do not have any other options.
6. High risk for POF (when significant loss of ovarian follicles is anticipated with cancer therapy).
7. Informed consent should be the must.
8. Informed consent from parents/guardians as well as informed assent from minors, if the patient is less than 18 years.
9. Patients should be physically and mentally healthy enough for surgery.
10. Patient should have the desires to have a child in the future (preferably before the age 50).
11. Thorough patient counseling is mandatory. Currently available fertility preservation options including embryo and oocyte cryopreservation, how to use cryobanked ovarian tissue for fertility restoration should be explained clearly.
12. Patient should understand the experimental nature and potential risks of cancer cell transmission.

INDICATIONS FOR OVARIAN CORTEX CRYOPRESERVATION

The treatment required for cancer (most of the types) occurring in younger women frequently involves removal of the reproductive organs or cytotoxic therapy that could affect reproductive function. This concern is also applicable to women who face gonadotoxic treatment due to other nonmalignant disorders (such as systemic lupus erythematosus). The possibility of long-term infertility after these types of procedures is a genuine threat, as shown recently by a prospective study assessing ovarian reserve in premenopausal women undergoing chemotherapy for breast cancer. In this series, Anderson et al. documented that both AFC and ovarian volume decreased with chemotherapy. They also showed a rapid fall in AMH and inhibin B concentrations during chemotherapy, although estradiol (E2) levels were maintained.[17]

Therefore, women diagnosed with these diseases during their reproductive period often have to consider not only the uncertainty of long-term survival but also the possible loss of fertility as a result of cancer treatment. In fact, there is ample evidence that females with cancer are highly interested in the topic of fertility preservation in their treatment regimens. Importantly, the reduced fecundity seen in older women is primarily related to the poor quality of aging oocytes and the decreasing number of oocytes (ovarian reserve).[2]

Oncological Medical Indication

Table 4 summarizes the most common oncological conditions requiring FP.[19,20]

Nononcological Medical Indications

FP options should also be discussed with adult and younger women and men affected by several nononcological medical conditions (Table 5).[19,20]

Table 4: Most common oncological conditions.[19,20]

Oncological medical indication	
Gynecological	Nongynecological
Breast cancer	Ewing's sarcoma
Vulvar carcinoma	Hodgkin's disease and non-Hodgkin's disease
Vaginal carcinoma	Leukemia
	Neuroblastoma
Cervical carcinoma	Bowel malignancy
	Wilms' tumor

Table 5: Most common nononcological conditions requiring FP.[19,20]

Nononcological medical indications	
Gynecological	Nongynecological
Uni/bilateral oophorectomy	Hematological diseases (Leukemia, aplastic anemia, sickle cell anemia, thalassemia major, aplastic anemia)
Risk of premature menopause	Behcet's disease
Benign ovarian tumor	Autoimmune disease • Systemic lupus erythematosus (SLE) • Behcet's disease • Granulomatosis with polyangiitis (formerly Wegener's granulomatosis) • Churg-Strauss syndrome (eosinophilic granulomatosis) • Steroid-resistant glomerulonephritis • Inflammatory bowel diseases • Rheumatoid arthritis • Pemphigus vulgaris
Severe endometriosis	Galactosemia
Mosaic Turner syndrome	Wegener's disease
BRCA-1, BRCA-2 mutations	Bone marrow transplantation

HISTORICAL BACKGROUND

In patients who have a high risk of ovarian failure after cancer treatment, ovarian tissue cryopreservation is an alternative strategy for FP. The studies of ovarian tissue cryopreservation and transplantation date back to 1950s. Although it is considered to be investigational by the American Society for Reproductive Medicine (ASRM), its apparent benefits have led to the increased use of this technology and promising results in recent years because of the ever-increasing research in the field of cryoprotectants and better cryofreezing equipment (Table 6).[21-29]

Table 6: Name of scientists and their respective studies.

Scientist name	Year	Scientific presentation
Leporrier et al.[21]	1987	Performed heterotrophic reimplantation of left ovary subcutaneously into the arm before the radiotherapy initiation in a Hodgkin's patient
Newton[22]	1996	Carried out studies showing primordial follicles and ovarian cortex could sustain cryofreeze procedure
Marconi et al.[23]	1997	Reported the accidental subcutaneous transplant of ovarian tissue was left in the subcutaneous area during laparoscopic resection of endometrioma
Oktay and Karilkaya[24]	2000	Performed the first orthotopic transplantation
Radford et al.[25]	2001	Reported ovarian cortical strips were grafted orthotopically in a 36-year-old patient who underwent right oophorectomy with cryopreservation of ovarian tissue prior to experiencing high-dose chemotherapy for a Hodgkin's lymphoma
Oktay et al.[26]	2004	Had performed heterotopic transplantation of fresh tissue to the forearm in two patients. He reported performing percutaneous oocyte aspiration with in vitro maturation and ICSI
Donnez[27]	2004	Published the first live birth in a patient with Hodgkin's lymphoma after autologous orthotopic transplantation from the frozen-thawed ovarian cortex. Ovarian cortex was cryopreserved before the gonadotoxic treatment
Hovatta[28]	2005	Validated that the human ovary is cryoresistant to the freeze-thaw protocol
Silber[29]	2007	Reported spontaneous pregnancy with live birth from transplantation of ovarian cortical graft in monozygotic twins was

OVARIAN TISSUE CRYOPRESERVATION TECHNIQUES

The viability of follicle and integrity of tissue compartments and cell-to-cell contacts must be ensured by the cryopreservation procedures.[28,30] Thus, studies investigating the most favorable cooling rates and dehydration times have been conducted. It is now well established that for obtaining satisfactory results, adequate penetration of cryoprotectant through the stroma and granulosa cells to the oocytes is required.[28] Choosing optimal freezing must minimize ice-crystal formation.

Collection of Ovarian Tissue

Tissue collection is best done during the early follicular phase to avoid large ovarian follicles/cyst or corpus luteum (Being hypervascular and space occupying, these cause anatomic distortion).

The tissues should be transported to the laboratory on ice, in a 4-(2-hydroxyethyl)-1-piperazineethane-sulfonic acid (HEPES)-buffered medium.

Ovarian tissue is collected by laparoscopy under general anesthesia. Electrocoagulation of the ovary can lead to primordial follicle loss of the remaining part of the ovary and is thus, avoided.

PREPARATION OF CRYOPROTECTANT

Dimethyl sulfoxide (DMSO), propanediol and ethylene glycol-based solutions are all equally effective for human ovarian tissue freezing. We do not add protein supplement due to its antigenicity.

Tables 7 and 8 encapsulate the preparation of the cryoprotectant requirements and preparation of ovarian tissue, respectively.

Histological Analysis

For every patient, one representative sample of the ovarian cortex, randomly chosen should be sent for histopathological examination. The specimens should be fixed in formaldehyde and embedded in paraffin.

5 μm sections are cut perpendicularly to the ovarian surface and stained with hematoxylin-eosin. All follicles are systematically counted. Serial sections are useful for follicle classification.

Table 7: Preparation of the cryoprotectant.

1. To DMSO 1.06 mL, sucrose 0.1 M solution 1 mL and patients serum 1 mL, add 6.94 mL of bicarbonate media to a final volume of 10 mL
2. This is then filter-sterilized through a 0.22 μm filter and cocktail is refrigerated
3. Pour 4 mL of cryoprotective solution in 60 mm dish and place it on the ice at least 30 minutes so that the solution is ice-cooled before the specimen is put in it for equilibration
4. Put 1 mL of the solution in cryovial and ice cool it

Table 8: Preparation of ovarian tissue for slow freezing.

1. After receiving the harvested tissue in the laboratory, the white tissue on the outer surface of the ovary should be removed as quickly and accurately as possible
2. Place the specimen in a dish containing HEPES media at 4°C temperature
3. Blade and forceps are used to separate the white, firm outer region from the underlying red tissue. It can be difficult to separate the two layers, but dissection can usually be achieved using a combination of sharp scissors, and surgical blades
4. White cortical tissue surrounding the ovary is smooth, elastic and tough and around 1 mm thick

FREEZING PROTOCOLS

Slow Freezing (Figs. 1 to 6)

Slow freezing has been the conventional method, despite reports of extensive loss of follicles and damage to stromal cells.[31]

Tables 9 to 11 summarize the equilibration procedure, cooling and seedling, and thawing procedures respectively.

The relatively poor survival of the ovarian stroma has been a concern of slow-programmed freezing.[32] This has been validated by transmission-electron microscopy, a method that precisely evaluates cryoinjury of membranes, mitochondria, and other organelles.[33]

Vitrification Technique (Figs. 7 to 13)

Cut the cortex tissue of each ovary into slices of 1 mm × 10 mm × 10 mm. The precise 1-mm tissue thickness is assured with a specially designed tissue slicer.

The tissue slicer is placed on the surface of the ovary. Then another plate is put over the tissue slicer, and the ovary is cut between the slicer and the surface

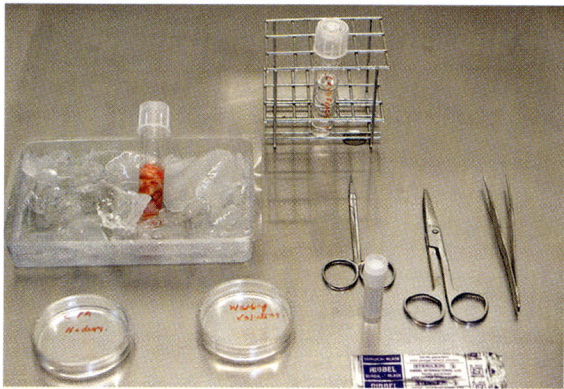

Fig. 1: The laboratory bench set up for slow freezing of ovarian cortex. Instruments, ovarian specimen and freezing cocktail have been kept ready. Note that the ovary has been kept on ice and freezing media consisting of DMSO and sucrose has been kept at room temperature.

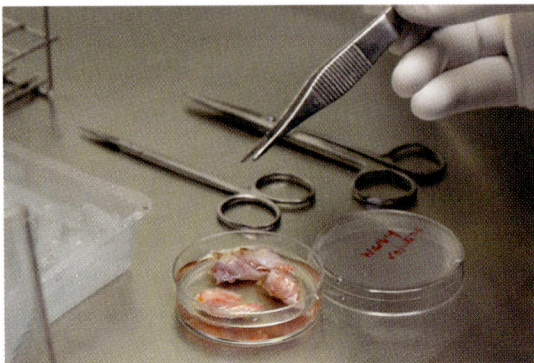

Fig. 2: Ovary specimen has been shifted to the 60 mm Falcon IVF plate containing HEPES buffered media at 4°C. Ovary has been bisected in two halves for easy handling.

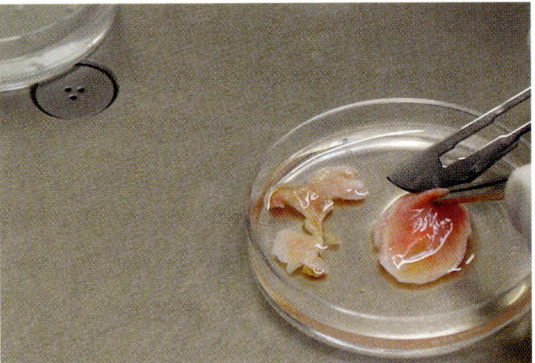

Fig. 3: Ovarian tissue is held carefully using a coarse dissecting forceps and medulla is gradually shaved off from the cortex. Ensure that the medulla is completely removed leaving behind white tunica albuginea.

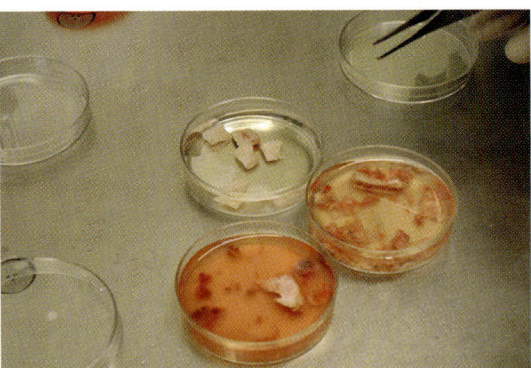

Fig. 4: The carved ovarian cortex bits are moved through different plates having washing media to clean all the debris and blood. After washing them thoroughly these are loaded in a cryovials containing the freezing media and kept at 4°C for 30–40 minutes for soakage. Use a shaker if available. Always send a small specimen of cortex and medulla each, for PCR and histopathological studies.

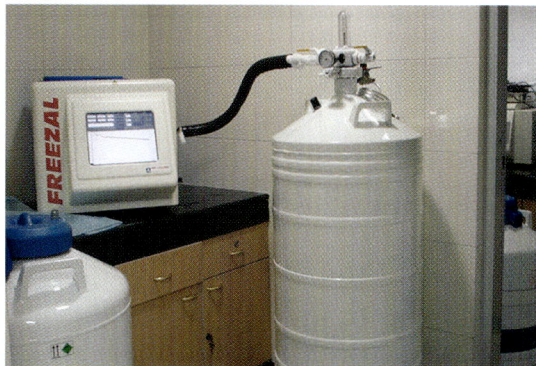

Fig. 5: Freezal cryofreezer. Prepare the slow freezer before starting the procedure. Check for LN_2 and electricity backup. Check the freezing program and manual seeding instruments if required.

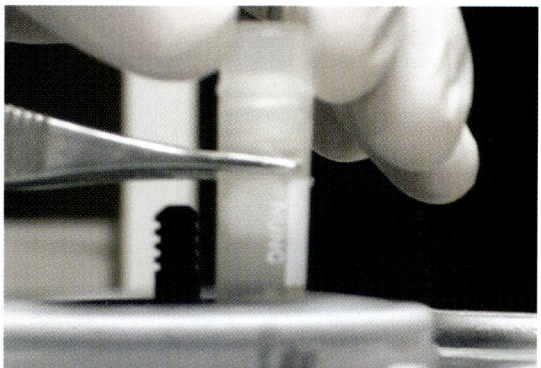

Fig. 6: Manual seeding is being carried out using a cooled forceps.

Table 9: Slow freezing-equilibration procedure.
1. After the tissue slices are ready, the pieces should be placed in the ice-cold cryoprotectant solution
2. Place the slices in 60 mm falcon dish filled with cold cryoprotectant solution
3. Every 5–10 min swirl the dish so that all pieces become exposed to the cryoprotectant
4. After 15–20 min take out the cortical slices and immerse them in the precooled cryoprotectant solution in the vials. The cryovial must be labeled before freezing commences
5. Keep the cryovial on the ice for 30–45 min on the ice. Meanwhile, run ovarian tissue freezing program on the cryologic machine

of the ovary using a sharp blade. The cortical ovarian tissue is thus cut into 1 mm × 10 mm × 10 mm pieces.

The ultra-thinness of the tissue is extremely important, not only for the cryopreservation but also for rapid revascularization after grafting. Tables 12 and 13 summarize the vitrification and thawing protocol, respectively.

Table 10: Cooling program and seedling protocol in slow freezing.

1. Run ovarian tissue freezing program on the cryologic machine. Initially cool at a rate of 2°C per min to –7°C
2. After 10 minutes of soakage of the specimen in the cryochamber at –7°C, manually seed the vials using a cotton wick or pair of precooled forceps
3. After the ice formation at the meniscus is confirmed put back the cryovials in the chamber immediately
4. The further cooling rate should be 0.3°C/min to –40 °C
5. Now cool at a faster rate of 10°C/min to –140°C and hold for 10 min
6. The vials can be plunged into liquid nitrogen, and placed on labeled canes for storage

Table 11: Thawing protocol in slow freezing.

Thawing (Slow freezing)

1. Remove the cryovial from the liquid nitrogen. Thaw the vials at room temperature for 30 seconds
2. Rapid thaw the vials by placing them in 37°C water bath for 2 minutes
3. Wash tissue in progressively lower concentrations of sucrose
4. Perform the last wash in 10% autologous serum
5. Cortex is ready for transplantation

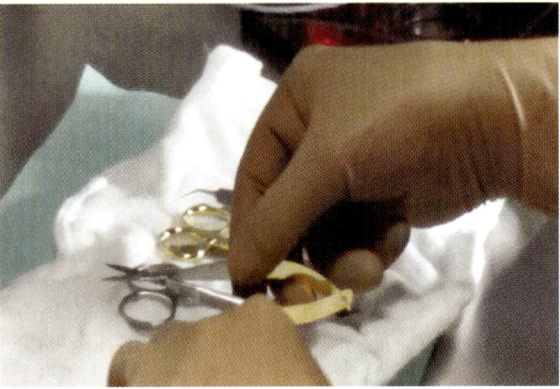

Fig. 7: Preparation for vitrification is more challenging. We use fine forceps and instruments.

■ SLOW FREEZING VERSUS VITRIFICATION

Although vitrification protocols have been described, to date, all reported live births are from ovarian tissue cryopreserved using slow freezing protocols, 60 versus 2.[34,35] Preliminary in vitro studies comparing slow-freezing and vitrification have yielded conflicting outcomes. While some investigators

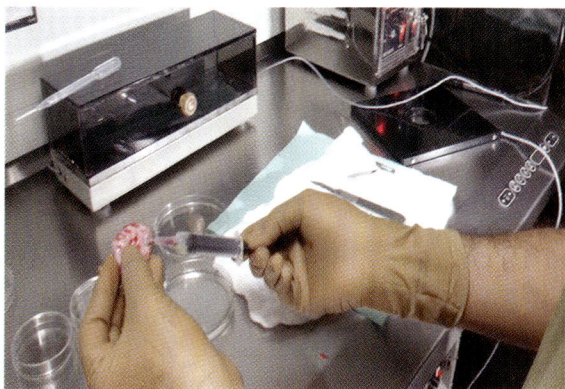

Fig. 8: The antral follicles on the ovaries are aspirated and if any immature oocytes are recovered they are cultured for in vitro maturation.

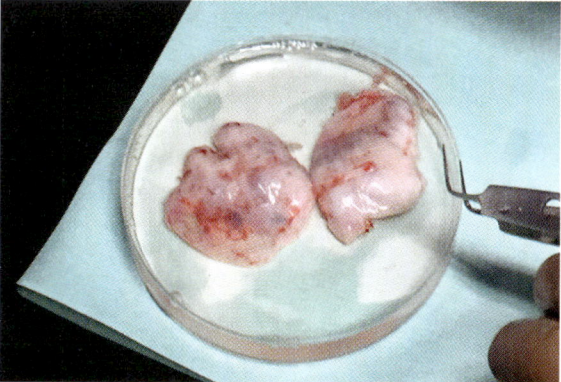

Fig. 9: The ovary is bisected in two halves for easy handling.

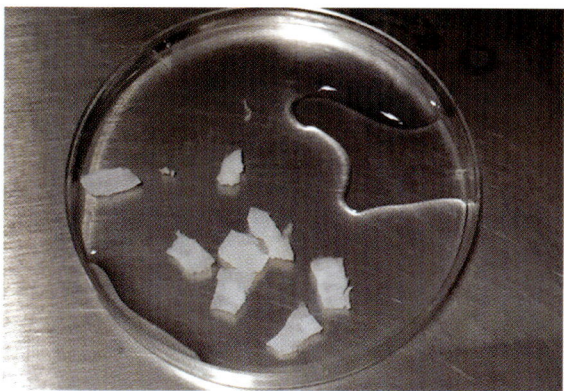

Fig. 10: Using fine instruments remove the complete medulla and at the end properly carved cortex should be thin and transparent.

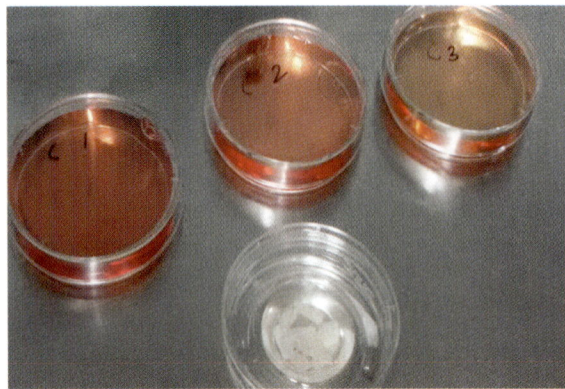

Fig. 11: Move the cortical bits through the Kitazato ovarian cortex vitrification media. Equilibrate the cortex in the media for 5 minutes each at room temperature.

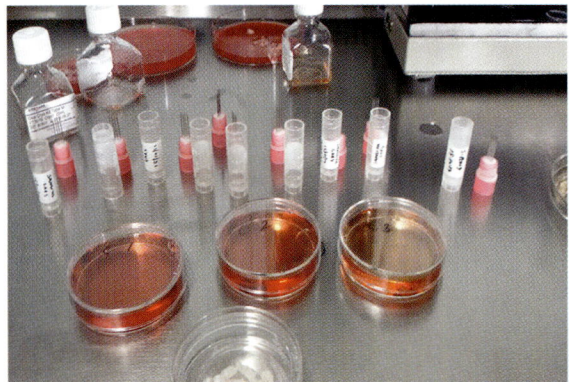

Fig. 12: Prepare the Cryo M devices for loading the cortex bits. Do proper labeling of the vials as these are to be cryopreserved for long duration of time.

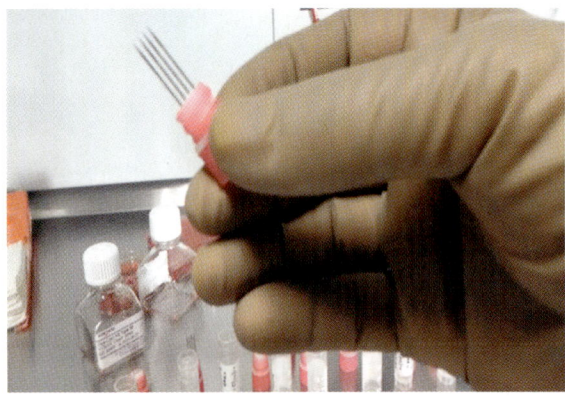

Fig. 13: Cryo M devices for loading the cortex bits.

Table 12: Vitrification protocol.

1. Ultrathin slices of the tissue are required for the cryopreservation, as well as rapid revascularization after grafting
2. Bring ES and VS to room temperature (25–27°C). Pour the full contents of ES vial (15 mL) into a 60-mm dish
3. Place the extracted tissue on the dish and wait for 25 minutes
4. Pour the full contents of VS vial (15 mL) into a 60-mm dish. Transfer the tissue in ES to the surface of VS using tweezers
5. Wait for 15 minutes
6. After the equilibration to VS, place the tissue on the Cryo M device Plunge the Cryo M device into fresh liquid nitrogen quickly
7. Check whether the tissue is translucent. Insert the cryo-tissue into the cap and twist it. Make sure if it is completely sealed
8. The cortical bits equilibrate in the media for 5 min each and then loaded on the Cryo device and then immersed in liquid nitrogen and store

Source: Kitazato ovarian cortex vitrification manual.

Table 13: Warming protocol.

Warming (Vitrification)

1. Take out the tissue from liquid nitrogen, quickly immerse it into thawing solution warmed to 37°C within 1 second
2. Leave the tissue in thawing solutions for 1 minute after immersing
3. Pour the DS (15 mL) into a 60 mm dish
4. Pour the TS with the tissue into a 90 mm dish
5. Transfer the tissue in TS to DS using tweezers
6. Wait for 3 minutes
7. Pour the WS1 (15 mL) and WS2 (15 mL) into 60 mm dishes. Do this preparation while waiting for dilution is done
8. Transfer the tissue from DS to WS1. Wait for 5 minutes
9. Transfer the tissue in WS1 to WS2. Wait for 5 minutes
10. After 5 minutes in WS2, immediately transplant or culture the tissues

Source: Kitazato ovarian cortex vitrification manual.

demonstrated excellent oocyte viability from vitrified ovarian strips and their ability to resume folliculogenesis,[36] others reported fewer primordial follicles and lowered AMH production from vitrified in contrast with slow-frozen human ovaries (Table 14).[37]

■ TRANSPLANTATION OF OVARIAN CORTEX

The primary objective of ovarian tissue storage is to reimplant a few thawed cortical strips into the patient (i.e. autotransplantation) once the patient

Table 14: Vitrification versus slow freezing.

Factors	Vitrification	Slow freezing
Time consumed	Less	More
Equipment	Inexpensive	Expensive
CPA concentration	High	Low
Cooling rate	High	Low
Ice crystallization	No	Yes
Mechanical damage	Lesser/none	More
Chemical damage	More	Less
Survival	Better	Poor

has completed cancer treatment, is disease free, and desires pregnancy.[38] Reimplantation of frozen-thawed ovarian tissue in the pelvic cavity is usually carried out by laparoscopy. The surgical technique is contingent on the presence (or not) of at least one ovary (Flowchart 1).[39]

Each site has distinct advantages and disadvantages. Orthotopic and heterotopic sites were studied for transplantation of frozen-thawed ovarian tissue. The existing menopausal ovary has been the popular site in orthotopic transplantation studies.[39,40]

Large strips (8–10.5 mm) and small cubes (2.2 mm) both were shown to restore ovarian endocrine function efficiently after orthotopic reimplantation. Transplantation of ultrathin slivers of thawed ovarian tissue termed "ovarian microorgans" has also been described, which achieved a successful live birth in a patient who previously failed to achieve pregnancy when conventional ovarian strips were used.[41]

■ OUTCOMES OF OVARIAN TISSUE GRAFTING

Endocrine indicators that the ovarian graft is functioning typically rise a few months after transplantation. The average time reported to first menses was 4.7 months, and the duration of graft functioning has varied from 9 to more than 86 months.[42] Pregnancies and live birth after transplantation were reported by natural conception[24] or after IVF.[43]

Ovarian function and spontaneous pregnancy in a 29-year-old female, previously treated with bone marrow transplantation were reported in 2006 by Demeestere I et al., after combined heterotopic and orthotopic cryopreserved ovarian tissue transplantation.[40]

Autologous heterotopic transplantation of ovarian tissue to a suprapubic site has also been reported by Oktay, resulted in spontaneous pregnancy and live birth.[44] The patient in this study had been menopausal for 2.5 years, get pregnant three months after the heterotopic transplantation. It has also been demonstrated in some patients that OTC during childhood was feasible and safe.

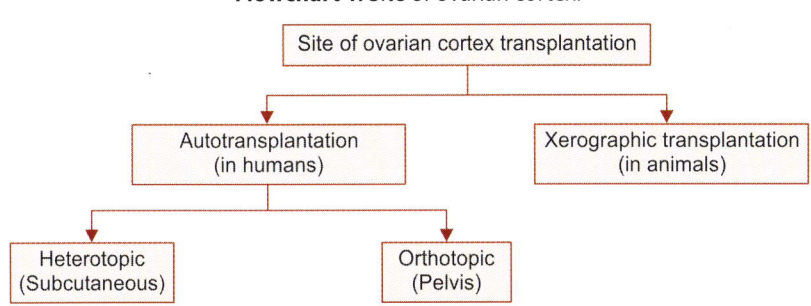

Flowchart 1: Site of ovarian cortex.

Refurbishment of Ovarian Activity

Oktay and Karilkaya documented the in vivo refurbishment of cryopreserved ovarian function and autologous transplantation. This orthotropic transplantation of ovarian tissue resulted in follicular development in response to menopausal gonadotropin stimulation. Subsequently, Oktay et al. reported heterotopic transplantation of the ovarian cortex to the forearm, after stimulation with gonadotropins, yields three oocytes.[24,26]

The reimplantation of cryopreserved ovarian cortex resulting in restoration of ovarian function, natural conception and successful pregnancy after hematopoietic stem cell transplantation for Wilms' tumor in a 32-year-old woman, has been reported by Dunlop CE et al., whose ovarian cortex was preserved 10 years before treatment of a high dose of chemotherapy. The patient underwent laparoscopic orthotropic transplantation of cryopreserved ovarian cortex to the original site of biopsy, on the left ovary. She ovulated 15 and 29 weeks postreimplantation with AMH detectable and conceived naturally following the second ovulation and gave birth to a healthy male infant.[45]

Potential Malignant Cell Contamination in Cryopreserved Ovarian Tissue

The potential for reintroduction of malignant cells is one of the major concerns of transplanting thawed ovarian tissue in cured cancer patients, which could propagate cancer recurrence. Preoperative imaging with ultrasonography and computerized tomographic scan can identify patients with overt ovarian involvement and hence, prevent unnecessary laparoscopies. Routine histology is used but usually does not identify malignant contamination of the tissue.

Live Birth from Ovarian Tissue Grafting

Revelli et al. reported the live birth after orthotropic grafting of the autologous cryopreserved ovarian issue and spontaneous conception in Italy.[46]

Prasath et al. reported first pregnancy and live birth achieved in 2014 from cryopreserved embryos obtained from in vitro matured oocyte after oophorectomy in an ovarian cancer patient.[47]

Recently, Jensen et al. reported approximately 86 live birth and nine ongoing pregnancies 95 children have been born or will get birth in the near future worldwide in women transplanted with frozen-thawed ovarian tissue.[48]

These data reassure and further suggest the cryopreservation of ovarian tissue is becoming an established fertility preservation method.

■ FUTURE OF OVARIAN CORTEX PRESERVATION

Women wishing to postpone maternity and transgender individuals before starting hormone therapy or undergoing surgery to remove/alter their reproductive organs should also be counseled accordingly. Embryo and oocyte cryopreservation are first-line FP methods in postpubertal women.

Ovarian tissue auto-transplantation in post-pubertal women is capable of restoring fertility with over 80 live births currently reported with a corresponding pregnancy rate of 23–37%. The recently reported successes of live births from transplants, both in orthotopic and heterotopic locations, as well as the emerging methods of IVM, in vitro culture of primordial follicles, and the feasibility of in vitro activation (IVA) propose new fertility options for many women and girls. Vitrification has also demonstrated successful live births and may be a more cost-effective method to freezing with less tissue injury.

Further, transplantation via the artificial ovary with an extracellular tissue matrix (ECTM) scaffolding as well as the effects of sphingosine-1-phosphate (SIP) and fibrin modified with heparin-binding peptide (HBP), heparin, and a vascular endothelial growth factor (VEGF) have demonstrated important advancements in fertility preservation.[49]

Whole-organ Freezing and Transplantation

The technique is limited by the ischemia that occurs at the time of thawing and reimplantation in the ovarian cortex. They are entirely dependent for their survival on time necessary for the establishment of neovascularization after grafting because these small cortical pieces are grafted without any vascular anastomoses. The cells in the graft may undergo significant ischemic damage as this process may require a minimum of 7 days, which results in massive loss of primordial follicles and drastically reduces the lifespan of the graft.[50-56]

To avoid these issues, whole-ovary freezing has also been investigated, with the aim of achieving vascular anastomoses after transplantation.[57]

Ovarian vascular transplantation using intact fresh ovaries has been shown to restore fertility in rats,[58] sheep,[59,60] and monkeys,[61] but a high rate of follicle loss is still a major concern.[62] A limited number of human studies with transplantation of fresh whole ovaries in orthotopic[62,63] and heterotopic[21] sites have been carried out with some success. The first live birth after transplantation of the whole fresh ovary between monozygotic twins discordant for premature ovarian failure was reported by Silber.[62]

In Vitro Maturation

Retrieval of immature oocyte from ovaries without ovarian stimulation followed by IVM and vitrification is a promising fertility preservation option for:
1. Pediatric patients (including prepubertal girls)
2. Women (both before and after cancer therapy, Abir R 2016)[64] who cannot delay their gonadotoxic cancer treatment and cannot undergo ovarian stimulation. Immature oocytes can be collected from the ovaries during both the follicular and luteal phases, which maximize the possibility for fertility preservation.

The combination of OTC with immature oocyte collection from the tissue followed by oocyte vitrification via IVM represents another promising approach to fertility preservation in young women with cancer.

Grynberg M et al. in November 2013 reported first live birth achieved after IVM of oocytes for a woman endowed with multiple antral follicles unresponsive to follicle stimulating hormone.[64-66]

Follicle Culture

Other than ovarian tissue cryopreservation, follicle culture can also be considered as the promising method in preserving fertility.

Especially for young patients without partners or who cannot undergo ovarian stimulation for oocyte/embryo cryopreservation and patients for whom the risk for reintroduction of malignant cells prohibit transplantation.

Follicle culture system can efficiently use all classes of ovarian follicles, derived from clinically cryopreserved ovarian tissue, as sources of gametes would maximize the reproductive potential for future fertility.[67]

■ ALTERNATIVE APPROACHES TO USE OF CRYOPRESERVED OVARIAN TISSUE

Alternative methods for the use of the cryopreserved tissue are theoretically possible: IVM of follicles isolated from the ovarian cortex to avoid transmission of malignant cells and the whole-ovary vascular transplantation to reduce follicular loss due to tissue ischemia.

These technologies, however, are experimental. Dr Balaji published the first report on pregnancy and live birth from frozen-thawed embryos obtained from fresh oocytes, harvested from the surgically removed ovary, after IVM and ICSI in a patient with advanced ovarian cancer.[168]

In contrast, autotransplantation of cryopreserved pieces of ovarian tissue is a relatively robust procedure that can be repeated over time, has relatively long graft survival, and has yielded the largest cohort of live births, making it the favored approach at this time.

CONCLUSION

Recently available data in the literature indicates that ovarian tissue transplantation is feasible and effective for preserving fertility. Thus, cryopreservation of ovarian tissue should be recommended to all adolescents and young women having to undergo highly gonadotoxic chemotherapy. However, the rate of survival of follicles after transplantation is still low and is yet to be improved. Although ovarian tissue harvesting seems to be safe, the risk of reimplantation of cancer from ovarian cortical transplants cannot be estimated at this time. Due to which, autotransplantation of ovarian tissue in women having suffered from systemic hematological malignancies is not recommended. In these situations, reimplantation of isolated ovarian follicles might represent an intriguing option in the future. In humans, research of whole-ovary freezing and transplantation is still at its initial stages.

KEY POINTS

- Ovarian tissue cryopreservation and transplantation is a feasible and effective method in preserving the fertility of prepubertal and pediatric patients as well as the patient with oncological and none oncological diseases.
- Primordial follicles can sustain the cryoprotectants as they are without zona and cortical granule.
- Several studies have been documented the successful pregnancies in post-therapy patients through transplantation of frozen-thawed tissue as compared to embryo and oocyte cryopreservation.
- IVM of follicles isolated from the ovarian cortex can be efficiently used to avoid transmission of the malignant cell.
- Successful live births from transplant of cryopreserved ovarian tissue in both orthotopic and heterotopic location have been reported.
- OTC can be performed at any time during menstrual cycle and no hormonal stimulation is required, thus no delay in chemotherapy.
- OTC can escape the cytotoxicity of the germline cells and the entire tissue can be returned to patients by grafting which can potentially restore both steroidogenic and gametogenic factors.

REFERENCES

1. Partridge AH, Gelber S, Peppercorn J, et al. Web-based survey of fertility issues in young women with breast cancer. J Clin Oncol. 2004;22:4174-83.
2. Meirow D, Nugent D. The effects of radiotherapy and chemotherapy on female reproduction. Hum Reprod Update. 2001;7:535-43.
3. Faddy MJ, Gosden RG, Gougeon A, et al. Accelerated disappearance of ovarian follicles in mid-life: implications for forecasting menopause. Hum Reprod. 1992;7:1342-6.
4. Bedoschi G, Oktay K. Current approach to fertility preservation by embryo cryopreservation. Fertil Steril. 2013;99:1496-502.

5. Cobo A, Serra V, Garrido N, et al. Obstetric and perinatal outcome of babies born from vitrified oocytes. Fertil Steril. 2014;102:1006-15.
6. The Practice Committee of the American Society for Reproductive Medicine. Ovarian tissue cryopreservation: a committee opinion. Fertil Steril. 2014;101:1237-43.
7. Meirow D. Reproduction post-chemotherapy in young cancer patients. Mol Cell Endocr. 2000;169:123-31.
8. Bath LE, Wallace WH, Shaw MP, et al. Depletion of ovarian reserve in young women after treatment for cancer in childhood: detection by anti-Mullerian hormone, inhibin, and ovarian ultrasound. Hum Reprod. 2003;18:2368-74.
9. Wallace WH, Thomson AB, Saran F, et al. Predicting age of ovarian failure after radiation to a field that includes the ovaries. Int J Radiat Oncol Biol Phys. 2005;62:738-44.
10. Meirow D, Biederman H, Anderson RA, et al. Toxicity of chemotherapy and radiation on female reproduction. Clin Obstet Gynecol. 2010;53:727-39.
11. Petrek JA, Naughton MJ, Case LD, et al. Incidence, time course, and determinants of menstrual bleeding after breast cancer treatment: a prospective study. J Clin Oncol. 2006;24:1045-51.
12. Goodwin PJ, Ennis M, Pritchard KI, et al. Risk of menopause during the first year after breast cancer diagnosis. J Clin Oncol. 1999;17:2365-70.
13. Isgro J, Sahadat K. Cyclophosphamide exposure in pediatric systemic lupus erythematosus is associated with reduced serum anti-Müllerian hormone levels. J Rheumatol. 2013:40(6):1029-31.
14. Roti Roti EC, Leisman SK, Abbott DH, et al. Acute doxorubicin insult in the mouse ovary is cell- and follicle-type dependent. PLoS One. 2012;7:e42293.
15. Perez GI, Knudson CM, Leykin L, et al. Apoptosis-associated signalling pathways are required for chemotherapy-mediated female germ cell destruction. Nat Med. 1997;3:1228-32.
16. Stumm S, Meyer A, Lindner M, et al. Paclitaxel treatment of breast cancer cell lines modulates Fas/Fas ligand expression and induces apoptosis which can be inhibited through the CD40 receptor. Oncology. 2004;66:101-11.
17. Anderson AR, Themmen A, Al-Qahtani NP, et al. Cameron the effects of chemotherapy and long-term gonadotrophin suppression on the ovarian reserve in premenopausal women with breast cancer. Hum Reprod. 2006;21(10):2583-92.
18. Kim SS. Recommendations for fertility preservation in patients with lymphoma, leukemia, and breast cancer. J Assist Reprod Genet. 2012;29:465-8.
19. Jacques D. Ovarian tissue cryopreservation and transplantation: a review. Hum Reprod Update. 2006;12(5):519-35.
20. Donnez J, Bassil S. Indications for cryopreservation of ovarian tissue. Hum Reprod. Update. 1998;4:248-59.
21. Leporrier M, von Theobald P, Roffe JL, et al. A new technique to protect ovarian function before pelvic irradiation. Heterotopic ovarian auto transplantation. Cancer. 1987;60:2201-4.
22. Newton H, Aubard Y, Rutherford A, et al. Low-temperature storage and grafting of human ovarian tissue. Human Reprod. 1996;11:1487-91.

23. Marconi G, Quintana R, Rueda-Leverone NG, et al. Accidental ovarian autograft after laparoscopic surgery: case report. Fertil Steril. 1997;68:364-6.
24. Oktay K, Karilkaya G. Ovarian function after transplantation of frozen, banked autologous ovarian tissue. N Engl J Med. 2000;342:1919.
25. Radford JA, Liberman BA, Brison D, et al. Orthotopic reimplantation of cryopreserved ovarian cortical strips after high-dose chemotherapy for Hodgkin's lymphoma. Lancet. 2001;357:1172-5.
26. Oktay K, Buyuk E, Veeck L, et al. Embryo development after heterotopic transplantation of cryopreserved ovarian tissue. Lancet. 2004;363:837-40.
27. Donnez J, Dolmans MM, Demylle D, et al. Live birth after orthotopic transplantation of cryopreserved ovarian tissue. Lancet. 2004;364:1405-10.
28. Hovatta O. Methods of cryopreservation of human ovarian tissue. Reprod Biomed Online. 2005;10729-34.
29. Silber SJ, Lenahan KM, Levine DJ, et al. Ovarian transplantation between monozygotic twins discordant for premature ovarian failure. N Engl J Med. 2007;356:1382-4.
30. Fuller B, Paynter S. Fundamentals of cryobiology in reproductive medicine. Reprod Biomed Online. 2004;9:680-91.
31. Fabbri R. optimization of protocols for human ovarian tissue cryopreservation with sucrose, 1,2 propanediol and human serum. Reprod Biomed Online. 2010;21:819-28.
32. Hreinsson J, Zhang P, Swahn ML, et al. Cryopreservation of follicles in human ovarian cortical tissue. Comparison of serum and human serum albumin in the cryoprotectant solutions. Hum Reprod. 2003;18:2420-8.
33. Keros V, Xella S, Hultenby K, et al. Vitrification versus controlled-rate freezing in cryopreservation of human ovarian tissue. Hum Reprod. 2009;24:1670-83.
34. Kagawa N, Silber S, Kuwayama M. Successful vitrification of bovine and human ovarian tissue. Reprod Biomed Online. 2009;18:568-77.
35. Sheikhi M, Hultenby K, Niklasson B, et al. Clinical grade vitrification of human ovarian tissue: an ultra-structural analysis of follicles and stroma in vitrified tissue. Hum Reprod. 2011;26:594-603.
36. Amorim CA, Dolmans MM, David A, et al. Vitrification and xenografting of human ovarian tissue. Fertil Steril. 2012;98:1291-8.
37. Oktem O, Alper E, Balaban B, et al. Vitrified human ovaries have fewer primordial follicles and produce less anti-Mullerian hormone than slow-frozen ovaries. Fertil Steril. 2011;95:2661-4.
38. Donnez J, Marie-Madeleine D, Diaz C, et al. Ovarian cortex transplantation: time to move on from experimental studies to open the clinical application. Fertil Steril. 2015;104(5):1097-98.
39. Kim SS, Battaglia DE, Soules MR. The future of human ovarian cryopreservation and transplantation: Fertility and beyond. Fertil Steril. 2001;75:1049-56.
40. Demeestere I, Simon P, Buxant F, et al. Ovarian function and spontaneous pregnancy after combined heterotopic and orthotopic cryopreserved ovarian tissue transplantation in a patient previously treated with bone marrow transplantation the Case report. Hum Repord. 2006;21:2010-4.

41. Meirow D, Baum M, Yaron R, et al. Ovarian tissue cryopreservation in hematologic malignancy: ten years' experience. Leuk Lymphoma. 2007;48:1569-76.
42. Janse F, Donnez J, Anckaert E, et al. Limited value of ovarian function markers following orthotopic transplantation of ovarian tissue after gonadotoxic treatment. J Clin Endocrinol Metab. 2011;96:1136-44.
43. Meirow D, Ben Yehuda D, Prus D, et al. Ovarian tissue banking in patients with Hodgkin's disease: is it safe? Fertil Steril. 1998;69:996-8.
44. Oktay K. Spontaneous conceptions and live birth after heterotopic ovarian transplantation: Is there a germline stem cell connection? Hum Reprod. 2004;21:1345-8.
45. Dunlop CE. Re-implantation of cryopreserved ovarian cortex resulting in restoration of ovarian function, natural conception and successful pregnancy after hematopoietic stem cell transplantation for Wilms tumour. J Assist Reprod Genet. 2016;33(12):1615-20.
46. Revelli A, Marchino G, Dolfin E, et al. Live birth after orthotopic grafting of autologous cryopreserved ovarian tissue and spontaneous conception in Italy. Fertil Steril. 2013;99(1):227-30.
47. Prasath, EB, Chan ML, Wong WH, et al. First pregnancy and live birth from cryopreserved embryos obtained from in vitro matured oocytes after oophorectomy in ovarian cancer patient. Hum Reprod. 2014;29:276-8.
48. Jensen KT, Fedder J, Ernst E, et al. 86 successful births and 9 ongoing pregnancies worldwide in women transplanted with frozen-thawed ovarian tissue: focus on birth and perinatal outcome in 40 of these children. J Assist Reprod Genet. 2017;34(3):325-33.
49. Ladanyi C. Recent advances in the field of ovarian tissue cryopreservation and opportunities for research. J Assist Reprod Genet. 2017;34(6):709-22.
50. Israely T, Dafni H, Nevo N, et al. Angiogenesis in ectopic ovarian xenotransplantation: multi parameter characterization of the neo vasculature by dynamic contrast-enhanced MRI. Magn Reson Med. 2004;52:741-50.
51. Israely T, Nevo N, Harmelin A, et al. Reducing ischaemic damage in rodent ovarian xenografts transplanted into granulation tissue. Hum Reprod. 2006;21:1368-79.
52. Qi S, Ma A, Xu D, et al. Cryopreservation of vascularized ovary: an evaluation of histology and function in rats. Microsurgery. 2008;28:380-6.
53. Oktay K. Ovarian tissue cryopreservation and transplantation: preliminary findings and implications for cancer patients. Hum Reprod Update. 2001;7:526-34.
54. Bedaiwy MA, Hussein MR, Biscotti C, et al. Cryopreservation of intact human ovary with its vascular pedicle. Hum Reprod. 2006;21:3258-69.
55. Martinez MB, Dolmans MM, Van Langendonckt A, et al. Freeze-thawing intact human ovary with its vascular pedicle with a passive cooling device. Fertil Steril. 2004;82:1390-4.
56. Gosden RG. Ovary and uterus transplantation. Reproduction. 2008;136:671-80.
57. Jadoul P, Donnez J, Dolmans MM, et al. Laparoscopic ovariectomy for whole human ovary cryopreservation: technical aspects. Fertil Steril. 2007;87:971-5.

58. Yin H, Wang X, Kim SS, et al. Transplantation of intact rat gonads using vascular anastomosis: effects of cryopreservation, ischaemia and genotype. Hum Reprod. 2003;18:1165-72.
59. Jeremias E, Bedaiwy MA, Gurunluoglu R, et al. Heterotopic auto-transplantation of the ovary with microvascular anastomosis: a novel surgical technique. Fertil Steril. 2002;77:1278-82.
60. Courbiere B, Caquant L, Mazoyer C, et al. Difficulties improving ovarian functional recovery by microvascular transplantation and whole ovary vitrification. Fertil Steril. 2009;91:2697-706.
61. Scott JR, Keye WR, Poulson AM, et al. Microsurgical ovarian transplantation in the primate. Fertil Steril. 1981;36:512-5.
62. Silber SJ, Grudzinskas G, Gosden RG. Successful pregnancy after microsurgical transplantation of an intact ovary. N Engl J Med. 2008;359:2617-8.
63. Mhatre P, Mhatre J, Magotra R. Ovarian transplant: a new frontier. Transplant Proc. 2005;37:1396-8.
64. Abir R, Ben-Aharon I, Garor R, et al. Cryopreservation of in-vitro matured oocytes in addition to ovarian tissue freezing for fertility preservation in pediatric female cancer patients before and after cancer therapy. Hum Reprod. 2016;31(4):750-62.
65. Chian RC, Uzelac PS, Nargund G. In-vitro maturation of human immature oocytes for fertility preservation. Fertil Steril. 2013;99(5):1173-81.
66. Grynberg M, Peltoketo H, Christin-Maître S, et al. First birth achieved after in-vitro maturation of oocytes from a woman endowed with multiple antral follicles unresponsive to follicle-stimulating hormone. J Clin Endocrinol Metab. 2013;98(11):4493-8.
67. Telfer EE, Zelinski MB. Ovarian Follicle Culture: Advances and Challenges in Human and Non-Human Primates. Fertil Steril. 2013;99(6):1523-33.
68. Meirow D, Levron J, Eldar-Geva T, et al. Pregnancy after transplantation of cryopreserved ovarian tissue in a patient with ovarian failure after chemotherapy. N Engl J Med. 2005;353:318-21.

CHAPTER
34

Role of Preimplantation Genetic Diagnosis and Comparative Genomic Hybridization in Healthy Outcome of ART

Dhiraj Gada, Shailaja Gada Saxena, Ritu Gada

■ INTRODUCTION

Infertility, defined as the inability of a couple to conceive despite trying for a year, affects approximately 12% of the reproductive population. Recent advances in assisted reproductive technologies (ART) like in-vitro fertilization (IVF), embryo transfer (ET) and intracytoplasmic sperm injection (ICSI) has helped to improve the success rate of infertility management. A critical step in these complex techniques is embryo selection. In most of the cases, embryo selection is done based on visual inspection of morphology of the embryo. Techniques such as preimplantation genetic diagnosis and screening (PGD/PGS) allow detection of genetic, numeric and/or structural chromosome aberrations. Several other methods collectively called as OMICS have been attempted that include measuring proteins, metabolic products and other factors that are released by the embryo into the culture media.[1] Other potential methods proposed for embryo quality assessment are measuring the mitochondrial activity and respiration rate of the embryos.[2,3]

■ PREIMPLANTATION GENETIC DIAGNOSIS SCREENING

Preimplantation genetic testing is an alternative used for prenatal diagnosis for couples who are at a high risk of transmitting genetic disorders to their children.[4] This method has one main advantage over traditional prenatal diagnosis approaches as it involves testing prior to the onset of pregnancy, hence avoiding affected pregnancy and termination. For this reason, testing the embryo at preimplantation stage is more ethically acceptable than the old methods that involved testing after pregnancy. The process of preimplantation testing involves testing of one or more cells obtained from the embryo at different stages of development. This testing in the embryo can be done in couples with an inherited genetic disorder or carriers of a structural chromosomal abnormality, and this is referred to as PGD. On the other hand, in infertile couples, screening of the embryo for possible de novo chromosome abnormalities when there are no known potentially inherited disorders it is termed preimplantation genetic screening or PGS. In this chapter, these terms have been interchangeably used.

Current PGD/PGS methods use the oocytes and embryos derived from ovarian stimulation and IVF to test for specific genetic abnormalities. The three main stages at which the genetic material can be sampled include the oocyte/zygote stage when by polar body biopsy[5] can be performed, the cleavage stage through blastomere biopsy[6] and the blastocyst stage by performing the trophectoderm biopsy.[7] Polar bodies (PB) can be biopsied sequentially, whereby the first PB is biopsied on the day of oocyte collection and the second polar body is biopsied postfertilization. The other option is to biopsy both the polar bodies simultaneously post fertilization.[5] Until recent past, the most widely used embryo biopsy strategy was to biopsy one or two blastomeres from a 6–10 cell cleavage stage embryo, on day 3. During this stage all the cells are totipotent that is they can give rise to any cell type or lineage.[6] The third option gaining more visibility is trophectoderm biopsy from blastocyst stage embryo. The herniating trophectoderm cells can be biopsied.[7] Like any technique, biopsy at any of these stages is associated with its own advantage and disadvantages.

When PGD was initially introduced, fluorescence in situ hybridization (FISH) and polymerase chain reaction (PCR) were the two commonly used first-generation technologies for diagnosis of genetic aberration. Generally, PCR-based methods were used for DNA based analysis for monogenic disorders, and FISH for aneuploidies or structural chromosomal aberrations. Use of whole genome amplification, next generation sequencing and comparative genomic hybridization assays are alternative modes of analysis, currently used widely for genetic analysis.

In this chapter we would focus on chromosomal aberrations, ways to detect these embryos in preimplantation embryos and the impact of these aberrations on outcome of ART.

Chromosomal Aberrations

Chromosomes carry the genetic information that dictates growth and development of embryos. A change in the number or structure of chromosome results in chromosomal aberration. Numerical chromosomal aberrations are associated with loss or gain of one or more chromosomes (aneuploidy) or entire set of chromosomes (polyploidy). The term aneuploidy refers to cytogenetic abnormalities whereby there is loss (monosomy) or gain of chromosome (trisomy). Aneuploidies may arise de-novo following meiotic or mitotic non-disjunction during gametogenesis or embryogenesis. Monosomies are usually not compatible with life. Trisomies of chromosomes 13, 18 and 21 are the common trisomies detected in live-births. The risk of trisomy 13, 18 and 21 increases with maternal age at pregnancy. Numerical abnormalities of sex chromosomes are more frequent, observed in 1 in 500 live births. This can be attributed to the fact that the abnormalities of sex chromosome have less severe clinical manifestations and are compatible with life. Polyploidies are numerical chromosomal abnormalities with changes in the number of complete sets of chromosomes, and are usually incompatible with fetal survival. Polyploidy include triploidy wherein the chromosome number is 69, and tetraploidy with 92 chromosomes per cell. Polyploidies are usually caused by dispermy, fertilization of single ovum by 2 sperms; diandry due to fertilization of a single ovum with a single sperm which has failed to undergo meiosis, or due to digyny as a result of failure of extrusion of polar body. On the other hand, structural chromosome aberrations arise due to errors in the exchange of genetic material between sister chromatids and homologous chromosomes during cell division. Such abnormalities arise due to chromosome break with subsequent reunion of the wrong segments of the chromosomes. Translocations associated with net loss or gain of chromosomal material which is unbalanced translocation, may lead to significant clinical consequences in the form of dysmorphic features and mental subnormality in the child. No loss or gain of chromosomal material, i.e. balanced translocation, may have no phenotypic abnormalities with normal mental and physical fitness in the child. Multiple generations of a family may have members with balanced structural rearrangements which may go undetected. The rearrangements could manifest in form of reproductive problems in the couple in the form of infertility, recurrent pregnancy loss or abnormal progeny. These reproductive problems can be attributed to meiotic events resulting in cytogenetically unbalanced conceptions. The various structural rearrangements include reciprocal and Robertsonian translocations, deletions, isochromosome, duplication, inversion, etc. It is estimated that 1 in 625 individuals carries a balanced chromosomal translocation. In couples with recurrent miscarriage, the incidence of structural chromosome abnormality in one of the partners is approximately 4–5%, mainly including reciprocal translocations and Robertsonian translocations.[8] Most numerical chromosome abnormalities detected in cleavage and blastocyst embryos are not compatible with implantation or birth, which negatively affects the success of assisted reproductive treatments. The detrimental effect of aneuploidy is illustrated by the high prevalence of chromosome abnormalities detected in spontaneous abortions. PGD provides an option to exclude the unbalanced embryos caused due to numerical and structural chromosomal aberration.

Detection of Chromosomal Aberrations

The most common methods used for detection of chromosomal aberrations are karyotyping or FISH. In PGD/PGS set up these are now being replaced by higher sensitivity techniques like comparative genomic hybridization (CGH) and array comparative genomic hybridization (aCGH).

Karyotyping allows analysis of all 46 chromosomes in a single test, giving a complete chromosomal picture. Karyotyping detects numerical and structural chromosomal aberrations and enables detection of gross errors involving 5 Mb regions. Karyotyping requires culturing of cells with longer turnaround time. Because of the need of culturing the cells, it is not the method of choice for PGD/PGS. Also, microdeletions and low grade mosaicism cannot be ruled out by karyotyping. On the other hand, FISH is a rapid test on interphase chromosomes that allows direct visualization of specific chromosomal targets using complementary DNA as a probe. The probe is composed of fluorescently labeled oligonucleotides (200–300 Kb) with differential absorption and emission spectra that are visualized using a fluorescence microscope as signals of different colors. FISH is used to detect aneuploidy and subtle chromosomal changes like deletions and duplications, suspected, defined and indicated in the patient.

Comparative genomic hybridization is a molecular cytogenetic method used for analyzing copy number variations (CNVs). It compares the ploidy level in the DNA of a test sample to a reference sample, thus giving information on gains or losses of either whole chromosomes or a part of the chromosome. As against karyotyping, the advantage of this technique that there is no need for culturing cells. In addition, CGH provides better resolution of 5–10 megabases compared to conventional cytogenetic analysis.[9] The DNA is extracted from sample to be tested and the reference sample. Both these are labeled with red and green fluorophores. Both the samples are mixed in 1:1 ratio to a normal metaphase spread. When the denatured sample and reference single stranded DNA are added to the metaphase spread, both the DNA bind to the locus of origin. Analysis is done using fluorescence microscope to identify chromosomal difference between two sources. When there is no loss or gain of chromosomal material, a neutral yellow color is observed under the fluorescent microscope. In case of gain of chromosome or chromosomal segment, one would see a higher intensity of the test sample color in a specific region of a chromosome, while a higher intensity of the reference sample color indicates the loss of material in the test sample in that specific region.[9] CGH is only able to detect unbalanced chromosomal aberrations like monosomies, trisomies, deletions and duplications, however, it cannot detect balanced chromosomal aberrations such as reciprocal translocations, inversions as there is no change in copy number in case of balanced rearrangements. The analysis of CGH results using metaphase chromosomes as the template, as described above, is time-consuming and labor intensive.

To improve the resolution of detection of chromosomal aberration up to a scale of 100 kilobase, DNA microarrays in conjunction with CGH techniques have been used, resulting in array CGH (aCGH).[10] These microarrays are made up of DNA sequences specific to human chromosomes spotted onto a platform, usually a glass slide. The principle is the same as metaphase chromosome CGH in that differentially labeled reference and test DNA are hybridized to the slide and differences in the fluorescence ratio are indicative of changes in DNA copy number. In case of array CGH, the use of metaphase spreads are replaced by 100–200 kb cloned DNA fragments known chromosomal location, thus allowing detection of aberrations onto the genomic sequence. Array CGH has proven to be a specific, sensitive, fast and high throughput technique making it more amenable to diagnostic applications.

Role of PGD and PGS for Detection of Chromosomal Aberrations and on ART Outcome

The success rate with ART is dependent on the age of the female partner as there is rapid increase in aneuploidies in the oocytes with advancing maternal age. Additionally, aneuploidy rates in the oocytes of infertile female patients seem to be even higher than those in the oocytes of women of the same age without fertility problems. Studies have shown high aneuploidy rate in human preimplantation embryos, practically involving all chromosomes.[11] It is difficult to obtain a comprehensive overview of chromosomes within in vitro cultured embryos because they have only a few cells and limited time available for establishing the diagnosis in the time frame of IVF cycle. Initial PGS strategies included FISH analysis with 5–12 probes. The 12 probe assay was able to detect more than 80% of chromosomally abnormal embryos.[12] Initial non-randomized studies utilizing FISH reported an improvement in implantation rates and fewer spontaneous abortions following PGS. However, similar positive results were not observed in later randomized studies.[12] These limitations entailed the need for a technique which would allow single cell 24-chromosomal analysis of preimplantation embryos. Recent innovation in comparative genomic hybridization and microarray technology has enabled the testing of all chromosomes in preimplantation embryos.

The detection of aneuploidy in single cells using metaphase-based comparative genomic hybridization (metaphase CGH) was developed to assess all chromosomes. Metaphase CGH was initially attempted for PGS for aneuploidies in single blastomeres and first polar bodies. However, the turnaround time for metaphase CGH was more than 3 days, necessitating the need for the embryos to be cryopreserved until a diagnosis is made followed by transfer in a subsequent natural cycle. This necessitated the need of better cryopreservation protocols. Introduction of better vitrification protocols provided the required solution and in conjunction with vitrification, CGH has been clinically applied to polar bodies through blastocyst biopsies. Simultaneously array CGH was introduced which proved to be much quicker.[13] The first successful clinical application of CGH in PGD was for a 38-year-old woman with primary infertility and recurrent implantation failure which resulted in the birth of a healthy female infant.

Most of the initial attempts with PGS using CGH/aCGH were on polar body biopsy as it provides more time for establishing the diagnosis. However, PGD using polar body is more expensive because of the requirement for separate analyses of the first and second polar bodies to obtain a precise prediction of the putative chromosomal aberration in the oocyte. To overcome this drawback, Feichtinger et al., (2015) attempted testing on pooled polar bodies and their results indicate that meiotic separation errors can be effectively detected in pooled polar bodies. Moreover, the live birth rate per transferred embryo strongly increased in couples following PGS of pooled polar bodies in comparison with a control IVF group without PGS.[14]

CGH has also been applied to day-3 embryo biopsies. However, many challenges were faced as the low survival rate with embryo freezing and thawing neutralized any beneficial effects of PGD, until the advent of vitrification. Although worldwide the trend is away from day-3 biopsy, many clinics continue using cleavage stage biopsy as the method of choice. This can be attributed to lack of expertise or proficiency with blastocyst culture and vitrification, additional cost associated with blastocyst culture and vitrification and patients prefer to have a fresh cycle.[13]

Most of the advanced centers in the US are now using day 5 biopsy combined with vitrification or replacement on the same cycle, either late day 5 or early day 6. In contrast, in European clinics the tendency is to go back to polar bodies. Studies have found that implantation and pregnancy rates for the patients with polar body biopsy were 11% and 21%, respectively, whereas for patients receiving blastocyst biopsy they were 58% and 69%.[1]

Apart from aneuploidies, aCGH can also be used for detection of structural chromosomal aberrations like translocations provided that the translocated fragment is more than 6 Mb. This is especially important in couples when either of the partners is the carrier of balanced chromosomal rearrangement, which in turn is the cause of infertility and repeated implantation failure. Using aCGH unbalanced structural differences between the normal reference and test sample can be shown with an added advantage of simultaneous aneuploidy screening of all 24 chromosomes. The only limitation of aCGH for translocations is that as mentioned earlier, it cannot differentiate normal from balanced embryos.

Many studies have reviewed the efficacy of aCGH screening of 24 chromosomes in terms of clinical and ongoing pregnancy rates for patients and shown significant improvement, thus proving the efficacy of the technique.[15,1]

Advantages and Limitations of CGH/aCGH

The advantage of using CGH/aCGH is that it allows analysis of all 24 chromosomes in one assay and both numerical and structural chromosomal aberrations can be simultaneously detected. Another advantage of array CGH is that it does not require preclinical validation before each IVF cycle, which is required for FISH. This avoids postponement of IVF treatment. In case of mosaicism, the error rate using FISH is estimated to be --7%, whereas with array CGH it is observed to be 2%.

As stated, aCGH easily detects chromosome imbalances such as aneuploidies, unbalanced translocations, deletions and duplications, however, diploidy cannot be distinguished from changes involving loss or gain of an entire set of chromosomes such haploidy or polyploidy. However, studies have shown that majority of 2PN embryos tested polyploid or haploid had additional abnormalities which were easily detectable by aCGH. Only a small 1.8% of all embryos are homogeneously polyploid or haploid. Furthermore, majority of the polyploid embryos arrest by day 4, leaving only 0.2% of developing embryos uniformly polyploidy or haploid that could produce a misdiagnosis.[1]. Next generation sequencing (NGS) has been used as an alternative to aCGH, which also allows simultaneous evaluation of single-gene disorders and abnormalities of the mitochondrial genome, from the same biopsy material.

CONCLUSION

Since the inception of PGD, the clinical applications for which PGD is being offered is gradually increasing. Simultaneously newer diagnostic techniques are being used for detection of genetic aberrations from FISH and PCR in the earlier years and now newer techniques like CGH, aCGH, NGS, etc. Each technique has its own advantages and disadvantages.

PGS, as is known does not improve the health of an embryo, rather it helps in accurate selection of embryo for transfer so as to achieve a healthy live birth and to reduce the risk of miscarriage. For detection of numerical and structural chromosomal aberrations CGH and aCGH have gained more importance against the earlier 5–12 color FISH testing, as these newer techniques can analyze all 24 chromosomes in a single assay. aCGH on blastomeres has provided new insights into the extent and frequency of chromosome abnormalities in preimplantation embryos, which would have been missed, if only FISH was used for testing. CGH remains technically challenging and, in its current form, is likely to be performed in only a few laboratories that have appropriate skill and expertise in molecular biology. Better and quicker aCGH is more widely used and holds great promise. However, it is important to remember that aCGH technique cannot be used to test balanced translocations (reciprocal or Robertsonian translocations, inversions and insertions) and some unbalanced translocations like point mutations, trinucleotide expansions, small deletions and duplications because they are beyond the resolutions of the method. In such cases, NGS based testing may prove to be a valuable alternative. Further research is required for choosing the most optimal method for diagnosis of aberration, detection of mosaic samples, etc.

KEY POINTS

- PGD/PGS can be performed at any stage of embryo development in form of polar body biopsy, cleavage stage embryo biopsy and blastocyst biopsy. Based on the method chosen for establishing the diagnosis, you can do the same cycle transfer or and frozen transfer in a subsequent cycle.
- CGH and aCGH allow study of all 24 chromosomes as against FISH.
- aCGH can pick up structural chromosomal aberrations along with detection of aneuploidy.
- 24-chromosome analysis is associated with improved implantation rate and ongoing pregnancy rate.

■ REFERENCES

1. Alfarawati S, Fragouli E, Colls P, et al. First births after preimplantation genetic diagnosis of structural chromosome abnormalities using comparative genomic hybridization and microarray analysis. Hum Reprod. 2011;26(6):1560-74.
2. Ao A, Wells D, Handyside AH, et al. Preimplantation genetic diagnosis of inherited cancer: familial adenomatous polyposis coli. J Assist Reprod Genet. 1998;15(3):140-4.
3. Cohen J, Wells D, Munné S. Removal of 2 cells from cleavage stage embryos is likely to reduce the efficacy of chromosomal tests that are used to enhance implantation rates. Fertil Steril. 2007;87(3):496-503.
4. Wells D, Fragouli E. Preimplantation genetic diagnosis. In: Textbook of Clinical Embryology. Cambridge: Cambridge University Press; 2013.
5. Verlinsky Y, Ginsberg N, Lifchez A, et al. Analysis of the first polar body: preconception genetic diagnosis. Hum Reprod. 1990;5(7):826-9.
6. Grifo JA, Boyle A, Fischer E, et al. Preembryo biopsy and analysis of blastomeres by in situ hybridization. Am J Obstet Gynecol. 1990;163(6 Pt 1):2013-9.
7. Veiga A, Sandalinas M, Benkhalifa M, et al. Laser blastocyst biopsy for preimplantation diagnosis in the human. Zygote. 1997;5(4):351-4.
8. Saxena GS, Desai K, Shewale L, et al. Chromosomal aberrations in 2000 couples of Indian ethnicity with reproductive failure. Reprod Biomed Online. 2012;25(2):209-18.
9. Weiss M, Hermsen M, Meijer G, et al. Comparative genomic hybridization. Mol Pathol. 1999;52:243-51.
10. du Manoir S, Speicher MR, Joos S, et al. Detection of complete and partial chromosome gains and losses by comparative genomic in situ hybridization. Hum Genet. 1993;90(6):590-610.
11. Delhanty JD, Wells D. Preimplantation genetic diagnosis: an alternative to prenatal diagnosis. Expert Rev Mol Diagn. 2002 Sep;2(5):395-9.
12. Munné S. Preimplantation genetic diagnosis for aneuploidy and translocations using array comparative genomic hybridization. Curr Genom. 2012;13(6):463-70.
13. Brezina PR, Anchan R, Kearns WG. Preimplantation genetic testing for aneuploidy: what technology should you use and what are the differences? J Assist Reprod Genet. 2016;33(7):823-32.
14. Feichtinger M, Stopp T, Göbl C, et al. Increasing live birth rate by preimplantation genetic screening of pooled polar bodies using array comparative genomic hybridization. PLoS One. 2015;10(5):e0128317.
15. Rubio C, Rodrigo L, Mir P, et al. Use of array comparative genomic hybridization (array-CGH) for embryo assessment: clinical results. Fertil Steril. 2013;99:1044-8.
16. Greco E, Bono S, Ruberti A, et al. Comparative genomic hybridization selection of blastocysts for repeated implantation failure treatment: a pilot study. Biomed Res Int. 2014;2014:457913.
17. Yang Z, Zhang J, Salem SA, et al. Selection of competent blastocysts for transfer by combining time-lapse monitoring and array CGH testing for patients undergoing preimplantation genetic screening: a prospective study with sibling oocytes. BMC Med Genomics. 2014;7:38.

CHAPTER 35

Purpose of an Animal Laboratory in Research: Outcomes in the Avenue

Pratip Chakraborty, Sakuntala Banerji, Gunja Bose

■ INTRODUCTION

Research in biomedical science is required for improvement of the quality of human life. This improvement stems in part from progress in ameliorating human disease and disability, in part from advances in animal health, and in part from broadening our understanding of complex and intricately connected biological systems of human and animal physiology and its disorders. The *Animal House* must be registered with the Committee for the Purpose of Control and Supervision of Experiments on Animals (CPCSEA), Ministry of Environment and Forests, Govt. of India bearing a Registration number, e.g. 473/PO/Re/S/01CPCSEA and has an established Institutional Animal Ethics Committee (IAEC)[1] that advises the students, teachers/researchers on facilities, policies and practices concerning the care and use of animals. On a whole, the animal house facility should be available to boost the teaching, training and research facilities and to meet the growing demand for high quality laboratory animals in the ever-advancing field of reproductive endocrinology herein. The laboratory of Institute of Reproductive Medicine houses rats and mice. Each species of animals is housed in barrier maintained individual rooms to avoid disease transmission and interspecies conflicts. All efforts are made to maintain the animals under controlled environmental conditions [temperature (22–26°C), relative humidity (60 ± 10%), 12 hr alternate light and dark cycle] with 100% fresh air exchange in animal rooms and uninterrupted power and water supply as per the regulations of CPCSEA.[1]

■ ANIMAL LABORATORY AND ASSISTED REPRODUCTIVE TECHNIQUES

Last two decades there is an exponential growth of infertility clinics in India. However, the training of the assisted reproductive techniques (ART) personnel/s is not adequate at times. The need of an animal laboratory will establish to offer training for clinicians and embryologists in *advanced reproductive technologies*. The training team will include specialists in embryology who are able to culture animal oocytes into embryos and blastocysts and allied fields which will share their clinical expertise and knowledge to the students in the laboratory of the training and research institute. The clinical scientists who work in clinical embryology are involved in in-vitro fertilization (IVF) treatment and reproductive research and are known as clinical embryologists. In IVF, the job revolves around the collection of human eggs to preservation of gametes for future use. In line to understand the basics of human reproductive physiology, the ART workforce need to be trained through theoretical and practical understandings of human reproductive science such as reproductive biology, embryology, infertility, and different assisted reproductive procedure or techniques. At the same time the embryologists must keep themselves up to date with the legislations and regulations in applying their knowledge of these subjects. It is to be noted that animals used in research have short lifespan and reproduce quickly which means that researchers can test how a medicine interacts in a living organism over a whole lifetime or whether any effects are passed on to their offspring. Tests are now required to be done on pregnant animals, provided the permission from CPCSEA in the hope of preventing the diseases which may arise after pregnancy in case of human.

■ BENEFITS OF ANIMAL HOUSE LABORATORY

The fruits from animal house laboratory have acquired honor in the meetings of ESHRE and ASRM which dated from 2013 onwards. Meeting of ESHRE 2014 have witnessed the effect of maternal hyperhomocysteinemia (HHcy) on embryo quality in mice (Figs. 1 and 2).

As it is well known that HHcy reduces embryo mitochondrion membrane potential ($\Delta\psi m$), induces embryo endoplasmic reticulum (ER) stress condition and alters expressions of stress and development genes, we investigated on the future embryo quality in hyperhomocysteinemic mice. We established information on the mechanism by which homocysteine promotes poor embryo quality simultaneously increasing the understanding of the genetic pathways involved in the pathogenesis of HHcy (Figs. 1 and 2).[2]

A year later in 2016, we documented the report of overactivity of sFlt-1 in unexplained miscarriage which may switch on oxidative stress thereby initiating the intrinsic pathway for apoptosis simultaneously down regulating VEGF (Figs. 3A to C).[3]

Since, hyperhomocysteinemia, oxidative stress and thrombosis are inter-related, the directionality of the association was somewhat clear but still further studies of the molecular and cellular mechanisms underpinning the connection between disordered homocysteine metabolism and thrombosis are warranted.

The animal house of the institute received a project from Department of Sciences and Technology (DST), Govt. of India titled *"Exploration of molecular*

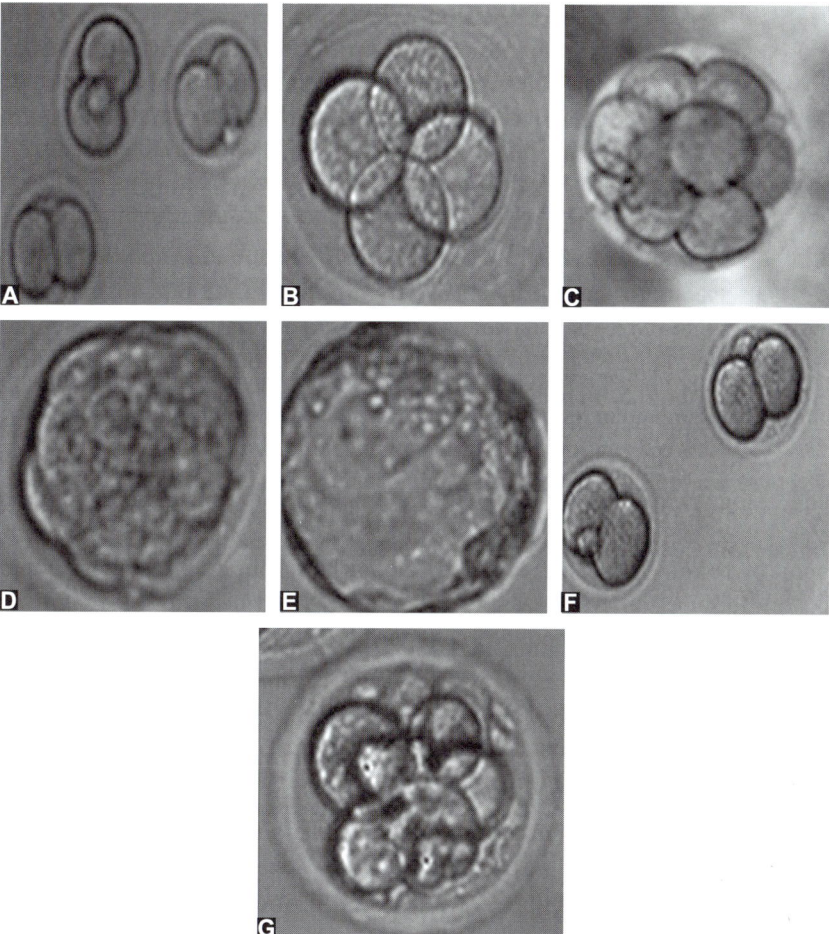

Figs. 1A to G: Effect of homocysteine on oocyte quality: imaging of in vitro fertilized mouse embryos at different stages of development with or without homocysteine (A) 2-cell, (B) 4-cell, (C) 8-cell, (D) compacted morula and (E) blastocyst in the control group. Homocysteine treatment resulted fragmented 4-cell embryo showing damage to embryonic development (G), however, no alteration at 2- cell stage (F). The scale bar indicates 100 mm.

cross-talk involved in the roadmap to hyperhomocysteinemia-induced pregnancy loss" which reported a pathway-based microarray approach (Fig. 5) to identify a distinct profile of miRNAs that carries signature to attest the pathway linking hyperhomocysteinemia-associated miscarriage (to be published). This is the first report that PKM2 is aberrantly expressed in miscarriage. The findings provide evidence that an oxidative stress-mediated placental damage perhaps represents the pathogenesis of hyperhomocysteinemia-associated pregnancy loss, which may pave the path toward development of pathway-based therapeutic options for recurrent miscarriage.[4]

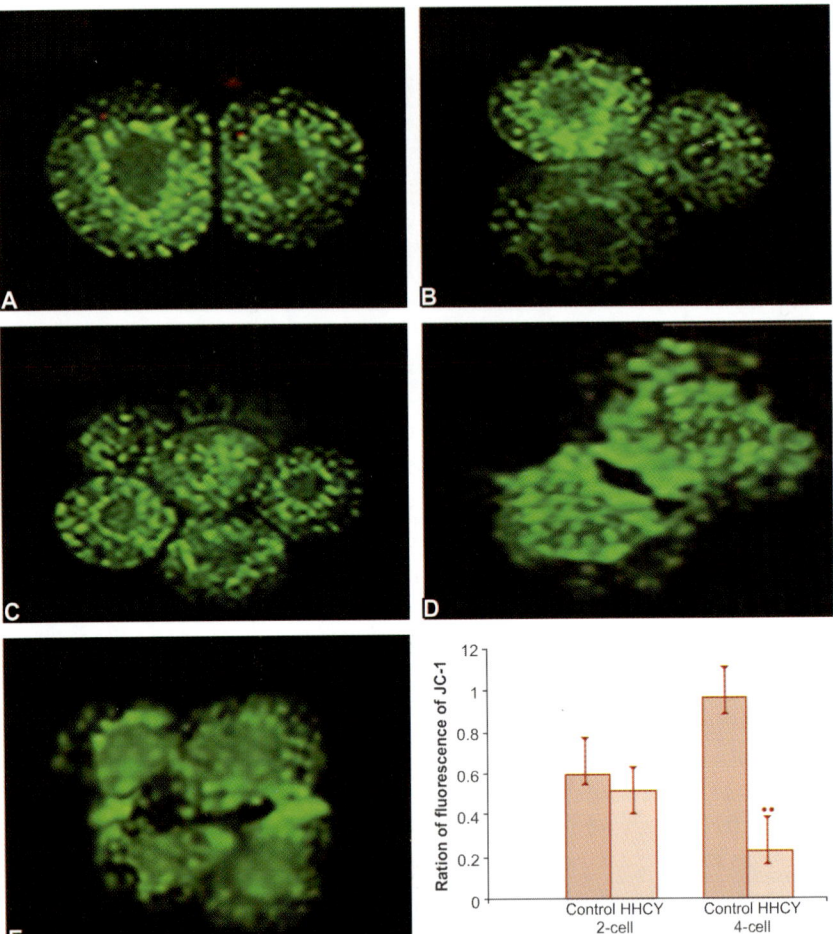

Figs. 2A to E: Effect of homocysteine on oocyte quality: representative images of mitochondrial membrane potential ($\Delta\Psi m$) in control (A to C) and hyperhomocysteinemic (D and E) embryos at different stages of development. The control set reveals cross-over of the dye over mitochondrial membrane and the staining is punctate. However, diffuse green cytoplasmic staining has been observed signifying no or very less $\Delta\Psi m$ at the 4-cell stage of the hyperhomocysteinemic set. Panels A to E were stained with JC-1 and images were captured at 529 nm. The scale bar indicates 100 µm. Ratio of JC-1 staining during mouse embryonic development. Above ratios were computed through obtaining a ratio of J-aggregate to J-monomer staining for five individual embryo section, averaged per embryo and then averaged among embryos from the same stage of development.

The role of culture media and cumulus cells in spontaneous maturation of zona-intact murine oocytes has been studied extensively.[5] Different workers have considered divergent aspects of IVM in mammalian oocytes.[6-8] However, in the majority of the studies, the basic medium is supplemented with varied

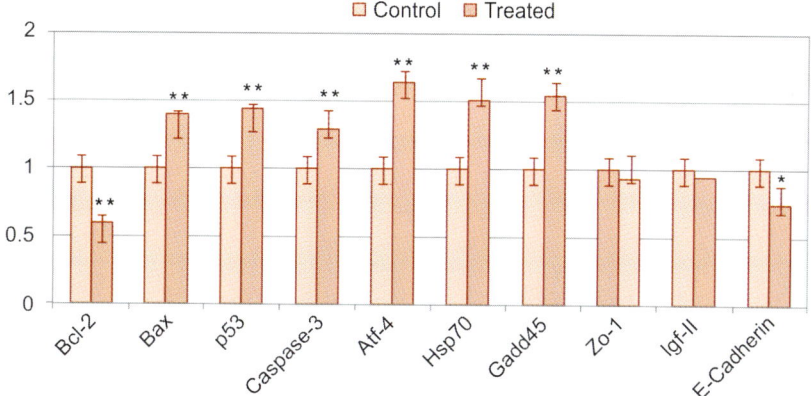

Fig. 2F: Effect of homocysteine on oocyte quality: qRT-PCR image/s of different stress related, developmental and apoptotic genes in the control and homocysteine treated cohort.

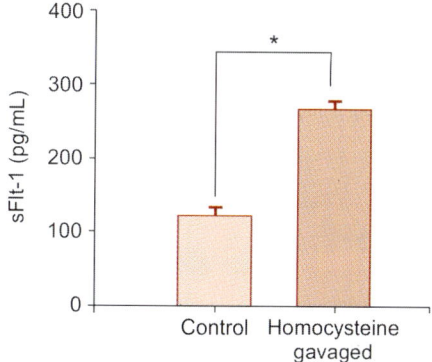

Fig. 3A: Elevated levels of sflt-1 may turn on the caspase cascade through downregulation of VEGF in hyperhomocysteinemia. The plasma sFlt-1 levels in homocysteine treated. A vs. B rats were significantly higher (p<0.0001) compared with those in control.

concentrations of hormones and serum. We have established a low cost IVM medium and assessed its efficacy in culturing the immature oocytes in a murine model in our animal house laboratory. Germinal vesicle breakdown (GVBD) of oocyte granulosa cell complexes (OGCs) have been achieved in 80% of IVM[7](equipped with protein factors extracted from human placenta) among which 70% reached up to fully mature Metaphase II stage and none was degenerated. 10% remained at Metaphase I (MI) stage. Fertilization rate was 60% altogether. This cues at the novelty of the culture medium as a support for growth and maturation (Figs. 6A to F).[9]

Beside basic research work, the animal house also gives ample chance to the fellow trainees and in-house doctors to handle and expertise themselves

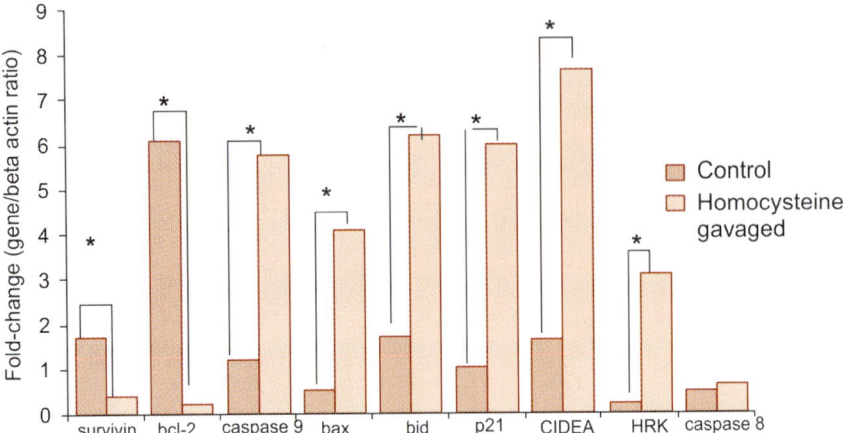

Fig. 3B: Elevated levels of sflt-1 may turn on the caspase cascade through downregulation of VEGF in hyperhomocysteinemia: Caspase cascade in the homocysteine treated pregnant female rat. While survivin and Bcl-2 were found to be downregulated, expressions of caspase9, Bax, Bid, p21, CIDEA, HRK were up-regulated by 3-fold. Dysregulated genes were revalidated by IHC as shown. (40X magnification; scale bar: 300 mm).

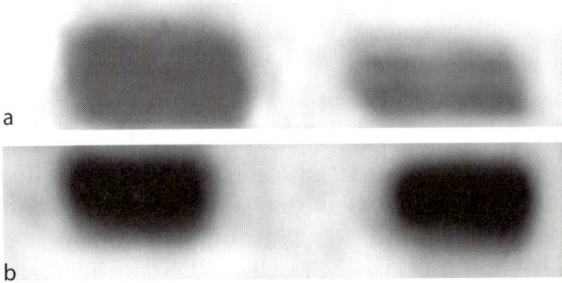

Fig. 3C: Elevated levels of sflt-1 may turn on the caspase cascade through downregulation of VEGF in hyperhomocysteinemia: Western blot analysis of VEGF in the placental tissues from saline-control; (a) homocysteine-treated, (b) pregnant rats. Immunoblot was quantified and expressed actin: $p<0.01$ as the densitometric ratio of VEGF/β-actin.

in rodent IVF and assisted reproduction. The students who want to be clinical embryologists cannot perform gamete collection, maintenance of viability of gametes, tissues and embryos, micromanipulation, cryopreservation, embryo culture and having knowledge of quality control, ethical issues and regulations surrounding gamete and embryo handling without training. During training period the students should involve themselves in clinical embryological work with mouse oocytes, experimental work and research studies in the animal laboratory (Figs. 7A and B).

Starting from the unicellular organisms, a variety of animal species contribute each year to medical breakthrough that save millions of human

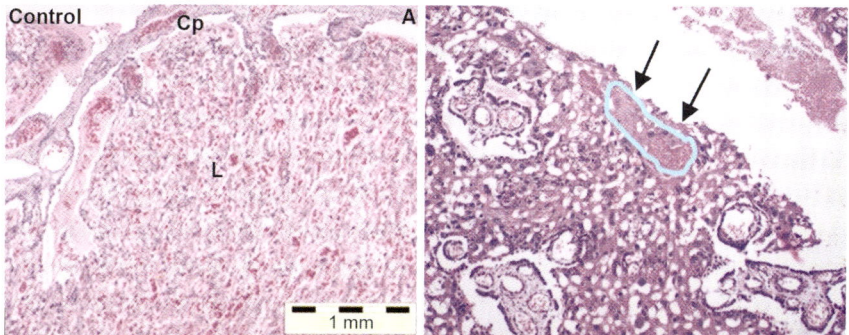

Fig. 4: Representative picture of placental histological observation by hematoxylin and eosin staining in GD18.5 in control (A) (n=5) and HHcy (B) (n=8) rat. Control placenta: normal labyrinth (L/Lab), chorionic plate (Cp); (H&E, 20×). Treated placenta: The histological observation showed the placental thrombus and atrophy of junctional zone in approximately 50% of hyperhomocysteinemic rats. (H&E, 20×). [Arrows: thrombi. Thrombus enlarged at junctional zone (H&E, 200×). Scale bars = 100 μm.]

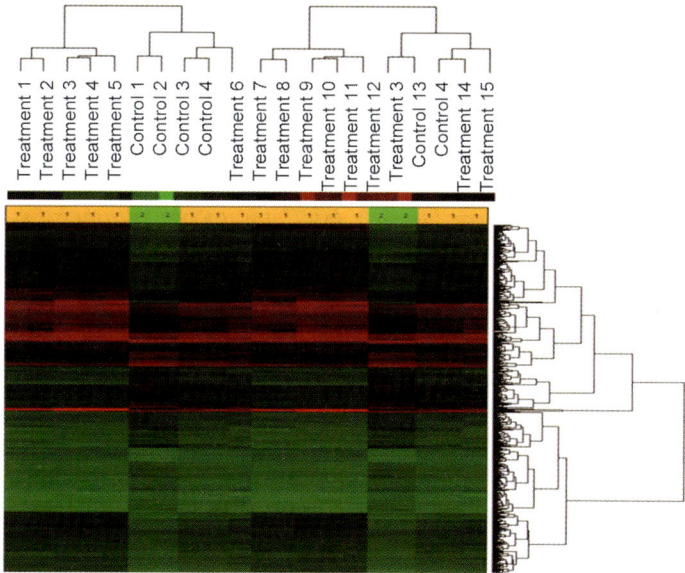

Fig. 5: Heat map illustration of phylogenetic tree of selected differentially selected genes. The genes (rows) and participants (columns) were grouped according to level and nature of gene expression and subjected to hierarchical tree clustering. The color code for signal strength in the classification scheme is as follows; induced genes are indicated by shades of red while repressed genes are indicated by shades of green. Black represents absent data.

lives each year. Through research on animals, scientists have discovered cues and preventions for a number of human and animal ailments. It is to be remembered, that fundamental principle is that animals must not be subjected

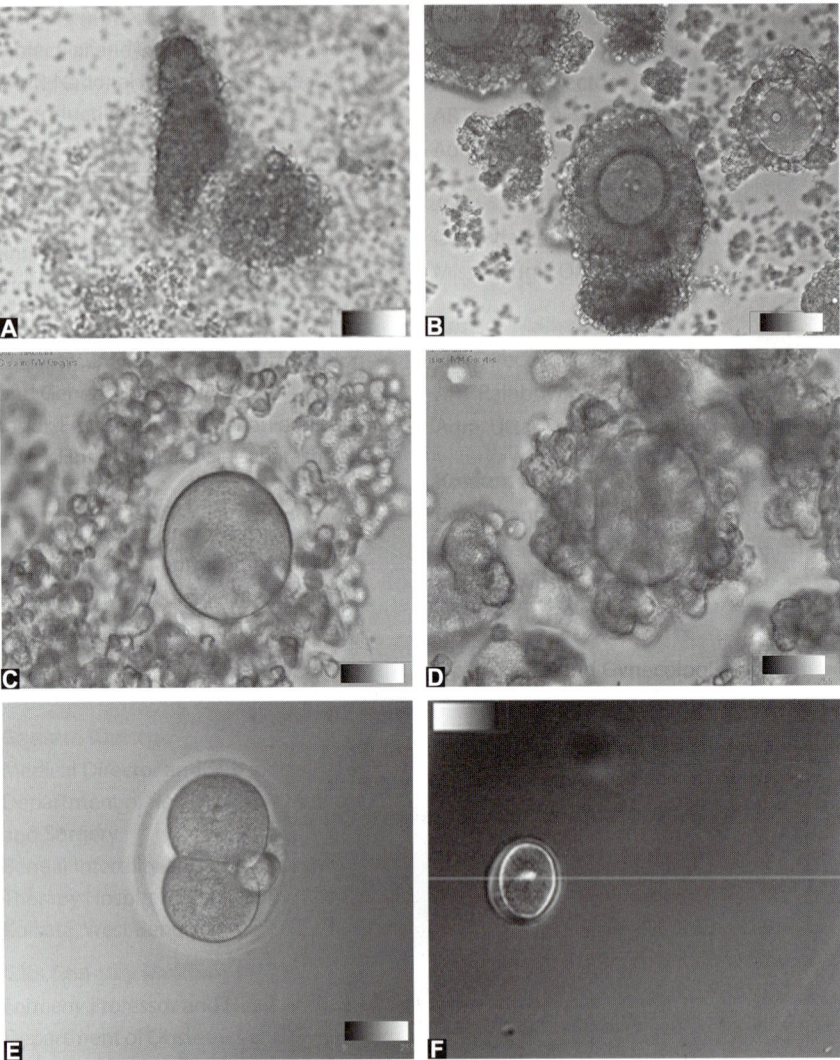

Figs. 6A to F: Steps of maturation of mice oocyte by in-vitro maturation medium prepared in the laboratory: (A) Immature GV stage at Diplotene stage of meiotic maturation; (B) GV stage oocytes with prominent nucleus in the center. The oocytes released some pregranulosa cells. (C) GVBD has taken place. The oocyte is at metaphase I with clear homogenous cytoplasm and no polar body. (D) Metaphase II oocyte matured in IVM7 medium (lab medium) with prominent Polar Body (PB) and homogeneous cytoplasm. (E) The oocytes matured in the media (IVM7) were inseminated (IVF) and 60% oocytes were fertilized and gave nice 2-cell embryos. (F) The intact spindle is shown by Oosight Meta Imaging System in an oocyte matured in IVM7, which indicates the good quality of the oocyte.

to avoidable distress or discomfort.[1] The other major responsibility of the animal house barring helping in research, is to ensure the persuasion of 3Rs of animal experimentation and the ethical principles of animal use are followed as per CPCSEA guidelines.

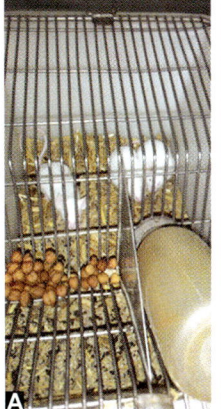
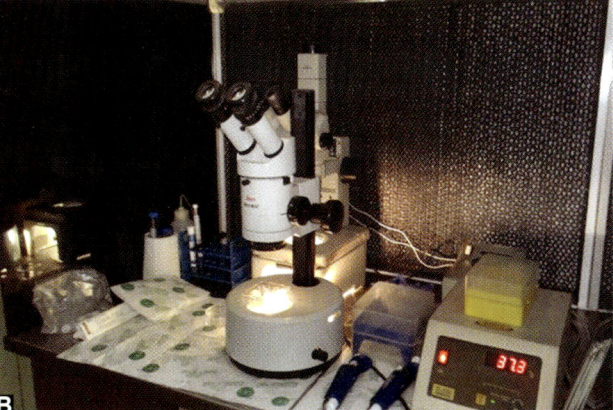

Figs. 7A and B: (A) Animal incubation in animal laboratory; (B) Oocyte identification in animal laboratory.

KEY POINTS

- Research in biomedical science is required for improvement of the quality of human life.
- Fundamental principle is to ensure the persuasion of 3Rs of animal experimentation and the ethical principles of animal use are followed as per CPCSEA guidelines during research so that the animals must not be subjected to avoidable distress or discomfort.
- If properly nurtured, the animal house of an establishment can give rewarding academic results as well as help the clinician/s to perform the diagnosis in any particular pathology.

REFERENCES

1. CPCSEA guidelines for laboratory animal facility. Ind J Pharmacol. 2003;35:257.
2. Chakraborty P, Yasmin S, Chattopadhyay R, et al. Effect of maternal hyperhomocysteinemia on embryo quality in mice. Hum Reprod. 2014;29:177-8.
3. Chakraborty P, Yasmin S, Goswami SK, et al. Hyperhomocysteinemia induced soluble fms-like tyrosine kinase over-activity leads to pregnancy loss in rats. Hum Reprod. 2016;30:187.
4. Chakraborty P, Banerjee S, Chatterjee S, et al. Attenuated pyruvate kinase M2 signaling pathway: the missing link in hyperhomocysteinemia-associated pregnancy loss. Hum Reprod. 2017;29:86.
5. Miao LY, Liu YX, Wu-T Q, et al. Cumulus cells accelerate aging of mouse oocytes. Biol Reprod. 2015;73:1025-31.
6. Wani NA. In vitro maturation and in vitro fertilization of sheep oocytes. Small Rumin Res. 2002;44:9-95.
7. Roa BS, Naidu KS, Amarnath D, et al. In vitro maturation of sheep oocytes in different media during breeding and non-breeding seasons. Small Rumin Res. 2002;43:31-6.
8. Kharche SD, Sharma GT, Majumdar AC. In vitro maturation and fertilization of goat oocytes vitrified at germinal vesicle stage. Small Rumin Res. 2005;57:81-4.
9. Banerji S, Chakraborty P, Debnath SS, et al. Development of a new in vitro maturation media to culture the immature mouse oocyte. Afr J Biotech (accepted). 2017.

CHAPTER 36

Third-Party Reproduction: From Embryologist's Point of View

Nivedita Shetty, Suparna Banerjee, Debhashree Ganguly, Srinivas MS

■ INTRODUCTION

The word "third-party reproduction" refers to involving someone other than the individual or couple who is planning to raise the child by the process of assisted reproductive technology (ART). This involves using donated eggs, sperm, or embryos and gestational-carrier arrangements, in which the pregnancy is carried by someone other than the intended parents. Surrogacy, also sometimes referred to as traditional gestational carrier, is a particular type of gestational-carrier arrangement where the woman who carries the pregnancy also provides the egg. Unless specifically indicated, the term gestational carrier in this chapter will refer to a woman who carries a pregnancy, but has no genetic link to the fetus.

Third-party reproduction can be socially, ethically, and legally complex. As egg donation has become more common, there has been a reconsideration of the social and ethical impact—this technology has had on prospective parents, their offspring, and the egg donors themselves. Surrogacy arrangements are controversial, and are subject to both legal and psychosocial scrutiny. This chapter will discuss the options for third-party reproduction, reviewing sperm donation, egg donation, embryo donation, and gestational-carrier arrangements.

■ DEFINITION

Third-party reproduction refers to a process, where a third person, other than the couple, provides sperm or eggs or *embryos* or where another woman provides her uterus, in order to help them reproduce.

However, the third-party's involvement is limited to the reproductive process and does not extend into the raising of the child.

It involves the following:
1. Sperm donation
2. Egg donation

3. Embryo donation
4. Surrogacy.

SOURCING THE DONORS AND SURROGATES

Types of donors in general:
1. Volunteer donors *(donation without financial reward—altruistic)*
2. Commercial donors *(donation with monetary compensation)*
3. Known donors *(donation to known recipients).*

Oocyte donors can be of two variants:

1. *Patient donors*: They enter an agreement with the infertility clinic to donate a proportion of their oocytes to others, in order to receive subsidized infertility treatment.
2. *Nonpatient donors*:
   – Volunteer donors
   – Known donors
   – Commercial donors.

SPERM DONATION

- Indications
- Evaluation of the sperm donor
- Evaluating the recipient couple.

Indications for Donor Insemination[1]

- The male partner has azoospermia or severe oligoasthenospermia and not willing for intracytoplasmic sperm injection (ICSI).
- The male partner has ejaculatory dysfunction [if not willing for testicular sperm aspiration (TESA) and ICSI].
- The male partner has a significant genetic defect.
- The male partner has a sexually transmissible infection that cannot be eradicated as in human immunodeficiency virus (HIV) (*relative indication as with ICSI the risk of transmission is very low*).
- The female partner is Rh-negative and severely Rh-isoimmunized, and the male partner is Rh-positive.
- Females without male partners, though in India the current draft (2014) of the ART bill, require the couple to be married for ART treatment.

Evaluation of the Donor—Evaluate for a Healthy Donor and Absence of Genetic Abnormalities

- Normal semen analyses.
- Screening for HIV, hepatitis B antigen, hepatitis C and venereal disease research laboratory (VDRL). After donation, anonymous donor specimens

must be quarantined for a minimum of 180 days. The donor must be retested after the required quarantine interval, and specimens may be released only if the results of repeat testing are negative.
- Genetic evaluation—detailed *personal and family history* for genetic disorders especially in parents, siblings and offsprings.

Some centers perform *karyotyping and genetic screening* according to ethnic background. In the north and certain western regions of India, thalassemia screening of donors is a must. The American Society for Reproductive Medicine (ASRM) guidelines recommend routine screening for cystic fibrosis carrier status in donors.

Evaluating the Recipient Couple

- Male partner—HIV, hepatitis B antigen, hepatitis C and VDRL.
- Female partner—HIV, hepatitis B antigen, hepatitis C and VDRL.

EGG DONATION

- Indications
- Evaluating the oocyte recipient and partner
- Evaluating the oocyte donor
- High success rate with donor programs
- Commercial egg banking.

Indications[2]

- Premature ovarian failure
- Iatrogenic ovarian failure due to ovarian surgery or radiation
- Menopause
- Risk of inheritable disease in child
- Poor responders or poor quality oocytes.

Evaluating the Oocyte Recipient and Partner

- Obtain informed consent from recipient and partner
- Semen analyses for the male partner
- Infection screening for both partners—sexual history, HIV, hepatitis B antigen, hepatitis C virus (HCV), VDRL.

Evaluating the Oocyte Donor

- Screening the donor for HIV, hepatitis B antigen, HCV, VDRL.

High Success Rate with Donor Programs[3,4]

- The *donor's age* is one of the most significant factors contributing to the high success rate. The recipient's age does not necessarily contribute to the prognosis.

- The most reliable predictive factors for pregnancy in oocyte donation cycles are the quality of the embryos and the recipient's midcycle endometrial thickness.
- The main reason for high pregnancy rates is the ovaries are not stimulated and hence the absence of very high estrogen levels affecting the endometrial receptivity.[3]

Egg Banking

- The first human birth from frozen sperm was reported in 1963[5,6]
- The first human birth from a frozen embryo was reported in 1984[7]
- In 1986, the first human birth from a frozen oocyte was reported.[8]

However, it is only now that, oocyte freezing is *no longer considered experimental*.[9]

The improved efficiency in oocyte freezing has made the concept of egg banking, as in sperm banking, a possibility.

Disadvantages to Fresh Oocyte Donation
- Long waiting lists due to difficulty in sourcing the donor
- Limited choice of donor
- No quarantine period (HIV and others infectious agents) as in sperm donation
- Supernumerary embryos cryostorage which increases the workload of the egg bank.

This improved efficiency in egg freezing combined with the disadvantages of fresh oocyte donation, has led to the emergence of a new phenomenon: "commercial egg banks (CEBs)",[10] although, still at an infantile stage in India.

- The reported pregnancy rate per oocyte was 7.5% using vitrification.
- The recommendation is to obtain a minimum of 6 oocytes (range of 4–7) per recipient considering oocyte survival on thawing, fertilization and cleavage.

ART GUIDELINES FOR DONOR GAMETES—2014 DRAFT[3]

- Known donors for either oocyte or sperm are not permitted.
- The ART clinics shall obtain donor gametes from ART banks only.
- Screening of gamete donors and surrogates; the collection, screening and storage of semen; and provision of oocyte donor and surrogates, shall be done by an ART bank.
- Nonspecific information in respect of donor of gametes including *height, weight, ethnicity, skin color, educational qualifications, medical history of the donor, including HIV/AIDS* should be provided but specific information like *identity* and *address* not to be provided. The age of the sperm donor should be between 21 years and 45 years of age.[3]
- The age of the oocyte donor should be between 23 years and 35 years of age.[3]
- Semen sample should be quarantined for at least 6 months before being used.

- The sperm of a single donor should not be used more than 25 times.
- The sperm donor, if married, requires the consent of his spouse.
- Mixing of semen from two individuals is not permitted.
- Oocytes from one donor can be shared between two recipients only provided that at least 7 oocytes are available for each recipient.

■ SURROGACY[11-14]

Surrogacy refers to a contract in which woman carries a pregnancy for another couple.

Terminologies[14]

- *Genetic couple or commissioning couple*—the couple who provides both sets of gametes or at least one set of gametes.
- *Surrogate*—the woman receiving the embryos created by the gametes of the genetic couple.
- *Traditional surrogacy*—in this situation the gestational carrier not only carries the pregnancy but also provides the oocytes. *This is not approved by the current ART guidelines in India.*
- *Gestational surrogacy*—in this situation the surrogate only carries the pregnancy and does not provide the gametes.
- *Commercial surrogacy*—when the surrogacy is paid for in addition to her medical expenses. This is not permitted in India according to the surrogacy (regulation) bill 2016.
- *Altruistic surrogacy*—when the surrogate is paid only for her medical expenses.

Indications for Surrogacy

- Absence of uterus.
- Presence of uterus with
  - Repeated miscarriages
  - Repeated implantation failure
  - Untreatable Asherman's syndrome.
- Medical conditions which make pregnancy life threatening.

Screening the Genetic Couple for Surrogacy

- Semen analyses and infection screening for the couple.

Screening the Surrogate

- Age—current guidelines—between 23 years and 35 years.
- Married and have at least a child of her own and also have consent of the spouse.
- Screen for infectious diseases—HIV, HBsAg, HCV, VDRL.

Taking consent from the surrogate and the commissioning couple along with the clinician.

ART Guidelines for Surrogacy—2014 Draft

- The commissioning couple and the surrogate shall enter into a surrogacy agreement.
- All expenses during pregnancy and delivery to be borne by the commissioning couple.
- The surrogate may also receive monetary compensation from the commissioning couple, for agreeing to act as surrogate.
- Surrogate mother should be a married Indian woman between 23 years and 35 years of age and shall have at least one live child of her own with minimum age of 3 years.
- No woman shall act as a surrogate for more than one successful live birth in her life and with not less than 2 years interval between two deliveries.
- Surrogacy for foreigners in India shall not be allowed but surrogacy shall be permissible to Overseas Citizen of India (OCI), People of Indian Origin (PIO), Non-Resident Indians (NRIs) and foreigner married to an Indian citizen.
- A commissioning couple shall not have the service of more than one surrogate at any given time.
- A couple shall not have simultaneous transfer of embryos in the woman and in a surrogate.
- A surrogate shall not act as an oocyte donor for the couple, as the case may be, commissioning surrogacy.

Surrogacy (Regulation) Bill 2016, as Introduced in the Lok Sabha

The salient features of the bill are:
1. To allow only altruistic ethical surrogacy to intending infertile couple.
2. The infertile couple should be between the age of 23–50 years and 26–55 years for female and male, respectively.
3. The intending couples should be legally married for at least 5 years.
4. The intending couple should be Indian citizens.
5. The intending couples have not had any surviving child biologically or through adoption or through surrogacy earlier except when they have a child and who is mentally or physically challenged or suffer from life-threatening disorder with no permanent cure.
6. The intending couples shall not abandon the child, born out of a surrogacy procedure under any condition.
7. The child born through surrogacy will have the same rights as are available for the biological child.
8. The surrogate mother should be a close relative of the intending couple and should be between the age of 25 years and 35 years.
9. She can act as surrogate mother only once.

GLOOM OF THIRD-PARTY REPRODUCTION

The needy infertile couple achieves their goal of having child by outsourcing the gametes, which is known as third-party reproduction. Third-party reproduction is a process wherein sperm or egg or embryo or uterus is obtained by third person other than infertile couple.

We have seen couple holding adorable infants created by third-party reproduction by means of ARTs. But one has to agree that third-party reproduction hides the highly profit making ART industry's bad secrets. Definitely it ignores what is required to create babies by third-party reproduction that is exploitation, risking the woman health who is donating the eggs. Hence, there must be honest look at surrounding the third-party reproduction before this is being considered to carry out in any organization.

EXPLOITATION OF WOMAN DONATING THE EGGS

Third-party reproduction involves procurement of gametes that is eggs from the woman and sperms by men. These gametes are artificially inseminated in the embryology laboratory in order to obtain the embryos. The embryos obtained by this method in the embryology laboratory can be cultured till blastocyst stage; thereafter, blastocyst must be transferred to the uterus of surrogate mother. When the pregnancy takes place, woman must gestate and give birth to the healthy baby. To carry out this entire procedure outside the human body by using medium made up of so many chemical and using an appropriate technology in order to get good quality embryos. Here, biology is not exactly fair, because semen is obtained through the process called male ejaculation, but it is a radically different situation when we wish to extract eggs from the superovulating ovaries. Here, woman donating the eggs must visit the ART unit daily to get administered painful injections of carcinogenic synthetic hormones and other drugs followed by operative procedure to retrieve the eggs from the well grown follicles of the ovary.

Generally during female menstrual cycle one or two eggs are produced, but during third-party reproduction more number of eggs will be obtained so there is eggs ploitation that is superovulating the ovary unnaturally, so that more number of eggs harvested from the healthy young woman. Obtaining embryos is not enough, we need to find out surrogate mother who will gestate and give birth to baby. She also undergoes similar regimen of painful procedure to prepare her body for implantation and gestation. All these events like egg donors and surrogates are subjected to short- and long-term health risks. The short-term risks are ovarian hyperstimulation syndrome (OHSS) characterized by difficulty in breathing, pelvic pains, swelling of limbs, severe abdomen pain, nausea, vomiting, weight gain, low urine output. Other short-term risks are ruptured cysts, ovarian torsions, blood clots, chronic pelvic pain, premature menopause and kidney failure.

The long-term risks include cancer, especially reproductive-ovarian, breast, or endometrial cancers and future infertility. Both egg donors and surrogate mothers will receive the Lupride injection which is known to pose side effects. Lupride also puts women at risk of intracranial pressure.

■ REGULATIONS AND THIRD-PARTY REPRODUCTION

There are no regulations for the ART industry to carry out third-party reproduction. However, guidelines are there and one has to follow this voluntarily. For this reason, it has become a popular destination for international fertility tourism. In India, initially third-party reproduction was allowed for all, but now it is only for Indians. Guidelines that are strictly voluntary and therefore unenforceable, for example woman should not undergo not more than 3–5 cycles of ovarian stimulation, yet woman may undergo more than what is mentioned in the guideline. There are no national registries to track the health of the women who sell their eggs or rent their womb as surrogates. After the procedure done, she is forgotten, even though she may suffer serious long-term health consequences. The most concerning is that there are not many peer-reviewed medical research studies on the long-term health safety effects of egg hyperstimulation or surrogacy.

What about the child produced by third-party reproduction? Women who have donated the eggs or became surrogate get rights of protection but the child born out of this method have absolutely none. For the sake of donor's privacy, the children do not have right to get information about their genetic history.

A 2001 study in the journal Human Reproduction concludes. "Disclosure to children conceived with donor gametes should be optional". This study extends strong support to the international response to the United Nations Convention on the Rights of the Child. This was mostly rapidly sighted human rights convention in the United Nations history. One of the fundamental rights included in the convention is the right to know one's parents. In the debate about donor/seller anonymity, this has been expressed as the Child's right to know the identity of his or her genetic parents. The increased knowledge and changing lifestyle may enable young people to have more strong moral claims to know their genetic identities. In future, these moral claims may be converted to legal rights.

■ REFERENCES

1. Practice Committee of American Society for Reproductive Medicine; Practice Committee of Society for Assisted Reproductive Technology. 2008 Guidelines for Gamete and Embryo Donation: A Practice Committee Report. Fertil Steril. 2008;90:S30-44.
2. The Assisted Reproductive Technology (Regulation) Bill, 2014. Government of India, Ministry of Health and Family Welfare, Department of Health Research.

3. Patki A, Sharma A. Oocyte and embryo donation. In: Rao K (Ed). Principles and Practice of Assisted Reproductive Technology (Vol. 1: Infertility). New Delhi: Jaypee Brothers Medical Publishers (P) Ltd.; 2014. pp. 791-7.
4. Noyes N, Hampton BS, Berkeley A, et al. Factors useful in predicting the success of oocyte donation: a 3-year retrospective analysis. Fertil Steril. 2001;76(1):92-7.
5. Sherman JK. Improved methods of preservation of human spermatozoa by freezing and freeze drying. Fertil Steril. 1963;14:49-64.
6. Trounson A, Mohr L. Human pregnancy following cryopreservation thawing and transfer of an eight cell embryo. Nature. 1983;305:707-9.
7. Chen C. Pregnancy after human oocyte cryopreservation. Lancet. 1986;1(8486): 884-6.
8. Practice Committees of American Society for Reproductive Medicine; Society for Assisted Reproductive Technology. Mature oocyte cryopreservation: a guideline. Fertil Steril. 2013;99:37-43.
9. Quaas AM, Melamed A, Chung K, et al. Egg banking in the United States: current status of commercially available cryopreserved oocytes. Fertil Steril. 2013;99: 827-31.
10. Cobo A, Meseguer M, Remohi J, et al. Use of cryo-banked oocytes in an ovum donation programme: a prospective, randomized, controlled, clinical trial. Hum Reprod. 2010;25:2239-46.
11. Potdar N, Gelbaya TA, Nardo LG. Oocyte vitrification in the 21st century and post-warming fertility outcomes: a systematic review and meta-analysis. Reprod Biomed Online. 2014;29:159-76.
12. Parmegiani L, Garello C, Granella F, et al. Long-term cryostorage does not adversely affect the outcome of oocyte thawing cycles. Reprod Biomed Online. 2009;19:374-9.
13. Goldman KN, Kramer Y, Hodes-Wertz B, et al. Long-term cryopreservation of human oocytes does not increase embryonic aneuploidy. Fertil Steril. 2015;103(3):662-8.
14. Malhotra J, Malhotra N, Patel N, et al. Surrogacy. In: Rao K (Ed). Principles and Practice of Assisted Reproductive Technology (Vol. 1: Infertility). New Delhi: Jaypee Brothers Medical Publishers (P) Ltd.; 2014. pp. 807-18.

CHAPTER 37

Understanding of ART Laboratory Work from Clinicians Point of View

Sunita Sharma, Gita Ganguly Mukherjee

■ INTRODUCTION

The in vitro fertilization (IVF) laboratory essentially takes over the role of a mother's womb in terms of being the environment for the growing embryo. It is the place where gametes and embryos are nurtured. The live birth rate following assisted reproductive technology (ART) has steadily improved from less than 1% to roughly 40% in 40 years. This has been possible due to better understanding of the biology of gametes and embryos which has guided the designing of better stimulation protocols, optimum culture conditions, and methods of cryopreservation. ART is a complex procedure with multiple factors affecting its outcome. Standardization of ART practices can decrease the variability in IVF outcome. The clinician in an ART clinic decides the best protocol for that patient based on the clinical parameters of the patient. Besides clinical practices, issues pertaining both to ART laboratory and to the personnel are critical in determining IVF success. A proper coordination of the clinician, embryologist, ART nurses, and paramedical staff is needed. This chapter focuses mainly on the importance of the clinician in the ART laboratory, how much he or she should know about the laboratory procedures and how to provide clinical decisions during trouble shooting situations.

■ AIM OF ART LABORATORY

An ART laboratory is one of the most important components in the treatment of an infertile couple seeking IVF. It comprises of various clinical treatments and laboratory procedures, including handling and manipulation of gametes and embryos. ART procedures include IVF, intracytoplasmic sperm injection (ICSI), preimplantation genetic diagnosis (PGD), gametes, and embryo cryopreservation. In human IVF, gametes and embryos are very fastidious in their requirement. There is a considerable awareness that the environment of the laboratory itself can alter the quality of the embryos and requires a multidisciplinary approach to optimize ART result. Therefore, the ART program should focus on generation of top quality embryos by optimizing embryo development milieu, selection of best quality embryo, and development of optimum cryopreservation methods for gametes and embryos.[1,2]

■ SERVICES OF ART LABORATORY

An ART laboratory offers the following services (Fig. 1):
- It offers semen analysis, sperm functional tests, semen preparation, and cryopreservation. It also provides donor semen and cryopreservation facilities to oncology patients. Surgical sperm retrieval procedure (epididymal and testicular sperm aspirations or testicular sperm extraction) is done and sample is assessed by embryologist for ICSI and/or cryopreservation.
- During the oocyte retrieval, the aspirated follicular fluid is handed over to the embryology team from which oocytes are separated and cultured. Depending upon the quality of semen sample, the oocytes are either inseminated or injected and incubated.
- Manipulation of oocytes, sperms, assessment of quality of oocytes, zygotes, and embryo (day 2/day 3 and blastocysts) is done to prepare them for transfer or cryopreservation.
- Good quality embryos are selected and loaded into transfer catheters for embryo transfer (ET) and clinician does the transfer.
- In the presence of thick zona pellucida or in couples with repeated implantation failures assisted hatching may be considered.
- Preimplantation genetic diagnosis may be offered to prevent serious inherited diseases and preimplantation genetic screening (PGS) for aneuploidy screening in recurrent implantation failures.

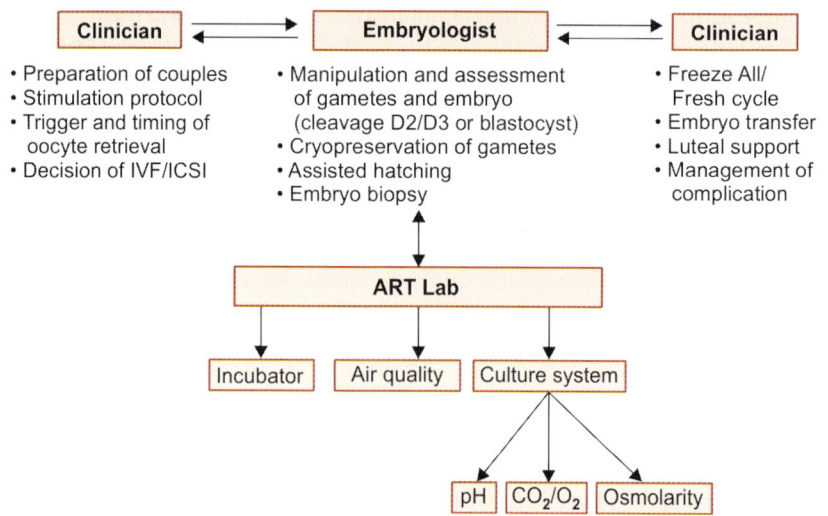

Fig. 1: Combination of clinical and laboratory perspective.
(IFV: in vitro fertilization; ICSI: intracytoplasmic sperm injection; ART: assisted reproductive technology)

Understanding of ART Laboratory Work from Clinicians Point of View

- Documentation and maintenance of records and results of all laboratory procedures are mandatory.

An ART clinician is a gynecologist who has interest in infertility and reproductive endocrinology and has knowledge in the hormonal control of the menstrual cycle and use of ovulation inducing agents. The responsibilities of the clinician would include the following:

- Initial history taking of the infertile couple
- Physical examination of the couple and advice of appropriate investigations
- Interpretation of results and treating them accordingly—either, expected management or carrying out procedures like intrauterine insemination (IUI), IVF, and ICSI.
- Pretreatment surgical procedures and surgical procedures before planning ART (for conditions like hydrosalpinx, polyp, fibroid, septum, and endometrioma)
- Proper record keeping.

Clinician in the IVF laboratory engages in a cycle of activities beyond the realm of clinical ART procedures. To name of a few such activities include consultation with the clinical embryologist and staff about the patient's treatment plan, ensuring that appropriate procedures are done, and proper identification of the patient or patient's specimens.

Along with preparation of the patient for IVF, the clinician should also have a thorough understanding of the laboratory equipment, culture medium, disposables, sterile culture conditions, and quality control of the laboratory equipment.

As the gametes and embryos are exposed to plastic wares with culture media within the incubator for most of the time, pH and temperature affects the embryo quality and thus the pregnancy rate. The clinician should be aware of the basic principles on which an incubator works. Knowledge of CO_2 and temperature calibration, pressure setting of CO_2 gas cylinder, the need to frequently clean the incubator, and change the water are also important. He should also make sure that in cases of power failure, the CO_2 incubator should have a backup power supply. The knowledge of the pressure settings for the flow, frequency for change of high efficiency particulate air (HEPA) filter, and the frequency for servicing of the unit is mandatory.

The basic operation of the micromanipulator along with the frequency of servicing, changing of lamp in case it burns out, is important to know. The clinician should know the method to focus the microscope and setting up of pipettes.

The clinician should have an idea of the different components of the culture media and the factors on which selection of proper media is done for each procedure like oocyte collection, sperm preparation, micromanipulation, embryo culture, blastocyst culture, freezing of sperm, and oocyte and embryo freezing (Fig. 2). It is also important to store the culture media properly by monitoring the temperature using thermometers in refrigerators and freezers.

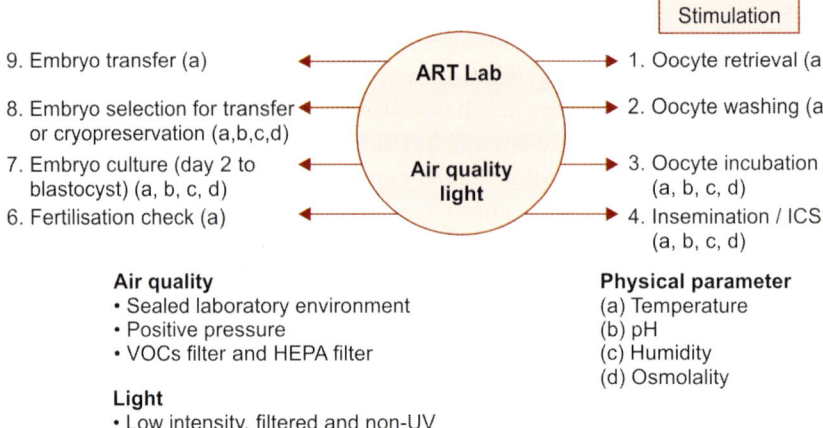

Fig. 2: Assisted reproductive technology laboratory procedures and control of physical parameters.
(ICSI: intracytoplasmic sperm injection; VOC: volatile organic chemical; HEPA: high efficiency particulate air; UV: ultraviolet)

It is important for a doctor to pay attention towards IVF laboratory cleanliness—the need for cleaning the IVF laboratory daily with a proper disinfectant that is nontoxic and odorless; CO_2 incubator cleanliness—regular cleaning and disinfection of CO_2 incubator; and asepsis while handling the gametes and embryos—washing of hands properly before handling the dishes containing embryos and wearing gloves while preparing the dishes and handling the culture medium. The clinician should change the cloth and slippers, cover hair, and put mask before entering the IVF laboratory.

Each ART laboratory should develop standard operating procedure (SOP) manuals in writing which should have a detailed description of the various procedures carried out in the laboratory step-by-step. While designing SOPs, the clinician should make sure that it addresses different clinical conditions and whether it can provide solutions in crisis situations.

How can Ovarian Stimulation Influence Laboratory Performance?

A clinician should know that a good stimulation with follicles more than 14 mm is expected to yield a well-expanded cumulus oophorus complex (COC) with higher number of MII oocytes whereas poor stimulation because of excess or suboptimal doses of gonadotropins or timing of trigger may result in abnormal COC morphology and fertilization and increased rate of aneuploidy. Age negatively affects the pregnancy rates in ART cycles, but as it is a nonmodifiable factor, we should pay more attention while designing our management strategies. Alpha and ESHRE surveys have shown that oocyte retrieval rate and oocyte maturation rate are important markers for quality of oocyte.[3] The optimum trigger to oocyte retrieval time is 34–38 hours. Higher oocyte maturation rate was observed more than 36 hours compared to less than 36 hours but fertilization rates and pregnancy rates were found to be similar.[4] So the response to ovarian stimulation is closely linked to the maturity and competence of the oocyte.

A Number of MII oocytes retrieved depend on the quality of stimulation (KPI) and presence of other pathologies like polycystic ovary syndrome and endometriosis. When we are dealing with women having endometrioma, there is a chance of mixing of endometrioma fluid with the oocyte which is detrimental to the oocyte quality. Embryologist should hence be careful while washing these oocytes.

The clinician and embryologist should have information regarding the clinical (dose of gonadotropin used, number of follicles developed, and IVF/ICSI) and embryology records (number of MII oocytes retrieved, number of good quality embryos, cleavage stage or blastocyst transfer, fresh or frozen transfer) of previous IVF cycles. So good communication about cycle planning and review of records between the ART laboratory and the clinician is crucial for successful IVF program (Von Vorheiss-KPI).

LABORATORY PROCEDURES AND SPERM PARAMETERS

There should be no specific cut-offs for semen characteristics to decide the procedure for the couple—IUI, IVF, and ICSI. A pretreatment "trial wash" will decide the definite procedure. The clinic should develop its own semen cut-off levels for deciding the treatment (Fig. 2).

Retrograde Ejaculation

This is a condition in which semen is released into the bladder during ejaculation. Medical management, urinary sperm retrieval, and surgical sperm retrieval (percutaneous epididymal sperm aspiration and testicular sperm aspiration) exist for the treatment of retrograde ejaculation. Post-orgasmic urine sample is collected either after voiding or after catheterization following alkalinization of the urine with oral sodium bicarbonate or increasing fluid intake. This specimen is then resuspended, centrifuged, checked for count and motility and accordingly used for the selected procedure either IUI, IVF, or ICSI.[5]

Nonobstructive Azoospermia

There are reports of presence of ejaculated sperm after letrozole in NOA patient.[6-8] For this group of patients, if semen analysis is done on the day of oocyte pickup, we can avoid unnecessary sperm retrieval procedure. In cases of primary testicular failure with NOA, medical treatment [clomiphene and human chorionic gonadotropin (hCG) or human menopausal gonadotropin] in men with NOA can improve surgical sperm retrieval.[9]

Assessment of Oocyte and Embryo

Of the oocytes retrieved for ART following ovarian stimulation, only 5% results in live birth.[10] Embryologist can select oocyte with good development competence by observing the expansion of cumulus in relation to COCs[11] and excluding cytoplasmic or extracytoplasmic anomalies such as increased cytoplasmic granularity, vacuolization, abnormality of first polar body, perivitelline space or zona pellucida. Presence of meiotic spindle and its position, observed with polarized light can also predict functionally superior oocyte.[12] Although, these criteria are not enough to select an oocyte with higher developmental competence, knowledge of such findings helps the clinician to modify stimulation protocol in subsequent cycle in cases of unexpected increase in abnormal oocyte.[13] Therefore, assessment of oocyte maturity is the combined work of both clinician dealing with ovarian reserve and stimulation protocol and the embryologist doing the morphological assessment of oocyte.

In routine practice, morphological assessment of pronuclear and embryo stage is considered gold standard to select embryo with higher implantation potential. Combination of several morphological criteria of embryo like symmetry of blastomeres, extent of fragmentation, multinucleation along with morphokinetic assessment by time-lapse technology and embryo metabolism help in embryo selection more accurately and may optimize the result of IVF cycles.[14]

Embryo Biopsy

Embryo biopsy can be done for embryo selection to identify affected embryos in couples susceptible to transmit specific genetic disorders or to screen for aneuploid embryos. Clinicians can suggest preimplantation genetic diagnosis (PGD) to couples at risk of transmission of a genetic disorder and thereby avoid the mental and physical trauma a woman has to undergo for termination of an affected pregnancy. Blastocyst stage biopsy has been found to be more useful than polar body or cleavage stage biopsy. Preimplantation genetic screening (PGS) with blastomere biopsy and fluorescent in situ hybridization (FISH) though reported encouraging results initially, failed to demonstrate promising outcome in further randomized controlled trials. Use of trophectoderm biopsy with array-based newer technologies which allows all chromosome testing can be a better option than usage of 9 chromosome FISH to improve IVF results.

Embryo Transfers

Embryo transfer technique is simple and yet a crucial step in ART program. ET done under ultrasound guidance gives better results than done blindly.

In difficult ET, pregnancy rate is reduced because of the trauma caused by the ET catheter or due to uterine contractions. Clinician decides the number of embryos (one to three) to be transferred depending on age of women, number and quality of available embryos, IVF cycles done earlier, and medical indication of the women.

If difficulty is achieved during transfer, physicians have the option either to go ahead with the ET with the additional maneuver like:

- After loading ET technique if preloading is done earlier. Outer sheath of ET catheter to be introduced first till the level of cervical internal os and then embryologist threads the inner catheter through the outer sheath into uterine cavity.
- If still resistance in negotiation through internal os, outer sheath along with stylet can be tried with or without tenaculum traction.

Clinician may proceed with embryo freezing, do the mock transfer reattempting before the actual ET.

- If needed do ET under anesthesia.
- When a difficult ET is anticipated, trial is done prior to the index cycle and embryologist should be informed about anticipated difficulty and additional measure to be taken during ET.

■ TROUBLESHOOTING IN ART LABORATORY

An ART laboratory and a clinician should have more frequent communication while dealing with few panic situations mentioned here:

- *Ovarian hyperstimulation syndrome (OHSS)*: If there is risk of ovarian hyperstimulation, laboratory should know about:
  - Type of trigger used—GnRH agonist/hCG
  - Prophylactic use of intravenous albumin or macromolecules
  - According to severity of symptoms of OHSS need of freeze all or fresh ET
  - Decision for blastocyst culture.
- *Poor response*: If there is no oocyte in follicular fluid:
  - Flushing of the follicle
  - Checking aspiration machine or aspiration pressure or flow rate
  - Stopping the procedure mid-way and checking compliance to hCG.

  If no sperm retrieved in case of NOA next step is:
  - Abandon the procedure
  - Use of donor sperm.

  If all sperms are nonmotile—hypo-osmotic swelling test is to be done to check vitality and ICSI can be performed.

  If patients fail to ejaculate:
  - Trial for collection of semen again
  - Testicular sperm aspiration
  - Cryopreservation of semen in advance.
- *Fertilization failure*: It can provide as a marker for a problem in gamete quality sperm function, oocyte activation, gamete receptors, sperm

processing, or in the number of spermatozoa used for insemination. In IVF cycles, failed fertilization rate should be less than 5% for stimulated cycles. Observed values above this rate should be reported and investigated. Successful fertilization depends on the inherent quality and cytoplasmic maturity.

If there is history of failed fertilization in the past, it is advisable to follow a few steps:
- Intracytoplasmic sperm injection for previous fertilization failure[15]
- Pre-IVF semen functional tests to be done—if high DNA fragmentation index above 30% antioxidant treatment and then ICSI
- Proper stimulation protocols
- Ca ionophore for assisted oocyte activation
- Selective utilization of relatively undamaged sperms (intracytoplasmic morphologically selected sperm injection, selection of hyaluron-bound spermatozoa—physiologic intracytoplasmic sperm injection, birefringence).

KEY POINTS

- In vitro fertilization success depends on proper coordination of the clinician, embryologist, ART nurses, and paramedical staff.
- Clinician should also have a thorough understanding of the laboratory environment, equipment, culture medium, and its quality control.
- Doctor should also have knowledge about laboratory SOPs.
- Good communication between clinician and embryologist will be deciding the best management strategy of the patient.
- For planning IVF cycle, the clinician and embryologist should be aware of previous records of infertility management.

REFERENCES

1. Janssens R, Guns J. Quality control: Maintaining stability in the laboratory. In: Gardner DK, Weissman A, Howles CM, Shoham Z (Eds). Text Book of Assisted Reproductive Techniques, 5th edition. CRC Press; 2017. pp. 10-16.
2. Sjöblom C. The assisted reproduction technology laboratory: Current standards. In: Gardner DK, Weissman A, Howles CM, Shoham Z (Eds). Text Book of Assisted Reproductive Techniques, 5th edition. CRC Press; 2017. pp. 17-36.
3. ESHRE Special Interest Group of Embryology and Alpha Scientists in Reproductive Medicine. The Vienna consensus: report of an expert meeting on the development of ART laboratory performance indicators. Reprod Biomed Online. 2017;35(5): 494-510.
4. Nogueira D, Friedler S, Schachter M, et al. Oocyte maturity and preimplantation development in relation to follicle diameter in gonadotropin-releasing hormone agonist or antagonist treatments. Fertil Steril. 2006;85(3):578-83.
5. Jefferys A, Siassakos D, Wardle P. The management of retrograde ejaculation: a systematic review and update. Fertil Steril. 2012;97(2):306-12.

6. Cavallini G, Beretta G, Biagiotti G. Preliminary study of letrozole use for improving spermatogenesis in non-obstructive azoospermia patients with normal serum FSH. Asian J Androl. 2011;13(6):895-7.
7. Selman H, De Santo M, Sterzik K, et al. Rescue of spermatogenesis arrest in azoospermic men after long-term gonadotropin treatment. Fertil Steril. 2006;86:466-8.
8. Kyrou D, Kosmas IP, Popovic-Todorovic B, et al. Ejaculatory sperm production in non-obstructive azoospermic patients with a history of negative testicular biopsy after the administration of an aromatase inhibitor: report of two cases. Eur J Obstet Gynecol Reprod Biol. 2014;173:120-1.
9. Shiraishi K, Ohmi C, Shimabukuro T, et al. Human chorionic gonadotrophin treatment prior to microdissection testicular sperm extraction in non-obstructive azoospermia. Hum Reprod. 2012;27:331-9.
10. Lemmen JG, Rodríguez NM, Andreasen LD, et al. The total pregnancy potential per oocyte aspiration after assisted reproduction-in how many cycles are biologically competent oocytes available? J Assist Reprod Genet. 2016;33(7):849-54.
11. Russell DL, Salustri A. Extracellular matrix of the cumulus oocyte complex. Semin Reprod Med. 2006;24:217-27.
12. Wang WH, Meng L, Hackett RJ, et al. The spindle observation and its relationship with fertilization after intracytoplasmic sperm injection in living human oocytes. Fertil Steril. 2001;75:348-53.
13. Martin Wilding, Loredana Di Matteo, Sonia D'Andretti, et al. An oocyte score for use in assisted reproduction. J Assist Reprod Genet. 2007;24(8):350-8.
14. Yanagida K, Fujikura Y, Katayose H. The present status of artificial oocyte activation in assisted reproductive technology. Reprod Med Biol. 2008;7:133-42.
15. Vanden Meerschaut F, Nikiforaki D, Heindryckx B, et al. Assisted oocyte activation following ICSI fertilization failure. Reprod Biomed Online. 2014;28:560-71.

CHAPTER
38

OMICS: Metabolomics, Proteomics, Secretomics and Genomics—Its Application in the Viability Score of Oocyte and Embryo

Bindu Chimote, Natchandra Chimote

■ INTRODUCTION

In the four decades after the first IVF baby was born, in spite of rapid, dynamic advancements in the clinical and embryological fields; the overall success rates in IVF have remained far from satisfactory. Enhancing live birth rates while at the same time minimizing multiple gestation rates and the complications thereof is the ultimate goal of every in-vitro-fertilization treatment protocol. In the entire cascade of events leading to successful implantation, by far the most important "rate limiting factors" are oocyte/embryo quality and endometrial receptivity. On the clinical side, application of customized stimulation protocols and use of adjuncts to improve endometrial receptivity are the current focus for clinical trials. The embryological factors that majorly influence success rates include use of optimized culture conditions, culture media and the quality of oocytes and embryos.

Conventionally, morphological scoring of oocytes,[1,2] cleavage stage embryos[3,4] and blastocysts[5,6] based on various parameters have been employed to evaluate oocyte and embryo viability and competence. However, the major disadvantage of these static, fixed time-frame assessment methods is that they are more liable to subjectivity and inter-/intraobserver, inter-center variations. Thus, dynamic morphokinetic method using time-lapse imaging was propagated. However, TLI has no standardized morphokinetic parameters, is not cost-effective and is more adept at de-selecting embryos rather than selecting the best ones. Moreover, it is felt that mere morphological assessment may not reflect the ploidy and viability status of oocytes and embryos.

■ OMICS APPROACH

The basis for the use of OMICS to assess viability status stems from the differential nutrient requirement/media composition for the growth and development of oocytes and embryos in vitro. During the course of this development, several energy substrates as well as micro-/macronutrients, among other components, at various concentrations are utilized; whereas some products are secreted into the culture medium. Culture medium drop is the dynamic microenvironmental milieu which is the site for transition from oocyte to zygote to embryo. Therefore, changes occurring at the metabolic, transcriptional, translational and genetic levels, as evaluated in spent culture-drops, could be valuable predictors of the oocyte and embryo developmental potential. The metric evaluation of uptake and production of components within the culture-media may be logically expected to vary as per the viability status and reproductive potential scoring of oocytes and embryos. Similarly, follicular fluid is the microenvironment where the oocyte undergoes the process of development and maturation. Evaluation of components within this milieu may reflect the oocyte viability status as well as early indicators of embryo viability and implantation potential. This article attempts to review available literature for various indirect and noninvasive in-vitro methods based on the OMICS approach.

OMICS, which comprises of metabolomics, genomics, transcriptomics, proteomics and secretomics is the systematic study of changes in the functional phenotype at cellular level via evaluation of the various metabolites, gene expression profile, transcriptomes (RNA molecules), protein profile and secretions, respectively. The methods employed for assessment of these components require high sensitivity as most of these molecules are present in minute (micro-, nanomolar) concentrations. Also, rather than group culture, it is advisable to do individual culture in small microdrops (20–40 μL volume) to be able to distinguish and trace the developmental profile of each oocyte/embryo. The most important consideration for the practical applicability of any of these methods is its speed, which would provide results within the time frame of the embryo culture.

■ TRANSCRIPTOMICS

The flow of genetic information follows the central dogma of molecular biology: DNA is transcribed to RNA, which is translated to protein. The total RNA content (m-RNA, t-RNA, r-RNA and mi-RNA) of a cell constitutes its transcriptome. The survival (viability) and function (competence) of the oocyte and embryos also relies on the timely activation of this molecular pathway. A continuous cross-talk between oocyte and somatic follicular cells is necessary for follicular development, oocyte maturation, cumulus expansion, and ovulation. Since cumulus and mural granulosa cells represent the characteristics of the oocyte; the transcriptomic approach in IVF (which enables monitoring of gene expression in somatic cells of the follicle, gametes, and embryos) provides a noninvasive means to assess oocyte viability and also a surrogate measure for embryo developmental and reproductive potential. Transcriptomics technology involves analysis of individual genes by quantitative reverse transcription polymerase chain reaction (qRT-PCR);

whereas whole genome transcriptomic profiling employs microarrays and high-throughput deep sequencing techniques. However, variations in the design and methodology of the microarray experiments and technological limitations complicate the interpretation of the results of microarray studies. Recent studies using qRT-PCR and microarray technologies have correlated changes in cumulus or granulosa cell gene expression with in-vitro embryo development potential and pregnancy rates.[7]

Micro-RNAs (miRNAs) are small non-coding RNA molecules that regulate the expression of several target genes. Interestingly, in blastocysts with the same morphological grading, the miRNA profile was observed to be significantly different between blastocysts from infertile and normal fertile patients.[8] In another study, three different miRNAs (miR-372, miR-191 and miR-645) were found to significantly differ in day 5 spent culture drops between embryos that led to a pregnancy and those that did not.[9]

Although results are encouraging, the actual clinical benefits of this technology to assess embryo viability need to be reaffirmed by randomized controlled trials.

Lower content of cell-free DNA (cfDNA) in follicular fluid has been correlated with lower fragmentation rates and higher quality embryos.[10,11] Recently, levels of mitochondrial (mt) DNA from blastocyst biopsy samples have been evaluated as markers of blastocyst viability status.[12] Higher than threshold levels of mtDNA was observed to have a 100% negative predictive value for pregnancy whereas normal levels of mtDNA were shown to offer an implantation rate of around 75% for euploid embryos. Similar findings have also been reported by Fragouli et al. 2017.[13] However, a retrospective study[14] involving next generation sequencing (NGS) and qualitative real time polymerase chain reaction (qrtPCR) of trophectoderm biopsies reported no significant difference in mtDNA content between blastocysts classified on the basis of age, implantation and ploidy status.

■ PROTEOMICS AND SECRETOMICS

The proteins that are translated from RNA constitute the proteome, whereas, when the proteins so produced are secreted by the developing embryo, they are referred to as the secretome. The proteome-secretome profile of the culture-medium is therefore logically, an index of the developmental stage and viability status of embryos.[15] Several constraints including use of protein (e.g. albumin) containing media, limit the measurement of the proteome-secretome profile by routine inexpensive methods;[16] since proteins which have molecular weights similar to that of albumin are rendered indistinguishable. Several proteins markers like platelet-activating factor, leptin, agrocranin, human leukocyte antigen G (HLA-G) and ubiquitin have been investigated in the embryonic secretion. Of these, sHLA-G appears to be the most promising biomarker for embryo viability.

s-HLA-G Fragment

The human leukocytic antigen (HLA) system consists of a group of genes residing on chromosome 6, that codes for proteins responsible for immune-regulation in humans. Several studies and meta-analysis have correlated elevated levels of sHLA-G fragments in spent culture medium with higher implantation potential.[17-20] An earlier study had also correlated content of s-HLAG secreted by embryo in day 3 culture media as an indicator of embryo competence.[21] By far, s-HLAG is the most efficient, standardized and applicable biomarker for embryo viability. However, this marker cannot be relied upon as a sole predictor because different culture conditions and patient populations have been shown to affect the proportion of s-HLA-G positive samples and their concentration in the culture medium.[22,23]

The proteomic profile is now being obtained by use of advanced techniques like mass spectrometry (MS). Using this method, the protein Jumonji (JARID2) which is known to regulate gene patterning of embryos has been found to be predictive of successful IVF outcome.[24] By this same method (MS), levels of another protein, Apolipoprotein A1, have been detected to be higher in spent culture drops of blastocysts with top grade morphology than those with poor or abnormal morphology.[25] Conversely, low levels of ApoA1 in the day 2/3 cleavage stage secretome were shown to correlate with positive pregnancy outcome.[26]

The protein-hormone human chorionic gonadotropin, a long-standing obstetric gold standard for implantation, has also been evaluated in the embryo secretome by MS.[27] Gene expression and immunoassay techniques coupled with MS have revealed that even early (2-cell stage) embryos secrete the b isoform of HCG in culture medium. On the other hand, presence of the h isoform in media has been associated with embryos with pathology/abnormal fertilization patter (3ProNuclei). Mass spectrometry-based proteomic analysis is less time-consuming compared to other routine methods like immunoassays and therefore can be more applicable in IVF where quick results are desirable.

The proteomic approach has been applied to follicular fluid (FF) components as well. Levels of different cytokines and chemokines in follicular fluid have been explored as biomarkers for oocyte/embryo development and implantation potential. Higher levels of Interleukin-2 (IL-2) and interferone gamma (IFN-γ) in FF have been associated with fast cleaving embryos. However, higher levels of IL-12 have been linked to greater degree of fragmentation in embryos.[28] The same authors also evaluated GCSF in individual follicular fluid as a significant biomarker of embryo quality and implantation potential. Chimote et al. in two different studies[29,30] analyzed endogenous levels of GCSF in pooled follicular fluid and GMCSF in day 3 spent culture drops as robust biomarkers of embryo viability. Three other studies established FF DHEAS, FF AMH and FF IGF-1 levels as markers of oocyte maturity, oocyte viability and embryo viability status respectively.[31-33]

METABOLOMICS

A metabolome represents the product of gene-expression and metabolomics helps associate the genotype with the corresponding phenotype. Metabolomics deals with diverse classes of metabolite molecules, such as amino acids, oxidation products, carbohydrates and carboxylic acids[34] which are then identified via their functional groups like carboxylic acids, ketones, aldehydes, alkenes or alkynes.

Amino acids, which are present in oviduct and uterine fluids in-vivo, also form important constituents of culture media owing to their multifaceted roles in regulating osmotic pressure, maintaining pH, involvement in carbohydrate metabolism and in biosynthesis of cells. It is known that the nonessential amino acids affect the number of trophoblast cells and influence blastocyst hatching whereas essential amino acids cause rapid division of inner cell mass and enhance the fetal development after implantation.

The amino-acid profile has been reported to differ between follicular-fluid (FF) and plasma and also between women with different indications for infertility. The amino-acid serine in FF whereas methionine and phenyl-alanine in plasma have been reported to be potential biomarkers of oocyte quality.[35] Raman spectroscopy analysis has revealed that lower levels of sodium pyruvate and higher levels of phenyl-alanine in spent culture-drops correlate with embryo development potential with a high degree of specificity.

In a study[36] investigating amino-acid turnover by high performance liquid chromatography (HPLC), the consumption of higher amounts of leucine and higher secretion of alanine was demonstrated to be more conducive for formation of top quality blastocysts. Similarly, another study evaluating a mixture of 18 amino acids in spent culture medium found that the amino-acid turnover of Asn, Gly and Leu correlated with clinical pregnancy and live birth, independently of other female predictors like age, baseline FSH, number of blastomeres and embryo morphology.[37] The amino-acid turnover of asparagine, glycine and valine in day 2/3 culture media has also been depicted to differ significantly between genetically normal and abnormal embryos.[38]

The viability score of oocytes and embryos is also obtained by assessing the metabolic footprint/profile of the culture medium. Techniques like nuclear magnetic resonance (NMR), mass spectrometry (MS) and Raman spectroscopy provide a distinguishable spectrum for embryos that have implantation potential versus those that do not implant.[39] The same algorithm has predictive value for viability of both fresh and frozen-thawed embryos.[40] Near infrared spectroscopy (NIR) has also been employed to generate a viability score to distinguish between viable and nonviable embryos by measuring the vibrations of functional groups rather than measuring the whole metabolites.[41,42] NIR offers advantage over other techniques in being able to be applied to small sample volumes, with immediate results.

However, systematic RCTs and meta-analysis have not been able to confirm the effectiveness of these techniques in selecting high viability score embryos that had the potential to implant and lead to successful pregnancy.[43]

Oxygen Consumption

Monitoring of oxygen consumption patterns in human embryos in culture till day 3 cleavage stage has also been linked to embryo morphology, viability and implantation potential.[44-46] However, this method is not without drawbacks, since the oxygen consumption rates often vary with the ovarian stimulation protocol used.[47]

Higher oocyte respiration rates (0.48 nL and 0.55 nL O_2/h) have been found to significantly correlate with oocyte viability whereas lower rates correspond with immature or atretic oocytes.

The noninvasive targeted metabolite analysis of oocytes by ultramicrofluorimetry has revealed that higher consumption of glucose along with a higher production of lactate favors fertilization.[48] Pyruvate is the primary source during early cleavage stage,[49] whereas glucose is the primary energy substrate for embryos at the blastocyst stage.[50] Indeed, lower levels of pyruvate in day 3 spent culture drops have been observed to correlate with pregnancy signifying that more pyruvate is utilized from the medium during this stage.[51-53] Another study correlates higher pyruvate turnover with abnormal oocyte karyotype. Pyruvate, thus, is an indicator of oocyte viability and embryo vitality.[54]

It is known that in-vitro culture exposes the oocytes and embryos to oxidative stress that may affect their viability status, thereby influencing IVF outcomes. Oxidative stress markers have been evaluated in follicular fluid by several studies. One such study examined stress markers like thiobarbituric acid-reactive substances (TBARS), protein carbonyl, and thiol groups for lipid and protein peroxidation. Levels of TBARS and protein carbonyl groups were found to be double the quantity among nonpregnant as compared to pregnant women, thus reflecting the negative impact of oxidative stress on embryo viability and pregnancy outcome.[55,56]

■ GENOMICS

The deterioration in quality and the associated enhanced chromosomal abnormalities in oocytes have been implicated in reduced live-birth rates and/or recurrent implantation failures by several studies. Deciphering the oocyte genomic profile may help identify the ploidy status and hence the oocyte/embryo development and implantation potential. Multiple annealing and looping-based amplification cycle (MALBAC)-based sequencing technology have been employed to analyze the genome of single human oocytes.[57] The genome of first and second polar bodies as well as of the pronucleus in donor oocytes have been shown to accurately identify aneuploidy and single nucleotide polymorphisms (SNPs) in alleles associated with diseased states.

In a recent study,[58] the AMH-receptor II gene mRNA expression in cumulus cells was found to be higher in oocytes that remained unfertilized compared to those that had fertilized. A marked observation was the association of high expression of mRNA of AMH receptor II gene with a parallel high level of intrafollicular lactate dehydrogenase activity in these follicles. These results signify that high antioxidant activity as a defensive response to cytotoxicity in the follicle and changes in the AMH signal transduction are related to oocyte fertilization and further embryo development status. This parameter therefore promises to be an effective marker for oocyte competence and embryo viability status.

■ CONCLUSION

Several metabolite biomarkers have been extensively investigated to assess oocyte/embryo viability. However, neither any single metabolite nor any particular technique is an exclusive indicator of viability status. Biomarkers evaluated by the OMICS approach are not 'stand-alone' markers but are a significant adjunct to ocular morphological scoring methods. Several large scale multicentric studies with uniformly optimized, applicable protocols and systematic randomized controlled trials are needed to corroborate the efficiency of metrical measurements of biomolecules and metabolic intermediates as effective predictors of oocyte and embryo viability status.

■ REFERENCES

1. Wilding M, Di Matteo L, D'Andretti S, et al. An oocyte score for use in assisted reproduction J Assist Reprod Genet. 2007;24(8):350-8.
2. Lazzaroni-Tealdi E, Barad DH, Albertini DF, et al. Oocyte Scoring Enhances Embryo-Scoring in Predicting Pregnancy Chances with IVF Where It Counts Most PLoS One. 2015;10(12):e0143632.
3. Veeck L. An atlas of human gametes and conceptuses. Carnforth: Parthenon Publishing; 1999.
4. Racowsky C, Vernon M, Mayer J, et al. Standardization of grading embryo morphology. J Assist Reprod Genet. 2010;27:437-9.
5. Gardner DK, Schoolcraft WB. In vitro culture of human blastocysts. In: Jansen R, Mortimer D (Eds). Toward Reproductive Certainty: Fertility and Genetics Beyond 1999. UK, London: Parthenon Publishing Group; 1999. pp. 378-88.
6. Richardson A, Brearley S, Ahitan S, et al. A clinically useful simplified blastocyst grading system. Reprod BioMed Online. 2015;31:523-30.
7. Uyar A, Torrealday S, Seli E. Cumulus and granulosa cell markers of oocyte and embryo quality Fertil Steril. 2013;99(4):979-97.
8. McCallie B, Schoolcraft WB, Katz-Jaffe MG. Aberration of blastocyst microRNA expression is associated with human infertility. Fertil Steril. 2010;93:2374-82.
9. Rosenbluth EM, Shelton DN, Wells LM, et al. Human embryos secrete microRNAs into culture media—A potential biomarker for implantation. Fertil Steril. 2014;101:1493-500.
10. Scalici E, Traver S, Molinari N, et al. Cell-free DNA in human follicular fluid as a biomarker of embryo quality. Hum Reprod. 2014;29(12):2661-9.

11. Kassim HR, AL-Omary HL, Shayma'a J. Ahmed Evaluation of Cell Free DNA in Follicular Fluid and Embryo Quality in Poly Cystic Ovarian Syndrome of Iraqi Women IOSR. J Pharmacy Biol Sci (IOSR-JPBS). 2018;13(1):5-9. e-ISSN:2278-3008, p-ISSN:2319-7676.
12. Ravichandran K, McCafferey C, Grifo J, et al. Mitochondrial DNA quantification as a tool for embryo viability assessment: retrospective analysis of data from single euploid blastocyst transfers. Hum Reprod. 2017;32(6):1282-92.
13. Fragouli E, McCaffrey C, Ravichandran K, et al. Clinical implications of mitochondrial DNA quantification on pregnancy outcomes: a blinded prospective non-selection study. Hum Reprod. 2017;32(11):2340-7.
14. Victor AR, Brake AJ, Tyndall JC, et al. Accurate quantitation of mitochondrial DNA reveals uniform levels in human blastocysts irrespective of ploidy, age, or implantation potential. Fertil Steril. 2017;107(1):34-42.e3.
15. Katz-Jaffe MG, Gardner DK. Symposium: Innovative techniques in human embryo viability assessment. Can proteomics help to shape the future of human assisted conception? Reprod Biomed Online. 2008;17:497-501.
16. Mains LM, Christenson L, Yang B, et al. Identification of apolipoprotein A1 in the human embryonic secretome. Fertil Steril. 2011;96:422-7.
17. Vercammen MJ, Verloes A, Van de Velde H, et al. Accuracy of soluble human leukocyte antigen-G for predicting pregnancy among women undergoing infertility treatment: meta-analysis. Hum Reprod Update. 2008;14:209-18.
18. Kotze D, Kruger TF, Lombard C, et al. The effect of the biochemical marker soluble human leukocyte antigen G on pregnancy outcome in assisted reproductive technology—a multicenter study. Fertil Steril. 2013;100:1303-9.
19. Guo XY, Jiang F, Cheng XJ, et al. Embryonic soluble human leukocyte antigen-G as a marker of embryo competency in assisted reproductive technology for Chinese women. J Reprod Med. 2013;58:477-84.
20. Sallam HN, El Kafflsh DM, Ismail AA, et al. Embryo selection by measurement of soluble human leukocytic antigen-G levels in embryo culture medium in patients undergoing ICSI. Fertil Steril. 2016;105.
21. Desai N, Filipovits J, Goldfarb J. Secretion of soluble HLA-G by day 3 human embryos associated with higher pregnancy and implantation rates: assay of culture media using a new ELISA kit. Reprod Biomed Online. 2006;13:272-7.
22. Tabiasco J, Perrier d'Hauterive S, Thonon F, et al. Soluble HLA-G in IVF/ICSI embryo culture supernatants does not always predict implantation success: a multicentre study. Reprod Biomed Online. 2009;18:374-81.
23. Rebmann V, Switala M, Eue I, et al. Soluble HLA-G is an independent factor for the prediction of pregnancy outcome after ART: a German multi-centre study. Hum Reprod. 2010;25(7):1691-8.
24. Pasini D, Cloos PAC, Walfridsson J, et al. JARID2 regulates binding of the Polycomb repressive complex 2 to target genes in ES cells. Nature. 2010;464:306-10.
25. Mains LM, Christenson L, Yang B, et al. Identification of apolipoprotein A1 in the human embryonic secretome. Fertil Steril. 2011;96(2):422-7.e2.

26. Nyalwidhe J, Burch T, Bocca S, et al. The search for biomarkers of human embryo developmental potential in IVF: a comprehensive proteomic approach. Mol Hum Reprod. 2013;19:250-63.
27. Butler SA, Luttoo J, Freire MOT, et al. Human chorionic gonadotropin (hcg) in the secretome of cultured embryos: hyperglycosylated hCG and hCGfree beta subunit are potential markers for infertility management and treatment. Reprod Sci. 2013;20:1038-45.
28. Lédée N, Lombroso R, Lombardelli L, et al. Cytokines and chemokines in follicular fluids and potential of the corresponding embryo: the role of granulocyte colony-stimulating factor. Hum Reprod. 2008;23(9):2001-9.
29. Chimote NM, Nath NM, Chimote BN. Granulocyte colony stimulating factor (G-CSF) level in follicular fluid is a prognostic factor for embryo developmental potential in in-vitro fertilization cycles. Fertil Steril. 2015;104(3):e306.
30. Chimote NM, Nath NM, Chimote NN, et al. Cytokine GM-CSF in day 3 spent culture drops decides the fate of embryonic development to blastocyst stage and quality of blastocyst. Hum Reprod ESHRE. 2016;31(1):Poster No. P-218, p. i223.
31. Chimote NM, Nath NM, Chimote NN, et al. Follicular fluid dehydroepiandrosterone sulfate is a credible marker of oocyte maturity and pregnancy outcome in conventional in vitro fertilization cycles. J Hum Reprod Sci. 2015;8:209-13.
32. Mehta BN, Chimote MN, Chimote NN, et al. Follicular-fluid anti-Mullerian hormone (FF AMH) is a plausible biochemical indicator of functional viability of oocyte in conventional in vitro fertilization (IVF) cycles. J Hum Reprod Sci. 2013;6:99-105.
33. Mehta BN, Chimote NM, Chimote MN, et al. Follicular fluid insulin like growth factor-1 (FF IGF-1) is a biochemical marker of embryo quality and implantation rates in in vitro fertilization cycles. J Hum Reprod Sci. 2013;6:140-6.
34. Nagy ZP, Sakkas D, Behr B. Non-invasive assessment of embryo viability by metabolomic profiling of culture media (metabolomics). Reprod Biomed Online. 2008;17:502-7.
35. Kirsipuu T, Laks K, Velthut-Meikas A, et al. Comprehensive elucidation of amino acid profile in human follicular fluid and plasma of in vitro fertilization patients. Gynecol Endocrinol. 2015;31(1):9-17.
36. Houghton FD, Hawkhead JA, Humpherson PG, et al. Noninvasive amino acid turnover predicts human embryo developmental capacity. Hum Reprod. 2002;17:999-1005.
37. Brison DR, Houghton FD, Falconer D, et al. Identification of viable embryos in IVF by non-invasive measurement of amino acid turnover. Hum Reprod. 2004;19(10):2319-24.
38. Picton HM, Elder K, Houghton FD, et al. Association between amino acid turnover and chromosome aneuploidy during human preimplantation embryo development in vitro. Mol Hum Reprod. 2010;16:557-69.
39. Kirkegaard K, Svane AS, Nielsen JS, et al. Nuclear magnetic resonance metabolomic profiling of Day 3 and 5 embryo culture medium does not predict pregnancy

outcome in good prognosis patients: a prospective cohort study on single transferred embryos. Hum Reprod. 2014;29:2413-20.
40. Vergouw CG, Botros LL, Judge K, et al. Non-invasive viability assessment of day-4 frozen-thawed human embryos using near infrared spectroscopy. Reprod BioMed Online. 2011;23(6):769-76.
41. Ahlström A, Wikland M, Rogberg L, et al. Cross-validation and predictive value of near infrared spectroscopy algorithms for day-5 blastocyst transfer. Reprod Biomed Online. 2011;22:477-84.
42. Botros L, Sakkas D, Seli E. Metabolomics and its application for non-invasive embryo assessment in IVF. Mol Hum Reprod. 2008;14:679-90.
43. Vergouw CG, Heymans MW, Hardarson T, et al. No evidence that embryo selection by near infrared spectroscopy in addition to morphology is able to improve live birth rates: results from an individual patient data meta-analysis. Hum Reprod 2014;29:455-61.
44. Shiku H, Shiraishi T, Ohya H, et al. Oxygen consumption of single bovine embryos probed by scanning electrochemical microscopy. Analyt Chem. 2001;73(15):3751-8.
45. Agung B, Otoi T, Abe H, et al. Relationship between oxygen consumption and sex of bovine in vitro fertilized embryos. Reproduction in Domestic Animals. 2005;40(1):51-6.
46. Tejera A, Herrero J, Viloria T, et al. Time-dependent O_2 consumption patterns determined optimal time ranges for selecting viable human embryos. Fertil Steril. 2012;98(4):849.e1-857.e3
47. Tejera A, Herrero J, de los Santos MJ, et al. Oxygen consumption is a quality marker for human oocyte competence conditioned by ovarian stimulation regimens. Fertil Steril. 2011;96(3):U618-U141.
48. Preis KA, Seidel G, Gardner DK. Metabolic markers of developmental competence for in-vitro-matured mouse oocytes. Reproduction. 2005;130(4):475-83.
49. Brinster RL. Studies on the development of the mouse embryos in vitro. II. The effect of energy source. J Exp Zool. 1965;158:59-68.
50. Gardner DK, Leese HJ. Non-invasive measurement of nutrient uptake by single-cultured preimplantation mouse embryos. Hum Reprod. 1986;1:25-7.
51. Hardy K, Hooper MAK. Non-invasive measurement of glucose and pyruvate uptake by individual human oocytes and preimplantation embryos. Hum Reprod. 1989;4:188-91.
52. Conaqhan J, Handyside AH. Effects of pyruvate and glucose on the development of the human preimplantation embryo. J Reprod Fertil. 1993;99:87-95.
53. Zhao Q, Yin T, Peng J, et al. Noninvasive metabolomics profiling of human embryo culture media using a simple spectroscopy adjunct to morphology for embryo assessment in in vitro fertilization. Int J Mol Sci. 2013;14:6556-70.
54. Harris SE, Maruthini D, Tang T, et al. Metabolism and karyotype analysis of oocytes from patients with polycystic ovary syndrome. Hum Reprod. 2010;25(9):2305-15.
55. Borowiecka M, Wojsiat J, Polac I, et al. Oxidative stress markers in follicular fluid of women undergoing in-vitro fertilization and embryo transfer. Syst Biol Reprod Med. 2012;58(6):301-5.

56. Becatti M, Fucci R, Mannucci A, et al. A Biochemical Approach to Detect Oxidative Stress in Infertile Women Undergoing Assisted Reproductive Technology Procedures. Int J Mol Sci. 2018;19(2):592.
57. Hou Y, Yan L FW, Li R, et al. Genome Analyses of Single Human Oocytes. Cell. 2013;155:1492-506.
58. Revelli A, Canosa S, Bergandi L, et al. Oocyte polarized light microscopy, assay of specific follicular fluid metabolites, and gene expression in cumulus cells as different approaches to predict fertilization efficiency after ICSI. Reprod Biol Endocrinol. 2017;15:47.

Index

Page numbers followed by, *f* refer to figure, *fc* refer to flow chart, and *t* refer to table.

A

Acetaldehyde 172
Acetyl carnitine 110
Acetyl co-A succinate 4
Acid phosphatase 3
Acridine orange test 28
Acrolein 84
Acrosomal
    cap 3
    sac containing enzymes 3
    status 74
Acrosome 3, 72
    body 21
    forms 3
    reaction 25, 26, 68, 76, 80, 81
Adenoma, pituitary 121
Adenosine triphosphate 4
    efflux of 76
Adriamycin 161, 338
Adult spermatozoa, anatomical segments of 2
Advanced sperm selection techniques 64, 65
Agrocranin 259
Air fluid method 267
    demerits of 268
    merits of 268
Air handling systems 182, 204
Air purification system 182*f*
Air quality 194, 196, 215
    equipment 181*f*
Alanine 261
    higher secretion of 398
Albumin 85
Alcohol consumption 100
Alpha fibers 4
Altruistic surrogacy 380
Amenorrhea 337
American Society for Reproductive Medicine 39, 49, 189, 255, 313, 378, 381
American Urological Association 45
Amino acid 231, 310, 398
    depletion/appearance 262*f*
    profile 398
    serine 398
    transportation 231
    turnover 261
Androgen binding
    globulin 14
        transports testosterone 14
    protein 15
Anejaculation 152, 153

Aneuploid 309
    embryos 313
Aneuploidy 30, 360, 361, 363, 364, 399
    screening 386
Angiotensin converting enzyme gene 3
Aniline blue test 28
Animal house laboratory, benefits of 368
Annexin V
    binding buffer 102
    conjugated paramagnetic microbeads 68
    glass wool filtration 70
Anorgasmia 149
Anthocyanins 112, 113
Antidepressants 154
Anti-mullerian hormone 337
Antioxidant 85, 107, 110, 112, 122
    therapy 29
Antisperm antibody 23, 62
Antral follicle count 290, 337
Antral follicular development 230
Anucleate fragmentation, percentage of 240
Aplastic anemia 340
Apolipoprotein A1 397
Apoptosis 83, 101
    pathway of 101
Arginine 110
Array comparative genomic hybridization 361
Arsenic 119
ART laboratory
    basic components of 173
    troubleshooting in 208
Artificial insemination utilizing human sperm 158
Artificial manipulation 282
Assisted hatching 134, 277, 278, 280, 282
    methods of 279
    technology 134
    using partial zona dissection, technique of 279
Assisted Human Reproduction Act 189
Assisted reproductive technology 24, 36, 44, 103, 107, 128, 165, 171, 192, 208, 222, 238, 255, 271, 279, 291, 308, 320, 326, 337, 359, 367, 385, 386, 388*f*
    cycles 166
    laboratory 189
        aim of 385
    predicting success of 52
    procedures 128
    process of 376
    utilization 191

Assisted reproductive treatment 64
Assisted zona drilling 281
Astaxanthin 112
Asthenospermia 41, 62, 160
Asthenozooserpmia 20, 37, 61
Asynchrony 132
ATPase enzyme 4
Autoimmune disease 340
Autosomal gene mutations 39
Axonemal
    defects 37
    structure 109
Azoospermia 36, 39, 41, 49, 118, 153, 160-162, 165
    complete 51
    factor region 41, 49
    kinds of 165
    nonobstructive 40, 41, 45, 132, 165, 389
    obstructive 48*fc*, 49, 165
    permanent 161, 162
    temporary 161

B

Bacteriological incubator 57
Basal serum follicle-stimulating hormone 39
Basement membrane 12
Beckwith-Wiedemann syndrome 136
Behcet's disease 340
Benchtop incubator 177, 199*f*, 203*f*
Benzene 172
Beta-blocking drugs 155
Binocular compound phase contrast microscope 57
Birefringence 392
Birth weight
    low 330, 331
    very low 331
Blastocyst 173, 175, 241, 248, 277, 396
    biopsies 363
    cryofreezing, advantages of 321
    cryopreservation 314
    culture 307, 364
    damage 282
    development 240, 257, 309
        course of 196
    enhancement of 313
    formation 226, 279
        prediction of 248
    hatching of 281
    in vitro 308
    inner cell mass 321
    morphological assessment of 311
    morphology of 312
    prediction 250
    splits 312
    stage 220, 240, 256, 263, 272, 309, 311, 320, 399

embryos 272
    morphology 240
    transfer 309, 313
    transfer 258, 273, 389
        method 313
    vitrification 314, 315*f*
Blastomere 213, 272, 278, 360
Blastomeric synchrony 260
Blastulation rates 190
Bleomycin 161, 338
Blood 183
    clots 209
    flow studies 151
    vessels 150
Body
    fluids 183
    mass index 113, 290
    myopathy, heredity inclusion of 137
Bone marrow transplantation 340
Bowel malignancy 340
Breast cancer 340
Busulfan 161, 338

C

Cadmium 119
Calcium oscillation 6, 289
Canadian Fertility and Andrology Society 189
Cancer 33, 99, 164
    cell transmission, Risks of 339
    treatment 33, 337
        advancement in 336
Carbendazim 118
Carbohydrate 277
    metabolism, products of 261
Carbon dioxide 202*f*
    sensors 202*f*
Carboplatin 338
Cardiac disorder 137
Carmustine 338
Carnitines 85
Carotenoids 85
Catalase 85
Cells
    biology 221
    concentration 328
    cryopreserved 158
    dehydration of 159
    free deoxyribonucleic acid, content of 396
    solidification of 318
    type 360
Cellular debris, presence of 58
Central nervous system tumors 161
Centrifuges 179
Cervical carcinoma 340
Cesarean delivery 274
Chemotaxis 7
Chemotherapeutic drugs, low-risk 338

Chemotherapy 99, 336, 339
    drugs in 338t
Chlorambucil 161, 338
Chlortetracycline staining 26
Chromatin status, abnormal 288
Chromium 119
Chromosomal
    aberrations 360
        detection of 361
    abnormalities 40, 135
    analysis 40, 308
    aneuploidy rate 160
    material, gain of 361
Chromosome 13, 18 and 21, trisomies of 360
    gain of 360
    segregation 9
    set of 360
Churg-Strauss syndrome 340
Cisplatin 161, 338
Cleavage rates 190, 226
Cleavage stage
    embryos 175
        cryopreservation of 327
    morphology 240
Clinical pregnancy rates 226
Clomiphene 389
Clomipramine 153
Cold shock injury 159
Combined oral contraceptives, number of 209
Comparative genomic hybridization 329, 361
Completely immotile sperm 131
Computer-assisted sperm analysis 26
Conventional cryopreservation methods 317
Copper 77
Cortex tissue 343
Cortical granule 289
Crohn's disease 296
Cryobank 175
Cryo-devices 175
Cryoinjury 302
Cryopreservation 101, 166, 175, 278, 295, 311, 317, 372
    cycles 180
    method 306, 317
    protocols 302, 363
    techniques 326
    theory of 158
    unit 173, 174
        description and function 174
        location and relationships 175
Cryopreserved ovarian
    cortex, reimplantation of 351
    tissue, transplant of 354
Cryoprotectants 159, 302, 314
    concentration of 301, 306, 318
    nonpenetrating 159
    toxicity 302
    type of 318

Cryostorage vessels 205
Cryptorchidism 44, 107
Culture media, role of 370
Cumulative live birth rate 194
Cumulus cells 209, 210, 228, 231, 232
    apoptosis, prevention of 234
    coordinate follicular 230
    oocyte communication 229f
    role of 230
    small amount of 210
Cumulus expansion 395
    enabling factor signal 234
Cumulus oocyte 209
    communication 230f
    complex 209, 229, 230, 289, 290
    denudation of 210
Cumulus oophorus
    cells 130
    complex 388
Cyclic adenosine monophosphate 230
    inhibits 231
Cyclic guanosine monophosphate 230
Cyclophosphamide 161, 338
Cysteines 85
Cystic fibrosis transmembrane conductance
        regulator 48, 136
    gene mutation testing 49, 52
Cytarabine 338
Cytochrome C reduction 109
Cytogenetic
    abnormalities 360
    analysis, conventional 362
    disease 336
Cytokinesis 249
Cytoplasmic
    droplets 7
    factors 289
    inclusions 291
    maturation 210
    syngamy 6
Cytoskeleton 213
Cytotoxic therapy 339
Cytoxan 338

D

Dacarbazine 161, 338
Dactinomycin 338
Daunorubicin 338
Dehydration, stages of 315f
Density gradient 61
    technique 61f
Deoxyribonucleic acid 132, 176
    bind 362
    breakage, presence of 90
    damage 22, 82, 89, 97
    defects, type of 95
    eukaryotic 1

fragmentation 25, 27, 89
  amount of 98
  index 29, 94, 97, 98
  levels of 98, 100
  initiation of 289
  microarrays 362
  strands 9
Depolymerization 320
Desire disorders 155
Diabetes, medical history of 18
Dichlorodiphenyltrichloroethane 118
Dietary substance 107
Dimethyl sulfoxide 159, 302, 342
Diploid spermatogonial cell 8
Donor
  age 378
  cycles 296
  evaluation of 377f
  gametes, ART guidelines for 379
  insemination, indications for 377
  oocytes 227
  semen insemination 165
  thalassemia screening of 378
  types of 377
Double density gradient centrifugation 101
Double embryo transfer 270
Doxorubicin 338
Duchenne muscular dystrophy 137

E

Earle's balanced salt solution 58
Echotip soft catheter 266
Ectopic pregnancy 191
Egg
  banking 379
    commercial 378, 379
  donation 376, 378
  donors 383
  fusion 277
  hyperstimulation 383
  ploitation 382
Ejaculate volume 20
Ejaculation
  control 156
  deficiency in 153
  delayed 149
  premature 18, 149, 151, 152, 152f
  retarded 152, 153
  retrograde 389
Ejaculatory
  disorders 44, 152
  disturbances 152
  dysfunction 166
Elective single embryo transfer 270, 271, 326
  criteria for 271
  outcome of 272
Electron transport system 82
Electronegatively charged sperm 68

Electrophoretic system 65, 66t
Embryo 166, 173, 226, 238, 277, 309, 317, 319, 331, 337
  assessment of 390
  biopsy 390
  cryopreservation 131, 300, 320, 322, 326, 332
    indications 300
  culture 261, 372
    and transfer 171
  developments of 220
  differs 321
  donation 227, 377
  endometrium asynchrony 320
  endoplasmic reticulum 368
  freezing 296, 391
    techniques of 301
  glue 266
  implantable 238, 307
  in vitro 308, 394
  loading 266, 267
  metabolome, assessment of 261
  mitochondrion membrane potential 368
  morphokinetic markers 243
  morphology 398
    assessment, conventional 238
  preimplantation 363, 365
  quality 214
    biomarker of 397
  rate of 323
  respiration rate of 359
  secretome 259
  selection, noninvasive method of 255
  spent media 260
  stage of 318
  toxicity 172
  transfer 179, 208, 216, 266, 270, 279, 289, 307, 326, 386, 390
    technique 266
  utilization rate 190
  vitrification protocol 302, 303f
Embryogenesis 54, 310t, 360
Embryonic death 282
Endocrine
  control 15
  disruptors 118
  indicators 350
Endometrial development, advancement in 328
Endometrioma 387
Endometriosis 112
  severe 340
  symptomatic 319
Endometrium 111, 309
Environmental sensors 205
  carbon dioxide 205
  differential pressure 205
  liquid nitrogen 205

oxygen 205
relative humidity 205
room pressure 205
temperature 205
Eosin nigrosin suspension 25
Eosinophilic granulomatosis 340
Epididymal sperm 131
    aspirations 386
    percutaneous 389
Epididymal spermatozoa 15
Epididymides 37
Erectile dysfunction 151, 154, 154f, 155, 156
    tests for diagnosing for 151
Estradiol 339
Estrogen receptors 15
Ethylene glycol 302
Ethylenediaminetetraacetic acid 310
Etoposide 161
Euploid 51
    embryos 329
        risk of 322
European Academy of Andrology 45, 49
European Society for Human Reproduction and Embryology 39, 189
Ewing's sarcoma 340
Exocytosis 289
Extracellular
    fragments 280
    ice crystal formation 301, 314
    pH 198
    solution 318
    tissue matrix 352
Extra-testicular factors 99

F

Facility
    management system 205
    monitoring systems 205
Female fertility, preservation of 337
Female germ cells, number of 336t
Female infertility 112
    causes for 111
    idiopathic 111
Female reproductive tract 111
Fertile controls 76
Fertility
    impaired 162
    preservation 162, 164
        group 160
    restoration 339
    treatment 164
        group 163
Fertilization 94, 132, 212, 226
    abnormal 212
    artificial 24
    failure 212, 288, 290fc, 391, 392
    low 290fc
    morphological assessment of 7f

oocyte in 231
process of 288
rate 72, 146, 190, 211, 371
scoring for 171
total failed 213
Fetal heartbeat 190
Fibroid 387
Fibrous tail sheath 4
Fimbria 309
Fludarabine 338
Fluid-only method 267
    demerits of 267
    merits of 267
Fluorescent in situ hybridization 30, 137, 360, 390
Fluoxetine 153
Folic acid 110, 113
Follicle
    culture 353
    rupture 221
    somatic cells of 395
    stimulating hormone 14, 135, 212, 337
        serum 21, 45
Follicular
    development 351, 395
    fluid 183, 397, 398
    phases 353
Folliculogenesis 349
Formaldehyde 172
Fourier transform infrared spectroscopy 262
Fragile X permutation 296
Fresh embryo transfer 305, 332
Fresh in vitro fertilization embryos 330
Fresh oocyte donation 379
Frozen
    cycles 327
    embryo 136, 330
        transfer 326, 331, 331t
    oocytes 320
    thawed blastocysts 321
    thawed embryo 273
    thawed ovarian tissue, transplantation of 350
    transfer 389

G

Galactose, monosaccharides like 302
Galactosemia 340
Gametes 317, 395
    cryopreservation of 326
    deficiency of 107
    donation 107
    intracellular regions of 215
Gametogenesis 360
Gap junction plays 229
Gas cylinders 176f
Gemcitabine 338
Genetic 53

causes 155
defects, vertical transmission of 52
disease 159, 322, 336
information 4
role of 44
screening 331, 378
selection 322
test, advanced 107
Genitourinary infections 44
Genomic 395, 399
Germ cells 13, 160, 161
Germinal angiotensin-converting enzyme 3
Gestational sac 305
development 190
Glass wool filtration 70, 70*t*
Globozoospermia 38, 291
Glutathione 110, 111
reductase 85
Glyceraldehydes-3-phosphate dehydrogenase 82
Glycoproteins 277
Gonadotoxic
cancer treatment 353
chemotherapy 354
treatment 339
Gonadotropic therapy 161
Gonadotropin 121
releasing hormone 121, 329, 337
Graduated embryo scoring system 241
Granulomatosis 340
Granulosa 228
cell 130, 209, 228
Gynecomastia 19

H

Haber-Weiss reaction 77
Halo test 93
Hatching process 277
Heating surface 180*f*
Heavy metal toxicity 119
Hematologic disease 159, 162
Hemochromatosis 121
Hemorrhage, antepartum 330
Hemospermia 36
Hepa system 181
Hepatitis
B antigen 377, 378
C 377
virus 378
Heterogeneous gonadal disorder 336
Heterotopic transplantation 350
High efficiency particulate air 182, 204, 388
High performance liquid chromatography 261, 398
Hindering normal testicular function 160
Histone 54
octamers 2
replacement of 89

Hodgkin's disease 160, 161, 340
Hodgkin's lymphoma 341
Homocysteine metabolism, disordered 368
Hormonal
diseases 44
manipulation 122
treatment 121
Hormone analysis 21, 39
Human
chorionic gonadotropin 190, 122, 132, 210, 289, 390, 328
embryos 263, 320
follicular, biochemistry of 309
gametes 220
immunodeficiency virus 165
infertility therapy, flexibility in 317
leukocyte antigen 259, 397
oocyte 288, 320
cryopreservation of 319
placenta 371
preimplantation embryos 260
reproduction 220, 221
reproductive physiology, basics of 368
spermatozoa 1, 2*f*, 77
morphology of 3*f*
tubal fluid 59
Hyaluron-bound spermatozoa, selection of 392
Hyaluronic acid sperm binding test 71
Hyaluronidase 3
Hydrogen
peroxide 108
radicals 110
potential of 197, 202*f*
Hydrosalpinx 387
Hydroxyethyl 342
piperazineethanesulfonic acid 177
Hydroxyl ion 108
Hyperactivation 76, 80, 108
Hyperhomocysteinemia 368, 369, 371*f*, 372*f*
associated pregnancy loss, pathogenesis of 369
Hyperprolactinemia 155
Hypertension 330, 331
Hyperthermia, testicular 78
Hypogonadism 107
Hypoosmotic swelling test 25*f*
Hypotaurine 85

I

Idarubicin 338
Idiopathic infertility, medical management in 107
Ifosfamide 161, 338
Imipramine 153
Immature oocyte, retrieval of 353
Immotile cilia syndrome 37
Immotile sperms, selection of 70

Immunoassay techniques 397
Immunobead test 35
In situ hybridization 160
In vitro
    activation 352
    culture 188
        conditions 278
    fertilization 32, 64, 94, 98, 107, 128, 166, 171, 181, 182, 188, 197, 198, 199f, 205, 209, 220, 238, 255, 288, 290, 292, 300, 307, 317, 327, 359, 368, 385, 386
        conventional 142
        laboratory 171, 172f, 215
        program 204
        set up 180
        workstation 179
    manipulation 220
    maturation 230, 337, 347f, 353
    produced embryos, rate of 318
    produced oocytes, rate of 318
Incubators 177f
    temperature analyzer for 183f
    types of 178f
Infectious disease 336
Infertile male, physical examination of 34
Infertility
    causes for 108
    identifying cause of 51
    idiopathic 108
    treating 107
Inflammatory bowel diseases 340
Inner cell mass 312, 312f
Insemination concentration/density 292
Institutional Animal Ethics Committee 367
Interferone gamma 397
International Committee for Monitoring Assisted Reproductive Technology 191
International Embryologist Society 320
International Index of Erectile Function 151
Intracellular
    ice crystals 302
    ice formation 296
    pH 201
    reactive oxygen species 76
    stores 289
Intracranial pressure, risk of 383
Intracytoplasmic morphologically selected sperm injection 73, 134f, 142, 290-392
    technology 133
Intracytoplasmic sperm injection 8, 25, 49, 64, 92, 94, 98, 103, 128, 130, 130f, 132, 142, 149, 173, 198, 209, 210, 221, 239, 255, 288, 290, 296, 332, 359, 385, 386, 388
    advantages of 131
    consequences of 135
    embryo transfer 305
    evolution of 128
    indications for 131
    off-shoots of 137
    physiological 29, 291
    technique of 130
Intrauterine insemination 32, 56, 58, 64, 94, 98, 107, 387
Intravaginal ejaculatory latency time 152
Iron 77
Isochromosome 361
Isoprostanes 84
Itai itai disease 119
IVF set up, components of 173

J

Jaundice 36
Jumonji protein 260

K

Kallman syndrome 21
Karyotype 45
Kitazato ovarian cortex vitrification media 348f
Klinefelter's mosaics 51
Klinefelter's syndrome 19, 23, 40, 42, 45, 51

L

Laminar flow 57
Large-for-gestational age 327
Laser assisted
    hatching 134f, 281
    zona drilling 281
L-carnitine 110, 112, 113
Lead 119
Leigh syndrome 137
Lepidium 113
Leptin 259
Leukemia 160, 161, 340
Leukocytes 78, 278
    peroxidase-positive 35
    presence of 20
Leukocytospermia 21
    presence of 83
Lidocaine 156
Lipid peroxidation 76, 82, 84, 109
Liquid nitrogen 158, 179, 304
Live birth 190, 351
    rates 135, 323
Loading cortex bits 348f
Long chain fatty acids, role of 112
Luminol 84
Luteinizing hormone 12, 14, 39, 45, 119, 232
    pituitary 329
    serum 21
Lycopene 110, 111
Lymphoma 161
Lysins proteases 278

M

Magnesium 113
Magnetic activated
    cell sorting 68, 69f, 97, 101, 103, 103f, 291
        technique of 102f
    cell storing 290
    sperm sorting 104t
Magnetic cell sorting 68, 69f, 69t
Male gamete 1
Male infertility 39, 53, 107, 108, 117-119
    clinical evaluation of 44
    etiology of 119
    evaluation of 18, 19
    genetics of 39
    treatment of 121
Male reproductive oxidative stress
    management of 85
    prevention of 85
Male reproductive system 76
Male sexual dysfunction 149, 150f, 156
    causes of 149
    communication 156
    education 156
    hormones 156
    mechanical aids 156
    medical treatment 156
    medications 156
    psychological therapy 156
Malnutrition, malignancy-related 161
Malondialdehyde 82
Mammalian
    embryos 188
    oocytes 370
Mass
    spectrometry 260, 397, 398
    spectroscopy 261
Maternal
    hyperhomocysteinemia, effect of 368
    ribonucleic acid 289
    transcript accumulation, deficiency in 213
Meiosis 10
    phase of 9, 9f
Meiotic
    competence failure 289
    division 8
Melphalan 338
Membrane, inner acrosomal layers of 3
Mercury 119
Metabolomics 259, 260, 395, 398
    analysis 272
Metaphase chromosome 362
Methotrexate 338
Methylation status 289
Methylcobalamin 110
Microbial contamination, level of 194
Microfluidic sperm cell sorter 70, 71f, 71t
Microinsemination sperm transfer 129
Micromanipulation 372
Micronutrients, role of 109
Microtesticular sperm extraction 132
Miscarriage 191, 369
Mitochondria 72
Mitochondrial
    abnormalities 37
    activity 359
    capsule 79
    level 77
Mitotic
    chromosomes, deoxyribonucleic acid in 1
    proliferation 8
Mixed gonadal dysgenesis 40
Modern reproductive medicine 255
Molecular cytogenetic method 362
Monogenic disorders 360
Monosomies 360, 362
Monozygotic twins 282, 313
    formation of 282
Morphokinetic
    embryo selection on basis of 259
    evaluation 308
Morphological grading systems 242t
Morphology
    conventional 248, 249t
    embryo selection on basis of 256
Mosaic
    samples, detection of 365
    Turner syndrome 340
Motile
    male reproductive cell 1
    sperm organelle morphology examination 72
    spermatozoa 35, 145
Motility 20, 80
    enhancers 110
Multicellular embryos 322
Multiple gestations 323
    risk of 270
Multiple pregnancy 191
    rate 272, 309
Mural granulose cells 228

N

N-acetyl-cysteine 113
National Institute for Health and Care Excellence 313
Near infrared spectroscopy 398
Neck 4, 7
Necrozoospermia 37
    characteristic of 37
Neonatal intensive care unit 331
Nerves 150
Neuroblastoma 340
Neurodegenerative disease 159
Neuropsychiatric disorders 52
Next generation sequencing 365, 396

Index

Nicotinamide adenine dinucleotide 77
   phosphate 77
Nitric oxide 108, 118
Nitroblue tetrazolium 109
Nitrous oxide 108
Nitroxyl ion 108
Non-apoptotic spermatozoa, selection of 68
Noncontact laser systems 281
Nonenzymatic antioxidants 85
Non-Hodgkin's disease 161, 340
Non-Hodgkin's lymphoma 160
Nonmalignant disease 163, 164
Nonmotile sperm cell 1
Normospermia 41
Normozoospermia 110
Novel sperm preparation technique 97
Nuclear
   cap 3
   magnetic resonance 261, 398
   syngamy 6
Nucleolar precursor bodies 6, 239
Nucleotides 231
Nucleus 3
   elongation of 11
Nutraceutical, types of 107

O

Obesity 99, 155
Oligoasthenospermia 131
Oligoasthenoteratospermia 108
   severe 131
Oligoasthenoteratozoospermia 133
Oligoasthenozoospermia 22
Oligospermia 41, 62, 118, 120
   severe 41
Oligozoospermia 20, 37, 49, 136, 160, 163, 165
   idiopathic 110
   severe 159, 160, 161, 163, 164
Oncofertility 167
Oncotesticular sperm extraction 162
Oncovin 161
Oocyte 130, 131, 166, 173, 175, 198, 208, 210, 221, 231, 293, 297, 317, 319, 331, 337, 363
   absence of 209
   accumulation of 328
   activation 289
      assisted 392
   analysis of 399
   assessment of 390
   chromosome 130
   collection 387
   cryopreservation 295-297, 317-319, 332, 336, 339, 354
      indications 295
      program 295
      safety of 319
   cumulus
      complex 231
      gap junction 235
      insight 228, 234
      relationship 230
   cytoplasm of 130f, 319, 321
   cytoplasmic components 132
   denudation of 210
   donation of 319
   Donation Program 319
   donor 377, 378
   early denudation of 221
   factors 288, 289
   freezing 296, 297, 337
      advantages of 297
      techniques of 296
   grading of 238
   granulosa cell complexes 371
   immature 209, 221, 347f, 353
   in vitro maturation of 210
   inactivation 212
   incidence of 291
   insemination of 171
   karyotype 399
   manipulation of 386
   maturation 395
   morphological scoring of 394
   number of 340
   nutrition and metabolism 230
   paracrine signaling 233
   postmature 209
   rate of 323
   retrieval 171, 208, 239
   role of 233
   secreted factors 233
Oophorectomy
   bilateral 340
   unilateral 340
Oophoropexy 337
Ooplasm 94
Optimum testicular temperature 120
Orphan embryos 306
Orthotopic reimplantation 350
Osmotic stress 159
Ovarian
   activity, refurbishment of 351
   cortex
      bits 344f
      cryopreservation, indications for 339
      preservation, future of 352
      site of 351fc
      slow freezing of 343f
      transplantation of 349
   failure, premature 336, 337, 378
   follicles 337
   follicular microenvironment 228
   folliculogenesis 228
   function 350

graft 350
hyperstimulation 64, 319
    syndrome 191, 323, 328, 329, 331, 382, 391
    controlled 320
insufficiency, premature 336
reserve 340
specimen 343f
stimulation 319
    controlled 327
    influence laboratory performance 388
stroma 343
tissue 344f, 349
    autotransplantation of 354
    banking, guidelines for 339
    collection of 342
    cryobanked 339
    cryopreservation 337, 341, 342, 353, 354
    cryopreserved 351, 353
    for slow freezing, preparation of 343t
    freezing 336
    grafting 350, 351
    heterotopic transplantation of 350
    transplantation of 351
tumor, benign 340
vascular transplantation 352
Ovulation
    hormones for 107
    hyperstimulation protocols, controlled 270, 300
Ovum penetration test 25
Oxidative stress 76, 80f, 108, 368
    effects of 76
    embryo selection on basis of 263
    role of 111
Oxygen consumption 255, 399
    embryo selection on basis of 260
Oxygen derivatives 108
Ozone 108

P

Paraplegia 132
Paroxetine 153
Partial zona dissection 129
Passive microbial air monitoring 204
Pediatric cancer 162
Pemphigus vulgaris 340
Penile implants 156f
Pentoxifylline 85
Perinatal mortality 330
Peroxynitrite 108
Pesticides 118
Peyronie's disease 154
Phenylpropanolamine 153
Phimosis 19
Phosphate buffer saline 59
Phospholipase A2, deactivation of 81

Phospholipid phosphatidylserine 68, 97
Phosphorylates mitogen-activated protein kinase 81
Phosphotyrosine phosphatase 81
Piezo electric pulse 281
Piezo technology 281
Piperazineethanesulfonic acid 209, 342
Plasma membrane 3
Plastic industry toxin 18
Platelet activating factor 259
Polar bodies 360
Polyangiitis 340
Polyaromatic hydrocarbon 120
Polychlorinated biphenyl 18
Polycystic kidney disease 37
Polycystic ovarian syndrome 112, 319, 326
Polymerase chain reaction 360, 395
Polymorphisms 44
Polyp 387
Polyploidy 360, 361
Polyunsaturated fatty acids 76, 109, 120
Polyvinyl alcohol 302
Polyvinylpyrrolidone 130
    polymers like 302
Poor semen quality, incidence of 160
Postacrosomal lamina 72
Posthumous sperm cryopreservation 164
Postovum pickup 293
Postvitrification 227
Postwarm excellent morphology 305
Postzygotic chromosomal abnormalities 213
Potential malignant cell contamination 351
Prednisone 161
Pregnancy
    biochemical 226
    multiple 271, 307
    optimum 268
    rates 32, 181, 268, 271, 314, 364
    spontaneous 350
Preimplantation genetic
    diagnosis 48, 50, 137, 173, 191, 292, 311, 322, 359, 385, 390
    screening 48, 250, 292, 296, 311, 322, 329, 386, 390
    testing 137
Premature menopause, risk of 340
Primordial germ cells 98
Procarbazine 161
Progesterone 331
    elevated 330
Pronuclear
    scoring 239
    stage transfers 239
Pronuclei 212, 256
Propanediol 302
Prophylactic salpingo-oophorectomy 296
Prostaglandin endoperoxide synthase 232
Protamine 6, 11, 89

Index

Protein
  carbonyl groups 399
  hormone human chorionic gonadotropin 397
  kinase A, activates 80
  morphogenetic 233
  peroxidation 399
  tyrosine kinase, activate 81
Proteolytic enzymes 11
Proteomics 259, 272, 395, 396
Pubertal mumps orchitis 18
Puberty, onset of 19
Pycnogenol 113

Q

Qualitative real time polymerase chain reaction 396
Quarantine period 379

R

Radiotherapy 99, 336
Raman spectroscopy 398
Randomized controlled trials 112, 327
Reactive nitrogen species 108
Reactive oxygen species 30, 76, 77, 83, 89, 108, 119, 176
  effects of 79, 108
  exogenous sources of 78
  measurement of 109
  presence of 99
  types of 108
Real-time motile sperm organelle morphology examination 72
Reciprocal translocations 361, 362
Recurrent early pregnancy loss 29
Refractory male infertility problems 159
Rehydration 318
Remote monitoring systems 205t
Reproductive
  cells 171
  disorders 117
  endocrinology 221
  function 339
Resting cell 8
Resuscitation, cardiopulmonary 256
Resveratrol 123
Reticuloendothelial system 12
Retrograde ejaculation 152, 153
  management of 153
Rheumatic disease 159
Rheumatoid arthritis 340
Ribonucleic acid 231, 259
  microarray 234
  molecules 395
Ribosome 231
Ringer's lactate 59
Robertsonian translocations 40, 361, 365
ROSNI-round spermatid nuclear injection 12
Round spermatid injection 132

S

Salazopyrin 36
Sarcoidosis 121
Sarcomas 160
Scar tissue 154
Schermann's discoveries 158
Second meiotic division 9
Secretomics 395, 396
Selenium 110, 111, 113
Semen 58, 183
  analysis 19, 35, 56
    normal 377
    routine 83
  banking 158, 159
    benefits 159
    reason 159
  cryopreservation of 391
  deoxyribonucleic acid fragmentation in 109
  parameters 22, 162
    analysis of 83
  quality 167
  volume 35
Seminal
  elastase measurement 83
  fluid
    different parameters of 20t
    parameters 20
  fructose 35
  neutral glucosidase 35
  oxidation-reduction potential 84
  oxidative stress, evaluation of 83
  plasma 78
  zinc 35
  fluid 21, 22t
Sequential embryo morphology assessment 241
Serotonin levels 155
Sertoli cells 13
Sex determining region 45
Sexual disorders 149
Sexual dysfunction 149, 150, 154
Sexual maturity 162
Sexually transmitted diseases 18
Sickle cell
  anemia 340
  appearance 312
Sildenafil 156
Single blastocyst transfer policy 309
Single cell 322
  gel electrophoresis assay 28, 93
Single embryo transfer 238, 270
  economic aspects of 274
Single gel electrophoresis 101f
Single human oocytes, genome of 399

Single nucleotide polymorphism 250, 399
Single static embryo evaluation 239
Singleton pregnancies 271, 274
Slow freezing 343, 346, 350t
    equilibration procedure 345t
Slow frozen blastocyst transfer cycles 328
Small for gestational age 330, 331
Small noncoding ribonucleic acid 263
Smith classification 239
Society for Assisted Reproductive
        Technologies 189, 255, 270
Soft tissue tumors 160
Somatic cells 89
Sperm 1, 130f, 173, 227, 386
    abnormalities 7, 8f
    acrosome reacted 26
    acrosomeless 131
    agglutination 36
    aneuploidy 25
        assay 30
        screening 30
    banking, users of 159
    birefringence 73, 74
    capacitation 289
    cell, uniflagellar 1
    chromatin dispersion 93
        method 28f
        tests 28
    chromatin structure assay 28, 93, 101, 109
    concentration 20, 35
        meticulous recording of 292
    count, normal 118
    cryopreservation 162, 163, 313
        indications for 164t
        protocol 166
        techniques 24
    demonstration of 153
    deoxyribonucleic acid
        damage 78, 92, 109, 291
        fragmentation 89, 90, 92, 97, 98, 100, 105
        in fertility, role of 94
        integrity 29
    donation 376, 377
    donors 159
        group 159
    epigenetics 53
    factors 291
    function testing 24, 30
    head protein, type of 6
    immotile 70, 132
    improper zona binding of 288
    injection 73f
        technique 142
        untracytoplasmic 292
    maturation 76, 109
    membrane maturity 71
    morphology 20, 35, 36, 145, 291
        abnormal 160
        normal 65
    motility 20, 79, 91, 109, 118
        normal 143f
    nuclear annulus 2
    nucleus 3
    oocyte fusion 81
    organelles 72
    parameters 108, 389
    plasma membrane 77
    preparation 171, 387
        laboratory 57
        procedure 57
        technique 56, 58, 293
    proportion of 146
    quality 160
    samples, storage of 57
    selection 66t
        criterion 293
        using zeta potential method 67f, 67t
    seminopathy 56
    straws 167
    subzonal injection of 129
    thawing 166
    vacuolated 143f
    visualized 134f
    wash, normal 60f
Spermatic cord 85
Spermatid 3, 9
    injection, elongated 132
Spermatium 1
Spermatocyte, secondary 8
Spermatogenesis 7, 12, 12f, 107
    apoptotic functions of 99
    effect of temperature on 13
    endocrine control of 14, 14fc
    process of 119
Spermatogonial stem cell 8
Spermatozoa 3, 25, 77, 77f, 144, 221, 278
    acrosome reacted 73
    aggressive immobilization of 211
    apoptotic 101
    different segments of 5
    genetic testing of 53
    globozoospermic 291
    immature 78
    motility of 13
Spermatozoal maturation 79
Spermatozoon 1
    hyperactivated 81
Spermiation 38
Spermiogenesis 11
    phase of 8, 11
Spermotogonia, types of 8
Sphingosine-1-phosphate, effects of 352
Spinal cord injury 37, 165
Sports nutrition 107

Index

Standard operating procedure 185, 196, 323
Standardized Training Programs 192
Stereo zoom microscopes 178
Sterile cryovials 166
Steroid hormone 107
Steroid-resistant glomerulonephritis 340
Stimulation
    protocols 328
    quality of 389
Styrene 172
Subfertility, male factor 271
Sucrose 317
    concentration 319
Sulfasalazine 36
Superovulation 328
Superoxide 108, 110
    dismutase 77, 85, 111
        level of 112
Sureview soft catheter 266
Surgical sperm extraction 122
Surrogacy 107, 227, 377, 380, 381, 383
    ART guidelines for 381
    commercial 380
    gestational 380
    indications for 380
    screening genetic couple for 380
    traditional 380
Surrogate 380
    mothers 383
    screening 380
Swim up
    technique 60f
    with centrifugation 59
    without centrifugation 59
Systemic disease 121, 163
Systemic lupus erythematosus 340

T

Tenaculum traction 391
Teratozoospermia 38, 160
Terminal deoxynucleotidyl transferase 93
    mediated deoxyuridine triphosphate nick end labelling 101f
Terratozoospermia 62
Test tube
    baby 128
    warmers 57
Testicular
    biopsy 23
    blood supply 163
    cancer 117, 160, 161
        risk of 52
    failure 20, 39
    injury 18
    sperm 123, 131
        aspiration 30, 45, 52, 132, 377, 386, 389, 391
        extraction 386

steroidogenesis 119
temperature 89
tissue extraction 167
trauma 44
volume 19
Testis torsion 163
Testosterone 39
    deficiency 155
    serum 21
Thalassemia major 340
Thawed oocytes 319
Thawing 318, 346
    method 176
    protocol 304
Thermochemiluminescence 263
Thermochron
    buttons distributed over 199f
    devices 198, 199f
Thick zona pellucida, presence of 386
Thiobarbituric acid-reactive substances 399
Thrombosis 368
Toluene 172
Toluidine blue test 28
Top quality blastocysts, formation of 398
Total antioxidant capacity 84
Total fertilization failure 288
Total quality management system 323
Toxic chemicals 163
Toxic regimen 161
Toxins 118
Transcriptomics 395
    technology 395
Transmembrane glycoprotein 83
Trehalose 302, 314
Trinucleotide expansions 365
Triple gas incubator 177
Triploid embryos 213
Trophectoderm 278, 309, 321
    biopsies 396
Trophoblast cells, number of 398
Tunica albuginea 344f
Turner's syndrome 271, 296
Tyrode's acid 280

U

Ultra-high magnification sperm selection 143f
Ureaplasma urealyticum infection 83
Urethral orifice 19
Uterine
    cavity 308
        inadequate 331
    receptivity and compatibility 307
    transfer media 266

V

Vacuolar area 72
Vacuoles 145

Vaginal carcinoma 340
Varicocele 19, 44, 78, 85, 89, 98, 107
Vas deferens
   congenital
      bilateral absence of 49, 136
      unilateral absence of 49
Veins, pampiniform plexus of 85
Venereal disease research laboratory 377
Vertical laminar flow hoods 177
Vinblastine 161, 338
Vincristine 161, 338
Vitality tests 25
Vitamin 113
   B_{12} 110
      therapy, effect of 110
   C 110, 113, 114
   E 110, 111, 113, 114
      deficiency 155
Vitrification 301, 305, 307, 314, 318, 327, 346
   development of 314
   freezing 350*t*
   group 305
   of blastocyst 314
   preparation for 346*f*
   protocol 349*t*
   solution 303
   technique 343
Volatile organic
   chemical 388
   compounds 172, 182, 194, 197, 204, 224
Vulvar carcinoma 340

W

Warming protocol 349*t*
Wegener's disease 340
Wegener's granulomatosis 340

White blood cells 21
Wilms' tumor 340
World Health Organization 24, 107

X

X chromosome 296
XX karyotype 45

Y

Y chromosome 1, 23
   microdeletions 41, 44, 49
Y microdeletions 39, 40, 42

Z

Zeta potential method 65, 67, 74
Zika virus 331
Zinc 109-111, 113, 119
Zona
   binding
      assays 25
      capacity 38
   dissection, partial 279
   dissolution 278
   dissolves 280
   drilling 129
   fails 279
   free hamster oocyte 129*f*
   pellucida 25, 38, 81, 129, 277, 280, 282, 289, 390
      specific proteins 277
   thickness 278
Zygotes 212, 213, 238, 386
   population of 314
   transfer 239